HEALTH INFORMATION MANAGEMENT: WHAT STRATEGIES?

Proceedings of former conferences:

Christine Deschamps, Marc Walckiers (eds.), Medical Libraries: Cooperation and New Technologies. First European Conference of Medical Libraries, Brussels, Belgium, 22-25 October 1986. Amsterdam; New York; Oxford; Tokyo: North-Holland, 1987. (Contemporary topics in information transfer. Vol. 5)

David W.C. Stewart, Derek J. Wright (eds.), Health Information for All: A Common Goal. Proceedings of the Second European Conference of Medical Libraries, Bologna, Italy, November 2-6, 1988. München; London; New York; Paris: Saur, 1989.

Suzanne Bakker, Monique C. Cleland (eds.), Information Transfer: New Age - New Ways. Proceedings of the third European Conference of Medical Libraries, Montpellier, France, September 23-26, 1992. Dordrecht; Boston; London: Kluwer, 1993.

Tony McSéan, John van Loo, Euphemia Coutinho (eds.), Health Information - New Possibilities. Proceedings of the fourth European Conference of Medical and Health Libraries, Oslo, Norway, June 28 - July 2, 1994. Dordrecht; Boston; London: Kluwer, 1995.

HEALTH INFORMATION MANAGEMENT: WHAT STRATEGIES?

Proceedings of the 5th European Conference of Medical and Health Libraries, Coimbra, Portugal, September 18-21, 1996

Edited by

Suzanne Bakker

Library Director,
Central Medical Library,
University of Amsterdam,
Amsterdam, The Netherlands

on behalf of the

EUROPEAN ASSOCIATION FOR
HEALTH INFORMATION AND LIBRARIES

SPRINGER-SCIENCE+BUSINESS MEDIA, B.V.

A C.I.P. Catalogue record for this book is available from the Library of Congress.

ISBN 978-90-481-4848-6 ISBN 978-94-015-8786-0 (eBook)
DOI 10.1007/978-94-015-8786-0

Printed on acid-free paper

CONTENTS

Chapter 3: QUALITY MANAGEMENT & ECONOMICS

Chapter 4: ACADEMIC LIBRARIES

Chapter 5: INFORMATION MANAGEMENT SKILLS

Chapter 6: ELECTRONIC DOCUMENT DELIVERY

Chapter 11: BIBLIOMETRICS

Chapter 12: INFORMATION QUALITY

Chapter 13: HISTORY OF MEDICINE

CONFERENCE COMMITTEES

Local Organizing Committee

Antónia Pereira da Silva, Coimbra (chair)
Helena Donato, Coimbra
Maria Amélia Hungria, Lisbon
Maria do Rosário Leitão, Lisbon
Lucilla Paiva, Coimbra

Local Scientific Programme Committee

Isabel Andrade, Lisbon (chair)
Noémia Canas, Coimbra
Arminda Sustelo, Lisbon

International Scientific Programme Committee

Jean-Philippe Accart, France
Suzanne Bakker, The Netherlands
Maria Asunción Garcia, Spain
Arne Jakobsson, Sweden
Vincent Maes, Belgium
Otakar Pinkas, Czech Republic
Gabriella Poppi, Italy
Maria Francisca Ribes-Cot, Spain
Lubomira Soltésová, Slovak Republic
John van Loo, United Kingdom
Paul van Olm, The Netherlands

ACKNOWLEDGEMENT

The publication of the proceedings is a reference made to the conference, the organizers and to the contributors. Above all we have to thank the Local Organizing Committee for the work done to make this conference a success. Beyond doubt, the scientific programme is the core of a conference, but no less important are the social events, the exhibition, the continuing education courses and the characteristics of the Association membership.

Organizing conferences is rather dominant amongst the activities of the Association, but not less important for the prosperity of EAHIL is the continuity in the work of the Executive Board, the Council and the Editors of the Newsletter. For this part we are very grateful to have the very skilful support of Roselyne Hoet, the secretary general of EAHIL. Not in vain did I turn to Roselyne Hoet for editorial assistance with some of the French papers of this proceedings.

The many exhibitors and sponsors are kindly acknowledged for their financial and moral support to the conference. We all pay gratitude to the Ministers and Directors of the many Portuguese governmental, academic and commercial organizations and institutes for their hospitality to host this conference.

AUTHOR ADRESSES

E. Akre
Diakonhjemmets hospital, Medical library, Box 23 Vinderen, 0319 Oslo, Norway

V. Alberani
Servizio per le attività, Istituto Superiore di Sanità, Viale Regina Elene, 299, 00161 Rome, Italy

M.L. Antunes
Instituto de Clinica Geral da Zona Sul, Largo Prof. Arnaldo Sampaio, Centro de Saúde de Sete Rios, P-1500 Lisbon, Portugal

C.J. Armstrong
The Centre for Information Quality Management (CIQM), Penbryn, Bronant, Aberystwyth SY23 4TJ, UK

B. Aronson
Office of Library and Health Literature Services, World Health Organization, 121 Geneva 27, Switzerland

M. Ashcroft
Instant Library Ltd., 22 Frederick Street, Loughborough, Leicestershire, LE11 3BJ, U.K.

P. Bador
ISPB Faculté de Pharmacie, Université Claude Bernard-Lyon 1, 8, Avenue Rockefeller, 69373 Lyon Cedex 08, France

S. Bakker
Centrale Medische Bibliotheek, Academisch Medisch Centrum, Universiteit van Amsterdam, Meibergdreef 15, 1105 AZ Amsterdam, The Netherlands

M.P. Barredo Sobrino
Biblioteca Facultad de Medicina, Universidad Autónoma de Madrid, C/ Arzobispo Morcillo 2, 28029 Madrid, Spain

M.J. Barrulas
CITI - Centro de Informaçao Técnica para a Indústria, INETI - Instituto Nacional de Engenharia e Tecnologia Industrial, Estrado do Paço do Lumiar, 1699 Lisbon Codex, Portugal

D. Baudin
Documentation Department, Centre International de l'Enfance, Chateau de Longchamp, Bois de Boulogne, 75016 Paris, France

R. Bravo Toledo
Centro de Salud El Greco, Avda. Reyes Católicos s/n, 28904 Getafe, Madrid, Spain

A. Bekavac
Central Medical Library, Zagreb University, School of Medicine, Salata 3, 10000 Zagreb, Croatia

L. Bianciardi
Università degli Studi, Facoltà di Medicina e Chirurgia, Biblioteca Centrale, Centro Didattico "Le Scotte", 53100 Siena, Italy

B.S. Brunelle
Ovid Technologies, 333 7th Avenue, New York NY 10001, U.S.A.

M. Camerlingo
CINECA, Bologna, Italy

F.M.G. Campos
Instituto da Biblioteca Nacional e do Livro, Campo Grande 83, 1751 Lisbon Codex, Portugal

L. Cavazza
Soprintendenza beni librari e documentari della Regione Emilia-Romagna, Via Farini 28, 40124 Bologna, Italy

A.M. Cawasjee
Cairns Library, The John Radcliffe, Oxford Radcliffe Hospital, Headington, Oxford OX3 9DU, U.K.

G. Cognetti
Istituto Regina Elena, Biblioteca, Viale Regina Elena, 291, 00161 Rome, Italy

L.A. Colaianni
National Library of Medicine, 8600 Rockville Pike, Bethesda, Maryland 20894, U.S.A.

M. Colombi
Schering-Plough S.p.A., Via Ripamonti, 89, 20141 Milano, Italy

V. Comba
Biblioteca Centralizzata di Medicina, Corso Dogliotti 14, 10126 Torino, Italy

A.M.R. Correia
CITI - Centro de Informação Técnica para a Indústria, INETI - Instituto Nacional de Engenharia e Tecnologia Industrial, Estrada do Paço do Lumiar, 1699 Lisbon Codex, Portugal

J. Crespo
Serviço de Medicina III, Hospitais da Universidade de Coimbra, Portugal

M. Curti
IRCCS Policlinico San Matteo, 27100 Pavia, Italy

M. Della Seta
Biblioteca, Istituto Superiore Di Sanità, Viale Regina Elena, 299, 00161 Rome, Italy

A. D'Emanuele
Department of Pharmacy, University of Manchester, Oxford Road, Manchester M13 9PL, U.K.

J. Dijkman
Library KNAW, P.O. Box 41950, 1009 DD Amsterdam, The Netherlands

B.M. Doran
The Mercer Library, Royal College of Surgeons in Ireland, Mercer Street Lower, Dublin 2, Ireland

L. Egghe
Limburgs Universitair Centrum, Universitaire Campus, 3590 Diepenbeek, Belgium

U. Elsner
Informations- und Dokumentationsstelle Ethik in der Medizin (IDEM), Akademie für Ethik in der Medizin, Humboldtallee 36, 37073 Goettingen, Germany

R.L. Faraino
Ehrman Medical Library, NYU Medical Center, 550 1st Avenue, New York, NY 10016, U.S.A.

J. Farmer
School of Information and Media, The Robert Gordon University Aberdeen, Faculty of Management, Hilton Place, Aberdeen AB9 1FP, Scotland, U.K.

H. Fauré
Bibliothèque interuniversitaire de Médecine, 12 Rue de l'Ecole de Médecine, 75270 Paris Cedex 06, France

V. Ferguson
John Rylands University, Library of Manchester, Oxford Road, Manchester M13 9PP, U.K.

D. Flake
R.M. Fales Health Sciences Library, Coastal Area Health Education Center, 2131 South 17th Street, P.O. Box 9025, Wilmington NC 28402-9025, U.S.A.

R. Gann
The Help for Health Trust, Highcroft, Romsey Road, Winchester, SO22 5DH, U.K.

F. Grainger
Glasgow University Library, Hillhead Street, Glasgow G12 8QE, Scotland, U.K.

L. Haglund
Spri Library and Research Report Bank, Box 70487, 10726 Stockholm, Sweden

M. Haines
Library and Information Commission, 2 Sheraton Street, London W1V 4BH, U.K.

S. Hornby
Manchester Metropolitan University, Faculty of Humanities and Social Science, Department of Library and Information Studies, Humanities Building, Rosamond Street West off Oxford Road, Manchester M15 6LL, U.K.

L. Hrcková
Research Institute of Rheumatic Diseases, I. Krasku 4, 92101 Piestany, Slovak Republic

R. Iivonen
Veterinary Library, P.O. Box 57 (Hameentie 57), University of Helsinki, 00014 Helsinki, Finland

E. Jannès-Ober
Institut Pasteur, Bibliothèque Centrale, Centre d'Information Scientifique, 28, Rue du Docteur Roux, 75724 Paris Cedex 15, France

M. Jauhiainen
Information Service Centre, Finnish Institute of Occupational Health, Topeliuksenkatu 41 a A, 00250 Helsinki, Finland

M. Jordà-Olives
Unitat d'Informació, Agència de Recerca í Docència, Hospitals Vall d'Hebron, Pg Vall d'Hebron 119-129, 08035 Barcelona, Spain

C.C.P. Kluiters
Elsevier Science BV, P.O. Box 211, 1000 AE Amsterdam, The Netherlands

I. Laamanen
Finnish Institute of Occupational Health, Information Service Centre, Topeliuksenkatu 41 a A, 00250 Helsinki, Finland

J.P. Lardy
Université Claude Bernard - Lyon I, Laboratoire RECODOC, 43 Bd du 11 Novembre 1918, 69622 Villeurbanne cedex, France

A.E. Larsen
The Danish Veterinary and Agricultural Library, Bülowsvej 13, 1870 Frederiksberg C., Denmark

C. Lheureux
Centre de Documentation en Santé publique, Service de médecine préventive et sociale, Faculté de médecine St. Antoine, 27, Rue de Chaligny, 75012 Paris, France

H.C. Lombard
Frik Scott Medical Library, P.O. Box 2318, Bloemfontein, 9300 South Africa

V. Maes
Pfizer, 102, Rue Leon Theodor, 1090 Bruxelles, Belgium

E. Marinoni
Biblioteca Biologico-Medica, "A. Vallisneri", Universita' degli Studi di Padova, via Trieste 75, 35100 Padova, Italy

A. Martin
Service d'Information Médico-Pharmaceutique (SIMP) PCH/AP-HP, 7, Rue du Fer à Moulin BP 09, 75221 Paris Cedex 05, France

M. Mazzucchi
Biblioteca Centralizzata di Medicina Veterinaria, G.B. Ercolani, Università degli studi di Bologna, Via Tolara di sopra, 50, 40064 Ozzano Emilia, Bologna, Italy

L.W. McClure
164 Elmore Road, Rochester, New York 14618-3651, U.S.A.

T. McSeán
British Medical Association, Tavistock Square, London WC1H 9JP, UK

A.M.E. Miguéis
Av. Urbano Duarte, 92 1e Esq., 3030 Coimbra, Portugal

A. Miguel-Alonso
Universidad Complutense, Facultad de Farmacia, Biblioteca "Leon Felipe", Ciudad Universitaria, 28040 Madrid, Spain

R. Milne
Critical Appraisal Skills Programme, Institute of Health Sciences, P.O. Box 777, Oxford OX3 7LF, U.K.

G.F. Miranda
Sanofi Winthrop S.p.A., Research Centre, Sanofi Midy, Via G.B. Piranesi 38, 20137 Milano, Italy

C.C. Morais
FCCN, Av. do Brasil, 101, 1799 Lisbon Codex, Portugal

P. Morgan
Cambridge University Medical Library, Addenbrooke's Hospital, Hills Road, Cambridge CB2 2SP, U.K.

A.C. Munthe
Norwegian College of Veterinary Medicine, The Library, PO Box 8146 Dep., 0033 Oslo, Norway

C. Mutafov
Medical Information Centre, 1, G. Sofijski Str., 1431 Sofia, Bulgaria

M. Nardelli
Medical Information Group, Medical Department, ZENECA S.p.A., Palazzo Volta, Via F. Sforza, 20080 Basiglio (MI), Italy

J.S. van Niekerk
Medunsa Library, P.O. Box 156, Medunsa 0204, South Africa

O. Obst
ULB Münster, University of Münster, Krummer Timpen 3-5, 48143 Münster, Germany

J. Palmer
Health Libraries & Information Network, Health Care Libraries Unit, Level 3, Academic Centre, John Radcliffe Hospital, Headington, Oxford OX3 9DU, U.K.

F. Pasleau
Université de Liège, Bibliothèque de la Faculté de Médecine, C.H.U. Bâtiment B-35, 4000 Sart Tilman, Belgium

N. Pinhas
Réseau DIC-DOC INSERM, Hopital de Bicêtre, 94276 Le Kremlin-Bicêtre Cedex, France

O. Pinkas
National Medical Library, Sokolská 31, 12132 Prague 2, Czech Republic

E. Poltronieri
Istituto Superiore di Sanità, Biblioteca, Viale Regina Elena, 299, 00161 Rome, Italy

M. Prates
Faculdade de Ciências Médicas - UNL, Biblioteca, Campo de Santana, 130, Lisbon Codex, Portugal

I. Rabow
Lund University Library - UB2, Main Library for Technology, Science and Medicine, P.O. Box 3, 22100 Lund, Sweden

D. Reinitzer
Universitätsbibliothek, University of Veterinary Medicine Vienna, Josef Baumann-Gasse 1, 1210 Vienna, Austria

I. Robu
Biblioteca UMF, Str. A. Iancu 31, 3400 Cluj, Roumania

F. Rump
Library of the Veterinary School of Hannover, Postfach 711180, 30545 Hannover, Germany

K. Saarniit
Medical Information Centre, Tartu University Clinicum, Puusepa Street 8, 2400 Tartu, Estonia

C. Sawers
South Thames Library & Information Services, Education Centre, Royal Surrey County Hospital, Guildford, Surrey, GU2 5XX, U.K.

G. Schmid
Centre de documentation et recherche de L'Organisation Sociopsychiatrique Cantonale (OSC), via A. Maspoli, 6850 Mendrisio, Switzerland

E.J. Scott
Glaxo Wellcome plc., Greenford Road, Greenford, Middlesex UB6 OHE, U.K.

B. Sebastiani
Consiglio Nazionale delle Ricerche, Biblioteca Centrale, P.le Aldo Moro, 7, 00185 Rome, Italy

J.G. Shaw
SatelLife U.K., The Old Rectory, Shoscombe, Bath BA2 8NB, U.K.

I. Snowley
Library & Information Services, Department of Health, Room 151c, Skipton House, London SE1 6LW, U.K.

L. Soltésová
University Library of P.J. Safarik University, Medical Library, Trieda SNP 1, 04011 Kosice, Slovak Republic

M.R. Špála
Institute of Scientific Information, First Faculty of Medicine, Charles University, Kateřinská 32, 12801 Prague 2, Czech Republic

P. Spoor
Nuffield Institute for Health, University of Leeds, 71-75 Clarendon Road, Leeds LS2 9PL, U.K.

P. Stadler
Boehringer Mannheim GmbH, Zentralbibliothek, Dept. TF-MLB, Sandhoferstr. 116, 68298 Mannheim, Germany

J. Szabó Szávay
Central Library of the Semmelweis University of Medicine, Üllöi út 26, 1085 Budapest, Hungary

M. Thomas
Boehringer Mannheim GmbH, Dept. TF-ML, Sandhoferstr.116, 68298 Mannheim, Germany

J. Tsafrir
Medical Library, Chaim Sheba Medical Center, Tel Hashomer 52621, Israel

C.J. Urquhart
Department of Information and Library Studies, University of Wales Aberystwyth, Llanbadarn Campus, Aberystwyth SY23 3AS, U.K.

L. Vasas
Central Library of the Semmelweis Medical University, Üllöi út 26, 1085 Budapest, Hungary

J. Vasco Costa de Sousa
Centro de Saúde da Venda Nova, Rua João de Deus, Lote B/C, Venda Nova, 2700 Amadora, Portugal

L. Veloso
Biblioteca Geral da Universidade de Coimbra, 3049 Coimbra Codex, Portugal

L. Vercellesi
ZENECA S.p.A., Medical Information Group, Medical Department, Palazzo Volta, Via F. Sforza, 20080 Basiglio (MI), Italy

A.A.H. Verhoeven
Hamburgerstraat 2-B, 9714 JB Groningen, The Netherlands

M. Virágos
Central Library, Medical University, P.O. Box 12, 4012 Debrecen, Hungary

K.C. Wagner
Gundersen Lutheran, Health Sciences Library, 1910 South Avenue, La Crosse, Wisconsin 54601-9980, U.S.A.

M. Walckiers
Université Catholique de Louvain, Service d'études, Place de l'Université 1, 1348 Louvain-la-Neuve, Belgium

S. Welsh
National Institute for Medical Research, Library and Information Service, The Ridgeway, Mill Hill, London NW7 1AA, U.K.

M. Williams
Veterinary Medicine Library, University of Illinois at Urbana-Champaign, 2001 S. Lincoln Ave., Urbana, Il 61801, U.S.A.

T.D. Wilson
Department of Information Studies, University of Sheffield, Sheffield S10 2TN, U.K.

F.E. Wood
Centre for Health Information Management Research, Department of Information Studies, University of Sheffield, Regent Court, 211 Portobelle Street, Sheffield S1 4DP, U.K.

C.R. Zaher
BIREME/PAHO/WHO, Rua Botucatu 862, Via Clementino CEP 04023-901, São Paulo, Brazil

M.A. Zulueta
Centro de Información y Documentación Científica (CINDOC), Consejo Superior de Investigaciones Científicas (CSIC), Joaquín Costa, 22, 28002 Madrid, Spain

PREFACE TO THE PROCEEDINGS OF THE FIFTH CONFERENCE

Suzanne Bakker, Central Medical Library, Academic Medical Centre of the University of Amsterdam, The Netherlands

Introduction

The conference held in Coimbra, Portugal, was the 5th European Conference for Medical and Health Libraries (5ECMHL), and the fourth conference that has been organized by the European Association for Health Information and Libraries (EAHIL). The Association was constituted in 1987, being the result of cooperation between European medical librarians, who met in Tokyo in 1985 during the 5th International Congress on Medical Librarianship and who prepared the First European Conference of Medical Libraries in Brussels in 1986.

EAHIL aims *"to raise standards of provision and practice in health care and medical research libraries"* and *"to keep health librarians and information officers professionally informed."* It is in this respect that the continuing education courses contribute most to medical librarianship and professionalism. In Coimbra there were several courses on "Internet", on "Databases" and "Information sources in health economics" and on "MeSH indexing", "Document delivery", "Critical appraisal skills" and "Electronic information organization". European medical librarianship will benefit from these international courses, next and in addition to the many national initiatives.

The Association is founded by medical librarians convinced of the importance of European cooperation. The growth and health of the Association is dependent on the friendship and personal networks among its members. The greater was the sadness when we heard of the sudden death on July 17th 1996 of Deonilla Pizzi, member of EAHIL's Executive Board. Deonilla showed us how valuable it is to combine professionalism with joy and friendship and above all generosity. The Programme Committee received an abstract from Deonilla, promising a thought provoking and stimulating presentation. Therefore I decided to have this abstract follow the preface of this publication in order to keep her and her contributions to EAHIL in our lively memory.

Summary statement

The theme of the conference "Health Information Management: what strategies" indicates the shift that occurred in medical librarianship from "collection management" towards "information management".

The former conferences of EAHIL have been focused on: "Cooperation" (Brussels, 1986), "Spread and access of information" (Bologna, 1988), "Information transfer" (Montpellier, 1992) and "New possibilities" (Oslo, 1994). Although there are many parts in Europe where the availability of medical and health information is far below reasonable standards, we recognize that after solving the problems of accessibility, the problems of information overload and organization of information have to be faced.

Medical, healthcare and allied activities, e.g. veterinary and pharmaceutical sciences, are information-dense and knowledge-intense disciplines. The introduction of information technology contributes to this problem by allowing more data to be manipulated and taken into account. Information technology as such is not the solution to information needs, nor to the problems of information management. Tools developed in the long tradition of librarianship and documentation are necessary building blocks of any effective and efficient information management system, whether or not computerized.

During this conference we have learned from experiences and results out of projects and research done in the medical library field in Europe. In plenary sessions we heard the ideas of opinion leaders, in parallel sessions we discussed practical issues and at the exhibition we learned even more of new technological possiblities.

In the special interest group sessions of the pharmaceutical librarians, the topics included both the organization of the information and of the profession; topics like quality assessment of information services, tendering of subscriptions, electronic databases and full-text journals, the retrieval and (quality) filtering of information from the web and the distribution of information via the web were extensively discussed.

Our veterinary colleagues discussed their ways of improving services: e.g. experiences with new library services and new learning materials; the opportunities of a new library building; European cooperation in veterinary education, including the mutual use of information sources. Special attention is paid to tailor-made information sources, presentations of the library during veterinary meetings and in veterinary journals and the improvement of document delivery to individual practitioners, not the least by strengthening veterinary interlibrary loan and cooperation.

The changes in the environment of medical libraries affect our profession and professional needs, as illustrated by the developments in the Norwegian Association as well as by the fact that "health information" modules are part of library science curricula. End-user education is recognized as part of tasks of the library. By doing so, librarians experience the reward of keeping up-to-date with modern technology for information management.

Several quality aspects of the information transfer process were considered: e.g. (1) the value added by librarians, (2) the human brain as integrator of data, information and knowledge, and (3) how to improve the quality and usability of information sources. It is in this respect that the role of the medical librarian towards Internet sources has been extensively discussed, with the OMNI- en GALENO-projects being examples.

Evidence-based medicine is a very important issue to our customers: as the costs of healthcare rise, governments force the institutions to deliver more, better and faster services for a lesser price. The rationale is that treatment should only be given when there is evidence for the effectiveness. With reference to the (academic) medical centre with the profile of being a *"centre of excellence"*, the (academic) medical library may well be called a *"centre of evidence"*. Projects to estimate the value of (library) information services, and to measure the quality and benefit for patient care, are under study. Some research is done on the need of information from scientific literature for clinical practice: decisions, education and clinical protocols and guidelines.

In many countries, Consumer Health Information still is an underserved area, although the European citizen has "health and information rights". As some of the presentations have shown, librarians can play a very important role in building a suitable collection and offering services in this area.

Specialized literature and information sources, either national or European or on a specific subject, are built and facilitate the retrieval of the right information on the right moment.

Academic medical libraries in different circumstances plan as many different ways of improving services to their users, be it a more personal (subject area) approach, tailoring the collection to the information needs, user surveys, or integrating library activities into a integrated hospital information system.

New technology offers possibilities for new features to enhance the value and ease-of-use of information sources. Hypertext linking is the electronic answer to bibliographic coupling for tracing citations and references. The presentation of library services on the world-wide-web, lay-out, color and other features as well as integration of different media are under study and results were presented. Nevertheless, still very important is document delivery by photocopies or via electronics. AIDA and ARIEL, are the names of the promising goddesses of ILL. The internet is not only a superhighway but at the same time a playground or marketplace where medical librarians have to market, offer and trade their services.

In addition to all these developments, there are changes in the medical curriculum as well: problem-based learning together with library instruction needs special attention of the directors and reference librarians of academic medical libraries.

A neighbouring field of librarianship is bibliometrics and scientometrics. Scientometrics is of interest to understand the role of information and communication in medicine and to study the discipline of medicine. The use of scientometric and bibliometric data is growing in order to measure scientific output and to evaluate research performance. Serving policy makers and providing the information they need, can be an important strategy in library policy. Bibliometrics has at the same time a more practical side: management information can be generated and used for decisions in library management. Moreover, a better and more detailed analysis of what librarians are doing for whom and how is an essential part of improving the services of medical libraries and information centres.

The history of medicine, medical libraries and publishers, has always been part of the conference programme, representing an element of reflection on "Where are we", "where are we going to" and above all, "where did we came from?". By looking into the past, the past of medicine, medical books, publishing, and journals, librarians can learn and understand, in order to be better equipped for the changes we are confronted with.

Future conferences

We are heading for a larger, and - at the same time - smaller information world: there will no longer be geographical frontiers or barriers for medical information needs. Electronic networks are already heavily used and will be an essential link between professionals and data, no matter what the physical distance is. By tradition the library was holding the resources with the data and our customers came to the library to read the book or journal with the information needed. What will be the role of the medical librarians, when electronic networks will form the link between our customers and the (electronicly published) information? It is most likely that the next conference in Utrecht in 1998 will deal with this subject.

Notwithstanding the trend of growing availability of and easy access to computer networks for end-users, am I convinced that the number of medical librarians involved in organizing, retrieving and distributing information in electronic and in print versions, will grow in the coming years! So do expect to meet more colleagues in Utrecht than in Coimbra! The number of issues we have to discuss, seems unlimited; enough subjects are left for the coming conferences in Utrecht (1998) and London (2000) and the many years thereafter.

METHODOLOGY TO DESIGN AN EUROPE-ORIENTED INTEGRATED HOSPITAL INFORMATION SYSTEM

Deonilla Pizzi (1948-1996), Universita degli Studi di Siena, Italy

Integrated Academic Information System (IAIMS) for hospitals are well established in the U.S.A. starting from the 1982 NLM National Program; on the contrary most European countries seem to pay little attention to the development of such systems. The aim of this paper is to delineate the methodology of designing the broad lines of an information system which takes into account the characteristics of health care services and medical education in the European countries, that show more common features than differences: the cultural, historical and political differences between Europe and the United States prevent us from adopting the American IAIMS model.

Usually librarians' contributions to the information system in their medical school and/or hospital consist of their traditional knowledge of bibliographic and scientific information sources. However no other person in the hospital has a global vision of the information sources which are necessary to the working of the hospital seen as a firm. In other words, the librarian only has the attitude to evaluate information as a resource and to recognise those sources which are peculiar to the purpose and development of different activities performed in the hospital, such as management, research, teaching and health care delivery.

The paper will suggest a step by step methodology to design this kind of model:
1) the recognition of information as "invisible assets" of the hospital firm.
2) the identification of the three information flows: environmental, external and internal flow.
3) the identification of the different information needs in the health care, academic and research context.
4) the identification the different systems: clinical information system, scientific and bibliographic information system, managerial and legal information system.
5) the suggestion of how to integrate in the light of system theory the above mentioned systems into an effective/efficient Integrated Hospital Information System.

FUTURE SCENARIOS: THE CONTEXT OF STRATEGIC PLANNING

Tom D. Wilson, University of Sheffield, UK

The problem of forecasting

Attempts to forecast the future are always wrong: the probability of being right, at any detailed level, is very, very small. All we can do is guess, aided by more or less information about the present direction of the economy, technological development, the political stability of the country and the probable direction of policy, the possible environmental developments that may take place, demographic trends, and so on.

In other words, we can draw trend lines: we can look at what is happening now and project the possible future, if things continue as they are. In this way we get such absurd projections as the forecast that by the year 2000 the total connections to the Internet will exceed the world's population.

Trend lines present problems of two kinds: first, they tend to be linear projections of the present state of affairs, but the normal growth curve, which describes the life and death of plants, animals, and living systems in general is the so-called S-curve, which shows the progression from birth, through growth, to maturity, decline and death. We can think of trend lines as fragments of the growth curve at different points in time, but because the life-span of social phenomena is unknown to us, we cannot be entirely certain about which bit of the growth curve the trend line is describing.

In other words we can look at what is happening now and project the possible future, *if things continue as they are*. However, things never do continue as they are. For example, all projections of the growth in road traffic have proved to be under-estimates; and, thankfully, the forecasts of the growth of AIDS have not been realised, whereas no one, to my knowledge, suggested that there would be the decline in male fertility that we now know is taking place in developed countries.

Apart from simply getting it wrong, because we do not fully understand the causative factors in complex systems, the other difficulty is that *the unexpected always happens*: that is, our trend lines are thrown into confusion by *discontinuous change* — when sudden, unexpected events change the course of history. Herman Kahn's forecast for the world in the year 2,000[1] did not include the downfall of communism - a highly significant discontinuity. Anything we attempt to say, therefore, about future information needs and future information habits that will affect the way health-care information is produced and used is almost certainly be doomed to be wrong.

S. Bakker (ed.), Health Information Management: What Strategies?, 1-8.

Starting from where we are

If I accept that I cannot be absolutely right, it would be possible, even then, to make some forecasts on the basis of known trends. It is usual in these circumstances to refer to the STEP functions mentioned earlier: scientific, technological, economic and political factors. (Some writers add an additional E for *environmental* factors.)

But how much can we actually foretell? We can argue that science and technology are going to continue to bring developments that will see an increase in the impact of information technology in virtually all occupations — a growth in robotics in production, a growth in the home use of computers, a growth in network connections and applications, an increase in the accessibility of information over the international networks, and all this at a steadily reducing unit cost. Simple linear projections will tell us this much. But no one knows, how fast these developments will take place and how far they will be inhibited or encouraged by economic and political factors.

We also know that even predictable events may not be properly accounted for: the current problems over the change of the century in the year 2,000 is a case in point: everyone knew it was going to happen but thousands of computer programs were written without any reference to the change and are likely to result in costs of millions of pounds to remedy (in fact a recent estimate puts the probably cost at between $400 thousand million and $800 thousand million between now and the year 2000).[2]

A further problem is that specialised professions rarely look beyond their own narrow frames of reference: so, in library and information work today, the discussions revolve around such issues as the development of the Internet and the World-Wide Web, the digitisation of information resources and the emergence of the electronic library, networks, cyberspace and universal access to information. Clearly, these things are important in health information systems and services and, clearly, they will be part of the process of defining a new social function, or set of functions, over time.

However, health information service relates directly to health care, and the future of health information services must take into account possible futures for health care. Clearly, a number of factors determine the health of nations, but the most important are the pattern of population growth or decline, advances in medical science and associated areas such as nutrition and hygiene, advances in agriculture and food production generally, the state of the economy, and the direction of public policy in relation to health care.

Some fairly hard data on some of these issues are available to describe the possible future of health care.[3] One of the most telling of Kennedy's graphs (Fig.1) is from *The Economist*, which shows the growth in world population, divided between the developed and developing parts of the world, between 1750 and 2100. The picture is very clear: in the developed world, population growth is very flat, growing slightly to about 2050 and then beginning to decline. The reason for this is that in most developed countries the fertility rates have been declining, partly because this tends to happen as countries become more affluent, but also because, as recent news stories have suggested, the fundamental levels of fertility have been declining. The consequence of declining fertility is an aging population and that brings with it economic and political difficulties in supporting that population on the declining youth base.

The increasing population in the developing world, on the other hand, is the advance of medicine, hygiene, and nutrition in these countries. Paradoxically, these developments have been led through the intervention of the developed world to reduce

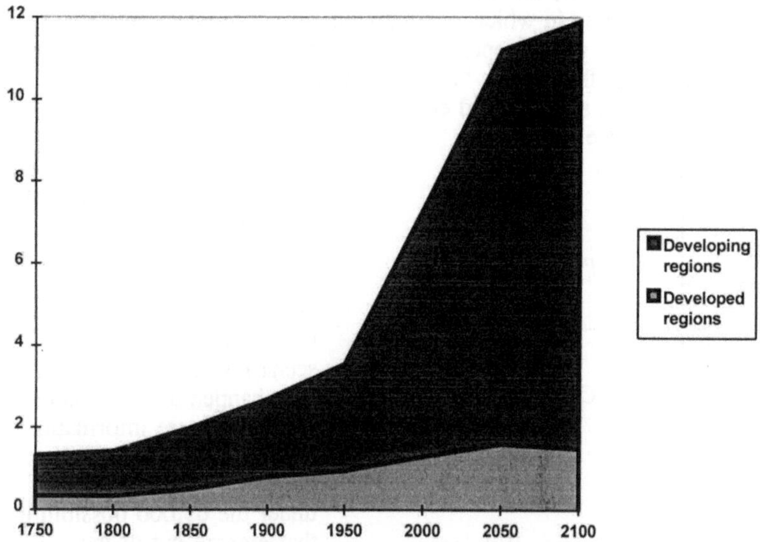

Figure 1: Population growth, 1750 to 2100 (Source: Kennedy, 1993)

infant mortality and improve living conditions generally. Populations in the developing countries have taken advantage of these developments not by stabilizing their populations but by increasing total family size, since, in agrarian societies, the number of family members available to work the land is a matter of importance. The past history of failure to have enough living children to provide the family workforce is a strong incentive to ignore pleas from international agencies and national governments to practice birth control.

It is evident, therefore, that a significant number of variables influence the demand for health services and the form that health care takes in different states. Trying to juggle those variables to provide some convincing view of the future is extremely difficult, since each represents a dimension of relevance and, depending upon the values of those dimensions, the possible futures are numerous. Just as an example: suppose we say that four dimensions are important: population growth, economic growth, advances in health care, and food production, and we assume for the sake of simplicity that each of these variables has four conditions - the total number of possible combinations that these four variables can take is then more than 63,000, i.e., more than 63,000 different possible futures - how, then, do we plot a line through these possible futures to give us the *most* probable future?

Scenario building

An alternative approach is to assume that certain underlying features of life are crucial to future development and that alternatives are offered, in broad terms, by considering the extent to which the future will be formed by the direction these key features take.

This approach is called *scenario building* and, quite by chance, as I was preparing this paper, a special issue of *Wired* came through the post, devoted to the future and with an article on building scenarios. The author, Lawrence Wilkinson,[4] posits two dimensions of importance:

individual vs. community, that is, the dimension of uncertainty about what kind of society we hope for — one in which our individualism triumphs over the community, or whether our group dependency will prevail; and

fragmentation vs. coherence, that is, the "uncertain character of social structure" — will society will provide stability and coherence, or will the centre fail to hold, and fragmentation take place?

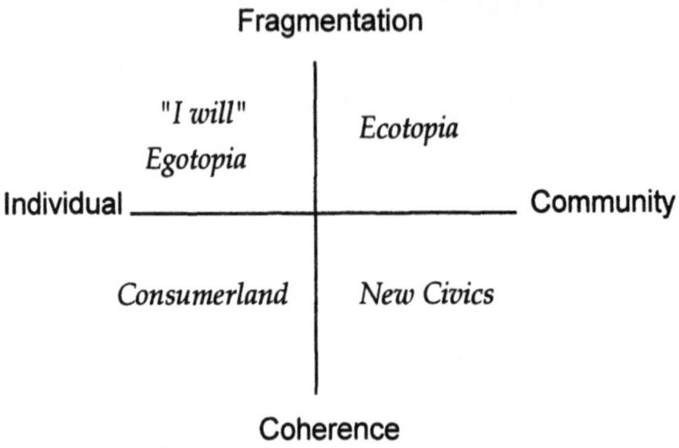

Figure 2: Possible scenarios (Source: Wilkinson, 1995)

Making these dimensions the axes of a matrix gives us the diagram shown Figure 2, with the terms attached to the quadrants assigned by Wilkinson. Perhaps we can explore the resulting scenarios in terms of what may happen to health care and health care information systems under these four possible futures, instead of under the 63,000 possibilities that emerge out of the previous analysis.

THE "EGOTOPIA" SCENARIO

Wilkinson names the first, upper left quadrant the "I will" scenario, but I have renamed it "Egotopia" to fit in with the names of his other scenarios. The consequences of this future are that work will be decentralised, communication systems (necessary to link the fragmented individuals) will dominate in society, and that the Internet (or whatever replaces the Internet) will become the space within which most people carry on their work. As a result of the fragmentation and the domination of an individualistic ideology, community infrastructures will decline.

What happens to health care under this scenario? The most obvious point is that health care ceases to be provided as a community 'good' (because the very idea of community declines) and responsibility for health care rests with the individual. Presumably, charitable and voluntary organizations will continue to provide some services, because general ethical principles of public service based upon either religious or other grounds, will continue to survive, but the individual, generally, will be responsible for his or her own health. In other words, health care will become more of a 'market' than it may be already and the health-care consumer will have to observe the principle of *caveat emptor* in this market as in any other.

How, then, will health information services function? If work becomes decentralized and teleworking becomes the norm, "virtual" libraries, with a vast increase in the range and variety of electronic information resources will be needed. The "electronic cottage" worker becomes the norm, working on a contractual basis for different kinds of organizations, connected to corporate databases and information files on-line.

The logical consequence of this is that the health information specialist, too, becomes a predominantly on-line worker, supporting the health specialist and the health-care consumer by similarly selling services and working to contract. Finding relevant information faster than competitors, faster than the not-information-worker can find it, and surviving on the basis of superior knowledge of the networks and of the information resources available through them.

Even in those institutions that persist (such as hospitals), it is likely under this scenario, that staff will be contracted for various purposes - to act as nurses, physicians, pharmacists, and so forth, on a competitive tendering basis. So, too, will information providers: even where the institution acts as the base for the service, and even when the service is delivered by staff belonging to the organization, the services will be sold and, of course, because the other staff are contract staff they will have the same kind of access to external information providers to satisfy their needs as any other health specialist not attached to the institution.

THE CONSUMERLAND SCENARIO

Wilkinson's Consumerland scenario is a view of the future in which people are consumers first and citizens second - if at all, and products are heavily personalized to fit individual demands. White-collar work becomes computerized and leisure increases, since the machine makes every worker much more productive in the time spent at work. There will be increasing privatisation, since the consumer is king and the market prevails.

The Consumerland scenario is different only in respect of its location at the coherence end of the scale, but it suggests that the stress on the individual will result in the replacement of community structures by privatised services, with individuals living not as citizens, but as consumers, pandered to by the manufacturers of products and services that are tailored to individual needs and to the changing fancies of the times.

The loss of white collar jobs to computers increases the number of people either fully occupied in servicing the leisure industries, and/or taking advantage of those industries as the need to work declines. How this is to be paid for will be one of the big debates of the 21st century, but the tendency towards coherence, rather than fragmentation, probably means that the politicians of the day will insist that the profit levels of multi-nationals and large businesses are reduced to transfer resources to the under-employed, so that the consumer society can be maintained - otherwise coherence could not be maintained.

This scenario suggests that health-care will have a predominantly community focus, but that its provision will be a matter of supply by private businesses. Those who can afford to pay for health-care will do so, either directly or through insurance schemes, but the community sense will be strong enough to ensure that the less well-off consumer will be provided for by the community - and it may be the local community, rather than the wider state.

The role of health information services in this scenario will be somewhat similar to that in Egotopia - the information broker and the cybrarian, selling highly individualised services to organizations and individuals, possibly (because of the social coherence dimension) grouped into cooperatives and, perhaps, forming companies to pursue an entrepreneurial role more effectively. If the coherence dimension is sufficiently strong, one might find cooperative health advice and information services which sell information services to companies (hospitals and clinics) and use part of their profits to provide similar services at lower cost, or completely free, to the ordinary consumer.

THE ECOTOPIA SCENARIO

Under this scenario, growth is slow because of the dominant community orientation. Business accepts civic responsibilities, which directs profits to community ends rather than to uncontrolled growth. Needless to say, community values prevail and access to networked information resources and communication systems becomes a subsidized right.

This scenario is closer to the generalized notion of a utopia, since it assumes a great deal of rational decision-making to conserve natural resources and to establish and maintain civic responsibility and community values. It is, perhaps, the ultimate extension of the ideals of liberal social democracy and, perhaps, in recent times, Sweden has come closest to realising that ideal. However, the trends of the past 15 years or so, particularly under the economic ideology of monetarism and the "free market" in many parts of Europe, has been against this possibility.

What is the future of health-care under such an scenario? In fact, it might not be so very different from the state of the National Health Service in the UK before the present government introduced the idea of an artificial "market" of purchasers and providers of health-care. That is, health-care provided as a community service, paid for by all and open to all. Of course, the "communities" could be either local or distributed and large or small. There are signs of this already in the USA where, for example, upper-middle class communities are being built, behind walls, with security personnel, so that the people within the wall can attempt to escape from the problems that bedevil the rest of society.

No doubt some health-care services would be marketed, as they always had been under the NHS, for example, physiotherapy, chiropractic services, and other types of care such as accupuncture and holistic medicine, but the services depending upon core clinical practice would be community provided or community purchased from health-care providers.

Given this scenario, health information services would clearly flourish and would be run by and for the medical institutions. However, because of technological developments, they would be rather unlike present services and might well be little more than nodes in the publicly accessible network, with little in the way of physical information resources, but employing people with many skills in discovering, indexing and cataloguing a burgeoning growth of networked electronic information.

Slow growth would also inhibit the pace of technological development and innovation and, while Net access might be a subsidized right, the resources on the Net and the extension of the network infrastructure to provide that access, might limit its usefulness. However, while business might not be so readily attracted to the Internet, community networks would flourish and libraries of all kinds would become connected to such networks to ensure fulfilment of their civic responsibilities. Slow growth might also limit the development of services, and restrict the groups that could be provided with free network access, delivering such access on a social priority basis, rather than ability to pay, but that would be the cost of community provision.

Again, therefore, we can see the development of the health information specialist as the network navigator, albeit in a rather different form from that envisaged under the Egotopia or Consumerland.

THE NEW CIVICS SCENARIO

The community and coherence of this scenario point to small group cohesion around the family, the tribe, or perhaps the neighbourhood, with shared values creating the cohesion. Electronic networks help to bind the groups together, even when they are separated by space and time. Wilkinson suggests that the groups will favour less government, but I doubt whether that is a necessary characteristic - certainly it does not accord with his suggestion that, in this scenario, public works will flourish.

It would seem logical to suggest that, under this scenario, health-care would be provided through mutual aid, either at the level of the community (in a geographical sense) or through the self-defined group, knitted together by common interests, ideologies or beliefs. Hospitals and clinics would tend to be small, with the larger specialised units provided through general taxation.

Again, this would seem to be a future in which health-care information services would flourish, although the settings might be very different from those we know now. We might expect that the values of community would support ideas of access to information, and the wide availability of knowledge. However, the small group focus of values might result in the fragmentation of existing systems, and there would be a need, consequently for managed collaboration among information providers. Given the general pervasiveness of networks, it might be that independent information brokers might also flourish, given that small units might not be able to support an information specialist of their own.

Because of technology, where physical information centres continued to exist, they would be very different, with less space for book and journal storage and display and more connections into the electronic networks, thereby providing community links for local health providers and consumers and network support for their efforts to access information.

Conclusion

Perhaps it is too obvious to state, but I'm sure you draw the appropriate conclusion from this analysis of the future - you will have seen that the prospect is that institutionally-based health-care services (or their successor systems) on something like their present model, will flourish if future society is one in which coherence and community are the dominant characteristics, while fragmentation can only be coped with if community persists. If fragmentation and a focus on the individual define the future, the present model (at least in some European countries) is likely to change.

Similarly, if we review the possibilites for health-care information services, we can see that, if coherence and community are the dominant characteristics, institutional-based services are likely to persist, while if an individualistic society develops, fragmentation of service will take place; information service will be delivered by a range of organizations and bodies, and the individual, networked information broker is likely to be an important part of the scene.

The role of social coherence in relation to health has recently been explored by Richard Wilkinson[5] who suggests that, in developed countries, "health is no longer affected very much by improvements in material prosperity" and who reports research showing that societies with greater equality are healthier societies. Thus, in the U.K., which has seen an intense, politically motivated attack on notions of equality over the past 17 years, the death rate of the poorest 10% of the population in the North of England is four times that of the richest 10%.

We can suggest, therefore, that if the blight of monetarist economic theory that has invaded not only the U.K., but also many other European states in recent years, continues to have its effect, European health is likely to decline, stress-related diseases will increase, and the pressure on health-care services will intensify. If, at the same time, "market forces" are allowed to determine the nature and extent, not only of health-care services, but also of information services, then the prognosis must be grim, since only those who can afford it will have access to health-related information and perhaps entire states will be unable to afford access to international medical databases.

I doubt whether any more persuasive argument can be found for the need for the European Community, which, through the redistribution of economic resources and its stimulus to the development of information systems and services in Europe, has done something to offset the harm done by income inequalities, dictatorships, and wars fomented on nationalist grounds. The Community is, perhaps, the best hope for a Europe in which health-care is genuinely free to all at the point of use, and in which information services are effectively developed to support that care. Within Europe organizations such as EAHIL and people like yourselves can play a significant role in ensuring that developments in information services will be such as to support the ideal of social coherence.

In the end the future role of health-care information services is going to be what you want it to become and I speak to those for whom the early years of the 21st century will be within their working lives. The younger you are, the longer you are going to work in the 21st century and the greater the impact you can have on the direction European society takes. While, inevitably, we are to some degree prey to the stronger forces of politics and economics, we can have some say in the kind of future that evolves. If we spot trends early enough, and move with them, we can be in advance of the general tendencies in society and in our professions, and if we embrace the excitement of change we can be part of the process of change and, to a degree, direct the course that events take. And, because the provision of health-care has that significant political dimension, we must also ensure that the politicians are aware of the power of our votes.

References

[1] Kahn H, Brown W, Martel L. The next 200 years. New York: Morrow, 1976
[2] Year 2000 promises strange days ahead. Byte 1996;21(2)
[3] Kennedy P. Preparing for the twenty-first century. London: Harper Collins, 1993.
[4] Wilkinson L. How to build scenarios. Scenarios: the future of the future. Special Wired ed. 1995:77-81
[5] Wilkinson R. Unhealthy societies: the afflictions of inequality. London: Routledge, 1996. (As reported by Kohn M. Unhealthy state of affairs. Independent on Sunday. 1996;(Sept.1):19)

THE HEALTH OF NATIONS ... THROUGH THE STRATEGIC DEVELOPMENT OF NETWORKING COOPERATION

Carlos Campos Morais, FCCN[1]/RCCN[2], Portugal

Introduction

To be an information professional means, at the end of this marveling century, to be professional, *tout court*, because of the prominent role of information nowadays. The coexistence of different individuals, e.g. professionals and citizens or rational and emotional personalities, is a dynamic balance between organisation and chaos. The same holds true on the levels of institutions, communities, nations or even in trans-national utopia. Although chaos could be set to order, with such an amount of *ex-formation* - using Gore's expression - and with information being tenuous and inaccurate, we might think of being right appealing to the need of order, rules, perfection. But this will not take into account the powerful laws and essentials of living matter: **health**. The health of a living being and, metaphorically, the health of any kind of structure that matches a similar function model, a nation, for example, assumes beforehand a normal evolution, the fulfilment of internal functionalities, the beneficial interaction with environment for the individual and for the species, the preservation and promotion of life and of its vital principles.

Health of nations

According to the World Health Organisation: *"in the context of health promotion (health) is the ability of an individual to achieve his potential and to respond positively to the challenges of the environment. (...) The basic resources for health are income, shelter and food. Improvement in health requires a secure foundation in these basics, but also information and life skills (..). The inextricable link between people and their environment constitutes the basis for a socio-ecological concept of health that is central to the concept of health promotion. Such a view emphasises the interaction between the individuals and their environment and the need to achieve some form of dynamic balance between the two."*

Considering either the individual, the organisation, or the nation as a system model, according to this concept, system inherent as well as environmental information and communication are necessary prerequisites and obligatory terms for self-regulation, which is mandatory to keep the system alive. Taking health as a resource and accepting in general that the living being strives to stay alive with some quality, i.e. to live with health, it is imperative that information/communication has

S. Bakker (ed.), Health Information Management: What Strategies?, 9-12.

adequate networks/channels and that the structured organism can, through his decisions centres, perform adequate self-regulation, whenever necessary.

Like for the individual, health -- as a resource of a nation -- demands the existence of a structure capable of developing and promoting its potentials: the economic, social and cultural development throughout resources in industry, education, defence, commerce, etc. and, last but not least, in health.

Well known is the technological panoply that allows the development of applications in this last field standing for either real or potential progresses in the various information access fields, in medical diagnosing, distant assistance to patients, prevention support campaigns to diseases, etc. Less known is the problem of health, generally speaking, for a big organisation like a nation, relating to its ability of structuring and interacting with its environment and to the networks that allow its information flows.

What kind of nations are we facing in this new/old reticulated world? The base of this new (not so brave) world is, recognisably, the accentuated and asymmetrical bi-modalism of the scarce very rich and the abundant very poor. This pattern, not only at the global scale, repeats like a fractal structure in smaller scales, for example in a urban structure of a great metropolis, New York, with the Bronx surrounding the wealthy apple stone ... Adam Smith, writing his book "The Wealth of Nations" two hundred years ago, would not recognise the result of his liberal utopia, and neither would Marx, in other different and devastated stops, of his utopia concerning the economical planning ruled by the State with a hand of steel. It is in this asymmetrical context, with the instability and turbulence that characterises the modern economy, that networks and the Internet have sprung out.

Internet at a glance

All the information about the Internet, disappearing, changing or growing, is found by definition in the Internet. The Internet was and is, an invention of academics, researchers, including the ones of the military phase. It is still the first anarchy in the power (a limited but not negligible disguised power) with well known ancestrals in other fields and ideologies, like the Commune or, less in the anarchic field and more in the one of the economic cooperation in network, the Hanseatic League.

Nobody leads, everyone cooperates, the State does not interfere, every kind of economy is possible. With these licensed anarchic/liberal recommendations was/is the Internet blessed. Business in its most various forms as the wheel for the large-scale or generally global development, is still not the predominant activity that takes place in the Internet: if we consider the yearly expenditure on advertisement in the USA, 60 millions of dollars is expended in the Internet, versus 140 millions in total. No doubt that advertisement will be one of the sectors of value creation in the Net.

In this rush to the West, permanently searching for new Eldorados, it is possible to envisage well known dipoles and alternatives aligned in a dynamic of opposites:

- anarchy *versus* organisation
- liberalism *versus* State interference
- creativity *versus* conservation
- liberty *versus* security

It doesn't seem possible to forecast the commitments and the balances that will be established between each of these poles but the fight is very blanched. On one side the academics and researchers, younger than priests in this very laic temple. On the other side the Administrations, the State, that always have had an attitude of distrust, bad will and envy, implacable priests of other leaden temples. In the middle, fortunately, the civil society, with excited citizens and businessmen, acting smartly and cautiously on trying to grab the chicken of the golden eggs, i.e. the organised anarchy. In a recent article in the Harvard Business Review, titled *Ruling the Net*, by Deborah Spar and Jeffrey J. Bussgang, it is argued that the informal rules, which have permitted the development of the Internet up until now, are not sufficient to fully attract the world of business. It is necessary to ensure more security in the transactions, to implement warrants related to the author rights, penalties for frauds and abuses, etc. The rules to be established will not come from a mandate of the government, but will, instead, be stated by the agents of the network community: Internet Service Providers, Information Providers, etc..

Health and diversity in functional networks

Coming back to normality, within the concept of health, it seems that it should be based on what is also common to the Gaussean statistical formulation: the coexistence of a majority which, in what concerns to living beings, corresponds to the development of a more usual genetic configuration (or of its morphology/ functionality/ most common structure), together with minorities that contribute to the growth of diversity. And we should take into account that, according to the Principle of the Requisite Variety by Ross Ashby, the decision, at a certain level, needs a greater level of variety than the levels that stand below.

Diversity reminds us of the many networks in our organism which are necessary to ensure the creation, maintenance and development of essential vital functions proper of the nervous system, the blood circulatory system, the reproductive system, etc. The health of the living being is related to the good and cooperative functioning of those networks that have, along with its functional specialisation, physiology and morphology, common principles in nature, at the level of the genetic code (would it be audacious to compare them to the communication network protocols?). When dis-functionalities occur, in one or more networks, the tissues loose structure and die -- *necrosis* occurs and could cause the death of the whole living organism. This notion and procurement for diversity is interesting -- a sustainable diversity from a simple and original soma, a collection of non-specialised cells. In several living organisms, more or less developed, diversity rebuilds itself and the functionalities get enabled again, when necessary, through organic, mechanic, electronic, etc. prosthesis, just like in the case of a transplanted organ, an artificial hand, a pacemaker, any other workmanship. This means that, in order to keep the health of the organism, to avoid necrosis that, in a last instance, can eradicate the individual's or even the species' life, a reintegration of functions in the affected networks takes place. Health and diversity of functional networks seem to be inseparable concepts for biological living beings or, in its more or less complex organisational metaphor, wherever they fit and cohabit, e.g. like in nations.

The real/face-to-face and the virtual

It is cautious to comment the level of commitment between the real/face-to-face/ and the virtual that turns out at each step in multiple activities taking place over a network structure: education, training, conferences and congresses, work planning, access to libraries, medical diagnosis, assistance to patients or elderly people, etc. In neither of these cases it is considered advantageous to follow a strictly technological guidance, only illusory attractive, through which the human being would be reduced to an autist computer key operator, physically confined and with a blistered brain. The great gain in productivity and communication, of multiplied access to the plenty new information sources, is a fundamental conquer as though the virtual activity always improves and expands the physical, sensorial, material activities. We can have better libraries as long as they correspond to better places to socialise and gain direct knowledge (either from people or information), with a strong potential to the virtual space, prodigalizing new information and creating new forms of relationship and groupwork, by using networks. We can take better care of patients in presence with more prepared and available teams when replacing the tedious and lengthy work by corresponding distant diagnosis activities, or distant vigilance, or medical prescription or conversation.

Consider this dichotomy made of the emergent dynamics between the face-to-face and the virtual and try to see the relation with another diade, typical of organisations with hierarchic levels of management and where distributed structures are considered. That's a local/not-local diade, where the not local can be regional or national or supra-national. In this diade we also must consider in the local pole what is face-to-face, material, close to the interest of the population. In the not-local pole should stay the more abstract activities headquarters (the ability to establish norms and regulatory principles) or the ability to ensure the global unit, accomplishing, for example, defence and military activities for the case of a nation. In some way there is a vector of conservation and stability, along the time, of radication and continuity - the local vector, equivalent to the face-to-face vector referred above. There is also a vector of modernity, contingency, that is an extension of the first, basic and fundamental: it is the one where some levels of decision related to the coherence of collection that demand a constant production of diversity in what respects to hierarchy functions.

Health of nations and strategic development of network cooperation

What kind of representation of a healthy nation is permitted? In order to stay out of the territory of wishful thinking we should conceive the health of a nation as a result of the conjunction of the following factors:

- The articulation of the local and face-to-face spaces with the global and virtual spaces by the potential mean of the use of networks and of the cooperative work
- The articulation of the local and operative space with the hierarchic spaces of superior level (regional, national) using networks to raise the increase of diversity at the different levels of decision
- The promotion of the citizens' health using the facilities mentioned above and the methods and methodologies, techniques and technologies suitable to the system.

This is my vision of healthier nations, using cooperation, networks and traditional face-to-face activity, with a better quality, for a little bit more happiness in our beloved mankind.

[1] FCCN-Fundação para a Computação Científica Nacional - National Foundation for Scientific Computation

[2] RCCN-Rede da Comunidade Científica Nacional - The Portuguese Academic Network

PROFESSIONAL DEVELOPMENT & MANAGEMENT STRATEGY: KEEPING UP-TO-DATE ON CHANGES IN RESOURCES

Lois Ann Colaianni, National Library of Medicine, USA

Great explorations

One of the classics in Portuguese literature is "The Lusiads" by Luiz Vaz de Camoes. "The Lusiads" is composed of ten cantos which celebrate the sixteenth century seafaring voyages of Portuguese explorers. The author has special significance to us because he attended the university at Coimbra in the 1540's. His life included an unfortunate love affair that led to his banishment from Lisbon; a father who was shipwrecked and drowned off the coast of Goa; the loss of an eye; imprisonment for a street brawl; and trips to China and India. The cantos are the story of one of the great explorations, Vasco da Gama's voyage to India. It is the story of the Portuguese people who in a little more than a century sailed over the globe, carrying their flag and their faith from Brazil to Japan, and "established not merely an empire but a new conception of empire based on mastery of the ocean routes."[1]

Many of you come from countries whose history includes brave and daring explorers who left their shores to learn about the world and often made themselves and their sponsoring countries rich. You may have studied Alexander the Great, Prince Henry of Portugal, Christopher Columbus, John Cabot, Jacques Cartier, Ferdinand Magellan, Vitus Bering, Leif Ericson, Francis Drake, Hernando Cortez, to name just a few.

World maps

At the beginning of the age of discovery world maps were based on the Ptolemy's descriptions. What would it have been like to have been an explorer in those days? Could the difficulties of ordinary living be overlooked in the excitement of participating in the voyages of exploration? Do opportunities for exploration exist today? Certainly! Explorations are taking place in space through the manned space craft and satellites which are exploring our universe. But there are other opportunities for exploration. You, like the Portuguese seafaring men, have an opportunity for some exciting voyages of discovery and fortunately you don't need to leave the comfort of your home or place of work.

Ptolemy's map showed the view of a world which was largely uncharted because travel by sea and by land was difficult. The view of the world has changed considerably. Today we are at the beginning of a great communication revolution. This is the map showing the Internet coverage of the nations that share this planet

S. Bakker (ed.), Health Information Management: What Strategies?, 13-17.

earth. This is your world to explore. By exploring this world you can bring back discoveries which can enhance your career and enrich your institution much as the early explorers created their reputations and enriched their countries.

SAILING

Early explorers had their ships. For your exploration you need a browser such as Netscape Navigator to access powerful search engines which will help you find locations of interest. Some of the top search engines and their World Wide Web addresses are:

InfoSeek (**www.infoseek.com**)
Lycos (**www.lycos.com**)
Excite (**www.excite.com**)
Alta Vista (**altavista.digital.com**)
Yahoo! (**www.yahoo.com**)
HotBot (**www.hotbot.com**)
Webcrawler (**www.webcrawler.com**)

If you know exactly where you want to go, you can use the location's address, Universal Resource Locator (URL), and set sail. If you don't know exactly where you want to go, but know what you want to find, you can search the Internet using one of the seven search engines I just mentioned to find a destination of interest.

I have time to mention only three locations to visit. The first is a virtual hospital in the state of Iowa in the U.S. [**http://vh.radiology.uiowa.edu/**]. One of the features at this site is a patient instruction book. A second is a subject index to biomedical information sources maintained by the Karolinska Institute in Sweden [**http://www.mic.ki.se/Other.html**]. The third is an attempt at distance learning in health sciences librarianship which is presented at a Johns Hopkins University site [**http://www.welch.jhu.edu/cthsl/**]. It will be interesting to see the use of newer technologies through this site.

In the sixteenth century only a few courageous individuals were discoverers. In order to be effective, each health sciences librarian must be knowledgeable about information resources in order to know what is available and to use resources effectively. I work at the National Library of Medicine in the U.S. Let me use NLM to illustrate my point.

Visit the National Library of Medicine

The Library has several products and services which are potentially useful to you. Some of these are the 40 databases, including MEDLINE; bibliographic records for many of the monographs and serials published throughout the world; biotechnology information resources; 59,000 images of prints and photographs from the History of Medicine collection; a controlled thesaurus of Medical Subject Headings (MeSH); data from the Visible Human Project, etc. Many of you may already use one or more of these. If a user asked you what process NLM follows to select journals for indexing in *Index Medicus* and MEDLINE, would you know the answer? If an editor receives a letter stating that his journal was just selected for indexing and wants to know when he can start searching and find citations to articles in the journal? Do you know how to find out? If a user asks if a particular journal is indexed, could you find out? If a user wants an article from a journal not available in your country nor in other resources you use for interlibrary loan, could you find out if NLM has it and the process to obtain it? If you acquire a biomedical journal published by a major publishing company in Japan or other country, where might you obtain a cataloging record? If a user needs help searching one of NLM's special toxicology databases, where would you go for assistance? If you are in a country without an International MEDLARS Center and a user with access to the Internet wants to search MEDLINE, could you tell him how? If you are asked about the number of gigabytes for the female in the Visible Human project, could you get the answer rapidly?

DISCOVERIES

If you have access to the Internet and a Web browser like Netscape Navigator, you can obtain the answers to all those questions using your computer. For example, let's start with the first question about the process used to get a journal indexed. NLM publishes its home page on the Web at the address: **http://www.nlm.nih.gov**. After accessing the home page you can search the section NLM Fact Sheets and obtain a fact sheet on the journal selection process. The fact sheet will explain that the Literature Selection Technical Review Committee reviews all new biomedical titles but editors and publishers and librarians can recommend titles by sending four recent issues in for review.

The List of Journals Indexed in Index Medicus. This list can be found through the NLM home page under NLM Publications. In this list, updated annually, titles are arranged alphabetically by abbreviation, by full title, by general subject category and by country of publication. Titles added during the year are printed in the NLM Technical Bulletin, also available on the home page. Titles recommended for indexing in 1996 will not be added until 1997 because of the backlog in data entry. The NLM Technical Bulletin is a wonderful publication about the NLM databases with all kinds of information about changes in the databases and search systems at NLM.

SERLINE. If someone wants to obtain an article from a journal not available in your country or in Europe, you could check the NLM database SERLINE or Locator to see if NLM acquires the title. Information on how to order a copy of an article can be obtained through the Interlibrary Loan Fact Sheet available on the NLM home page.

Catalog. Why spend time cataloging if someone following accepted standards has already done it? Use the Internet to search the NLM catalog by telneting to Locator at **locator.nlm.nih.gov**. You can print or download cataloging records for books and journal titles. If you forget the address, you can find it through the NLM home page.

Toxicology. There is increasing concern throughout the world about pesticides, toxic chemicals, and environmental hazards. You could search a number of useful databases. How do you find out about them? From the NLM home page you can link to the Specialized Information Services home page. The Registry of Toxic Effects of Chemical Substances might be a good resource to obtain the answer to your query.

Search interface. If a user wants access to NLM databases at NLM using a simple but powerful search interface, you could direct him or her to **http://igm.nlm.nih.gov**, the address for Internet Grateful Med. There the individual will find directions on how to register to obtain a code and password and arrange for billing the charges. Once the user takes a few minutes and registers, the individual can search MEDLINE, and eventually all the MEDLARS databases taking advantage of the 478,000 terms from 31 biomedical vocabularies in the Unified Medical Language System (UMLS). This is very useful for individuals who want to use French, Spanish, Portuguese, or German terms to search because MeSH has been translated into these languages and the terms are included in the UMLS. One can search on "coeur" and obtain all the articles indexed with the MeSH term HEART.

The Visible Human. One of the most exciting programs the Library has produced recently has been the Visible Human. The data for the male was released two years ago. This past fall, the data for the human woman was made available. If one of your users wanted to know how big the data set was for the female, could you find out quickly? The Visible Human Project Fact Sheet will give you that information and also the address of the FTP site where the user could find six full color anatomical images and an explanatory README file. Each image is over 7 megabytes in size. The data set for the entire female is 40 gigabytes, more than twice the size for the male, because the axial anatomical images were obtained at 0.33 mm intervals for the female instead of the 1.0 mm intervals for the male. If your user wants to obtain the data, you don't have to write NLM to find out how. The information on how to FTP the license agreement and costs is all available through the NLM home page.

History of medicine. Perhaps a user needs some pictures of persons famous in the history of medicine or wants some pictures to illustrate a lecture. You can access 59,000 images from the History of Medicine's Prints and Photographs collection at **http://wwwoli.nlm.nih.gov/databases/olihmd/olihmd.html**. A slide or print can be ordered for any of these images. The user can search the records to identify the images of potential interest and view them on his or her computer screen.

Resources

I hope that this quick overview of some of the NLM resources will encourage you to set sail on the Internet to discover new resources for your use and the use by your users. Show your users how to search the Internet. Show them how to locate sites with information of particular interest to them. Libraries are helping their users by producing lists of useful URL's with a brief description of the resources. Many are holding classes demonstrating some of the more popular ones.

At every meeting there is at least one librarian who doesn't have access to the Internet and feels that he or she cannot obtain access. This reminds me of the fable about the crow. A thirsty crow, seeking water in a garden, found a pitcher with a small amount of water in it. The crow tried, but he could not reach into the pitcher far enough to reach the water. The crow finally had an idea. He picked up a pebble in his beak and put it in the pitcher. One pebble after another was put into the pitcher until the stones had displaced enough water to bring the water level high enough for the crow to reach it with his beak. He drank his fill and then flew happily away.

If you want access to the Internet, you like the crow need to look around to find a source either in your institution or through a provider. Then you need to find the small things you need to do to get the Internet within your reach. This may be convincing an administrator or a researcher that the information resources are worth the cost. This may be convincing the computer department that the library needs access to this resource. Perhaps you can use an economic argument with administrators, showing that access to them would save time and money. You, like the early explorers, may need to find a sponsor, someone who knows about the value of Internet access to convince your administration.

VALUABLES

It is very important that health sciences librarians become familiar with the Internet and its resources. Health sciences librarians must become knowledgeable about the information tools they use. The least expensive way for most of us to do this is by regularly checking information on the Internet to see what new services are available and how tools are changing. This will take time and effort, but much less than the early explorers spent learning about their world. Health sciences librarians must be able to teach their users about available resources and how to both access and use them. Our profession deserves members who will keep up-to-date and be experts. As Camoes said in the tenth Canto about the explorers of the sea, *"Thus far o Portuguese, it is granted to you to glimpse into the future and to know the exploits that await your stout-hearted compatriots on the ocean that, thanks to you, is now no longer unknown."*[2] You can establish a new concept of health sciences librarianship based on the mastery of the telecommunication routes and the information resources accessible through these routes. May you sail safely and return to your shores bringing riches in information for your profession and the users it serves.

References

[1] Atkinson, William C. Introduction. Translation of the Lusiads by Luis Vaz de Cameos. Middlesex, England: Penguin Books, 1952. p. 7.

[2] Ibid. p. 246.

TOWARDS THE INFORMATION SOCIETY: THE NATIONAL UNION CATALOGUE IN PORTUGAL

Fernanda Maria Campos, Vice-President of the National Library, Portugal

Abstract

The paper presented a brief state-of-the-art concerning PORBASE - The National Union Catalogue on Line strengthening the importance of cooperation with special libraries, like the medical libraries.

The concept and the role of a "national union catalogue" has been analysed under the framework of the Information Society and with special emphasis on two important items: the explosion in electronic publishing anf the Information superhighways.

As a result, different network architectures or scenarios which may be used for the union catalogue were presented, briefly discussing the implications for the future of PORBASE.

S. Bakker (ed.), Health Information Management: What Strategies?, 18.

INFORMATION TEACHING: BEYOND CURRICULUM INTO LIFELONG LEARNING

Manuela Prates Caetano, Fac. de Ciências Médicas UNL, Lisboa, Portugal

Introduction

Invited to speak about "information skills in the curriculum" I chose this title because it was inspiring and it should reflect an ongoing reality in our area. The title stands as a true commitment of Health Sciences Libraries and a standing goal for Information Users' education.

The target user groups taken for this communication will be essentially Health Sciences' professionals - whether students, teachers, researchers or health care providers. There will be extensive reference to the medical field because it is heavily illustrated in the literature, although mentions to nursing, pharmacy and allied health experiences can also be found in published material.

The main global issues that have a profound effect in our subject are Information Technology, Education, Health Care and Economical issues.

- *Increased expectations from the public*, whether health or information consumers, come out of a higher level of information and education.
- *Growing professional dependence on technology* - Not mentioning our own, this evidence is so important in Health Sciences as to justify the increasing integration weight of "Medical Informatics" in the curricula of Medicine.
- *Ethical Issues* - although later than health professionals, librarians are becoming increasingly aware of the ethical implications of many decisions that were not viewed as sensible some years ago. Ethics are also involved in education when decisions are made in favour of some individuals/groups and against others.
- *Cost-containment issues* are affecting health care, downsizing libraries and giving indirect pressure towards issues of quality and excellence that both professional areas face nowadays.
- *Multisectorial environment and team-work with other specialities* - equally mentioned as vital to the profession, both by librarians and health sciences professionals.
- *Pressure for wider and more general professional roles* - world-wide recommendations to counteract the professional imbalance of medical specialists in relation to generalists, go in similar direction to our own claims of broader roles for the profession.
- *Need for self-directed, lifelong learning* - Inevitably all these issues call for changes, that - besides practice and policy actions - do lead to an educational response. There exists a clear universal move towards active, mostly problem-

S. Bakker (ed.), Health Information Management: What Strategies?, 19-24.

based learning. Instead of being teacher-centred it becomes learner-centred and its main goal is the individual being able to learn independently along his or her life. The fact that WHO, the European Union and National Governments do sponsor meetings in Medical Education, simultaneously highlights the effect that educational developments bring into practice and policies and, inversely, reflects the changing dynamics of health sciences and health care delivery over the past ten years.

This emerging scenario is deeply related with our own professional practices and goals. Not just because health sciences libraries are changing from print to digital. But mainly because the health sciences professionals' education is changing towards individual ability to access, evaluate and manage information all through their lifes.

Librarians seized this as a new professional opportunity and - while also being questioned in their traditional profile - embraced this role: "now education services can no longer be considered new or optional services - indeed they are considered standard public services offered in most health sciences libraries-..." (*Dimitroff*).

Library instruction

In 1996 *Earl* reported the results of a survey conducted in U.S. medical school libraries about "library instruction in the medical school curriculum" - the ETSU survey. Comparing to a similar study reported by *Martin* in 1975, the results showed that the number of schools offering instruction had increased from 18% to 74.5%. However only in less than half of these schools library instruction was a required part of the curriculum. This means that the goal of curriculum integration is not yet as significant as expected.

The range of programs currently offered in health sciences libraries (Fig.1) is not equally distributed in terms of frequency. All programs that libraries can manage by themselves, independently of the parent organisation are certainly the most used -- such as tours, point-of-need assistance and specific topic/product sessions. Other programs that involve some sort of collaboration with the parent institution, like class- or course-related instruction have been also regularly offered. If there is a formal mention to such programs in the curriculum it is mostly on an elective, optional basis.

Educational Programs
in Health Sciences Libraries

- Tours and Orientations
- Liaison and Clinical Medical Programs
- User Groups and Journal Clubs
- Consultation
- Outreach
- Point-of-need assistance
- Specific topic/product session
- Class- or Course- related Instruction
- Curriculum-Integrated Instruction

(adapted from Melanie Wilson et al., 1995)

• M Prates Caetano - EAHIL 96

Figure 1

Now we can question ourselves why isn't this scenario considered to be enough? What do we mean by curriculum integration? How can we achieve lifelong learning?

Curriculum integration and lifelong learning

There is curriculum-integration when 3 of the following criteria are met (*Burnham*):

1) the institution outside the library is involved in the design, execution and evaluation of the program.
2) the instruction is directly related to the students' course work and/or assignments.

3) students are required to participate.
4) the students' work is graded or credit is received for participation.
Those programs considered to be most effective are the ones that have been integrated in an obligatory basis into the course, and have required assignments.

As it stands, curriculum-integration answers to the required efficacy of the learning process but does **not** answer to the content issue, the one that gives relevance to the learning process and is directly related to lifelong learning.

Educational Services in health sciences libraries have been progressing from the traditional concept of Bibliographic Instruction (BI) to Information Management (IM) programs. IM is the content that allows information-seeking to be approached as a building process, with different levels of growing complexity being gradually introduced. IM is the content providing a direct answer to lifelong education needs referred by health sciences professionals.

Education, training and adult learning

Two other notions quite important to our educational purposes are the distinction between education and training, and the understanding of adult learners' characteristics.

Training	Education
-Develops proficiency in practice or application of knowledge and skills	-Wide cognitive perspective, deepening understanding of problems
-Goal directed	-Not necessarily important to everyday practice
-Circumscribed in its application	-Not directed to immediate effect
-Emphasizes procedures	-Emphasizes process

• M Prates Caetano - EAHIL 96

Figure 2

From the present distinction (Fig. 2) we can understand that Health Sciences librarians have been offering much more training than education and that lifelong learning stands as an educational objective exceeding much of traditional library skills training. Another important aspect to consider is the fact that our learners are adults and therefore share some specific characteristics - behavioral, emotional and cognitive - that absolutely need to be addressed. The perception that "adults learn faster and retain far more when they perceive a direct relationship between new information and present needs" (*Hubbard*) stands also a major reason for curriculum-integration.

A content analysis of the literature on libraries' educational programs seems a meaningful contribute to our present overview.

Zachert defined for any professional literature, 3 major categories of articles: description of personal or institutional experience, empirical research and finally theoretical formulation, representing a progression into the scientific approach of a subject.

The same author reported that, from 1975 to 1986, 70% of published articles on educational services in libraries were descriptions of experience of a single library, another 10.5% were reviews of the literature or descriptions of multilibrary experiences, and, finally, reports of empirical or theoretical research were lacking.

A similar approach was later used by *Dimitroff* when analysing 123 LIS articles from 1987 to 1994. The author states that "the percentage of articles describing educational services research is considerably lower than the percentage of research articles in any topic identified in other studies of the LIS literature" and considers that findings reported in 1991 are still the same in 1996.

Thus, while techniques and methodologies are available, the most pressing needs for research in this area have not yet been addressed. At this point it becomes also evident that librarians who take educational responsibilities should have any kind of understanding of educational theory besides possessing effective presentation skills.

Instructional-systems design

Let us review some important concepts behind the information teaching process: the instructional systems-design, with a particular focus on evaluation, and some topics on organisation and management of educational services.

INSTRUCTIONAL SYSTEMS-DESIGN

Instructional Systems-Design is the core element of scientific planning for educational services (*Allegri*).

- Target audience analysis - aims at group homogeneity so as to assure the most appropriate level of instruction.
- Needs assessment - is conducted to identify discrepancies between current and expected performance or knowledge levels.
- Goals and objectives - while the first focus on expected results at the ideal level, the second must be specific and achievable to help teachers attain the purposed goals.
- Content analysis - requires a subject matter expert and must take into consideration the hierarchy of learning.
- Delivery systems - would require knowledge of learning theory so as to identify a person's general approach to learning and therefore choose the most appropriate instruction method.
- Evaluation - is a critical process to the overall results once it provides information that contributes to improvement in both the teaching and the instructional design processes.

The frequently reported absence of accurate evaluation of whatever has been done in LIS educational programs - therefore basing most of our work in mere assumptions - is possibly one of the main causes of a less developed scenario than expected during the last years.

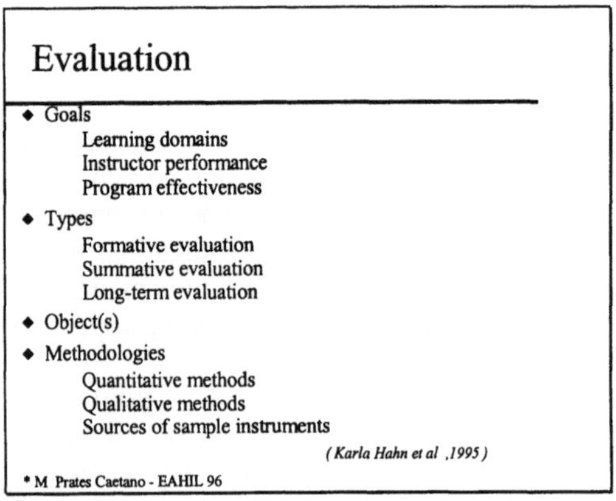

Figure 3

EVALUATION PROCESS

Main topics of an evaluation process (Fig. 3):

• The domains where to measure the learner's success in achieving the educational goals are directly related with the adult learner's characteristics mentioned before.

- <u>Psychomotor skills</u> are the skills used for physical and spatial tasks and relate to behavioural characteristics.

- Changing affective attitudes may also be the objective of some educational programs and these will be influenced by the emotional characteristics of learners.
- Cognitive skills deal with the recall of knowledge and the achievement of skills and is obviously related to the learner's cognitive characteristics.

• Types of evaluation:
- Formative evaluation focuses on program development, therefore being best activated at the beginning of the planning process.
- Summative evaluation is concerned with the overall effectiveness of a program or of specific instructional materials.
- Long-Term evaluation provides a means of tracking the success or failure of a program over time, being a mechanism for measuring the quality of instruction.

ORGANISATION AND MANAGEMENT

Educational Services
Organization & Management

- Organizational Structures
- Financial Issues
- Staff
    - profile
    - recruitment / training
- Support Structures
    - teaching/learning location & space
    - teaching/learning materials
    - scheduling
    - formularies & administrative documents
    - promotion policies

(adapted from Elizabeth Wood, 1995)

• M Prates Caetano - EAHIL 96

Figure 4

For any educational program to be adequately developed organisational & management issues must also be addressed (Fig. 4).

There are many different types of organisational structures supporting the various educational programs currently offered.

From the scenario that does not present any particular structure, to the one referring an Educational Department with a Department Head reporting to the Library Director, there is a whole range of possibilities.

Most of the times libraries do not have a clearly identifiable educational structure in the organisational chart, which seems natural to correlate to the more usual non-systematic approach in this matter.

After reviewing some of the factors considered to be necessary for a successful achievement in this field, we must recognise that there exists a great deal of libraries that cannot by any means develop neither one of the recommended steps for this process.

This acknowledgement does not mean that we should give up an educational role. There are a few simple hints that can help us achieve the possible educational programs in our organisation with some degree of success, whenever recommended approaches are not possible. These activities will contribute to the library's visibility, making it easier to proceed to more ambitious goals later on.

Institutional factors

Some key-factors to watch carefully in our parent institution, before starting:

• Our parent institution's mission statement can function as a sort of target analysis helping us define the main priorities.

• We usually receive many sorts of direct or indirect information and suggestions either from users and non-users of the library. Besides that we should discuss with them possible scenarios to answer to educational needs.

• The notion that we must establish and maintain good relations with other departments/units is not an accessory one. Many programs reported in the literature came out of invitations or were organised in conjunction with other specialists. This is particularly the case with the Departments of Informatics. This has been a very delicate relationship, sometimes with the Library assuring the maintenance of a Computer Centre, other times with a Library and an Informatics Unit equally positioned under a Resource Centre, some other times with a Department of Informatics leading the educational interventions referring to Information Management. These and many other existing models reflect a most familiar trend in our current professional history : the growing difficulty to define boundaries between two professions whose core knowledge-basis seems to overlap in some areas of Information Management and Medical Informatics.

• Our professional status is certainly a major issue in the definition of library-related educational programs. There are mentions in the literature referring the lack of academic required level as an identified barrier for curriculum integration, or for the exclusion from important Planning and Decision Committees. This may be so, but my deep belief is that more than a curricular status it is an individual high profile that is needed. How can we abandon a mere supporting role and achieve partnership with a low profile? This is very much the matter in our area.

• Resources - monetary, professional and administrative costs are to face. But it is questionable if current budget formulas are valid for educational services. Findings as those of the “Rochester study” can help us highlight cost-containment issues as a long-term effect.

Conclusion

One of the main goals of our profession nowadays is the development of "formalised instructional programs that will link individuals to information and to systems that provide them with personal memory extenders and lifelong learning support" (*Schwartz*). Libraries' educational programs must transcend the goal of training for proficiency in the use of tools and techniques, and - through Information Management education - enable health professionals to master problem-solving and use those tools and techniques for understanding, evaluating and managing the information process.

References can be requested from the author.
fax:+351.1.885.3420 / e-mail: prates@lila.fcm.unl.pt

GLOBAL KNOWLEDGE MANAGEMENT SYSTEMS: CHALLENGES FOR LIBRARIES IN THE DIGITAL ERA

Ana Maria Ramalho Correia, CITI/INETI, Lisboa, Portugal

Introduction

One of the characteristics of our contemporary society is the increasing importance of information. A society has always developed through the exchange of information and ideas, but the real benefits came when information was converted into digital format, that is, data in machine-readable format suitable for computer processing, network transmission and magneto-optical storage.

Once information could quickly and easily be transferred from one point to another, its potential could be exploited to generate a radical change in the culture of information use.

Information and its dissemination by means of Information and Communication Technologies (ICT), the enabling technologies, are central feature of contemporary society. One of the most important practical applications, arising from the convergence of the enabling technologies, is the loosely federated network of networks known as the INTERNET. This phenomenon has resulted in a dramatic increase in the amount of information available and supplied in digital format. This valuable resource can then be processed as required and delivered in whatever form is convenient for the client.

There has been a paradigm shift from local to global storage and retrieval of information. The resultant ease of access, to information services across the world, is determining the future shape and role of the library that wishes to remain the preferred point of access to information for citizens of the "Global Information Society", and that wishes to be prepared for the opportunities and challenges of the twenty-first century - the evolving "Digital Library".

Proper management of change should position the library at the focus of the information society providing a forum for information managers, information technology (IT) professionals, academics, students, researchers and citizens at large to access the Global Knowledge Management Systems.

Defining the Digital Library

It is difficult to know where to begin and end such a definition without creating a catch-all of indeterminate focus, hardly a rewarding undertaking. But we know that

S. Bakker (ed.), Health Information Management: What Strategies?, 25-30.

the digital library of the future has to be a know-how organisation and this is perhaps the most fruitful area in which to begin the search for a definition.

The *successful digital library* will have:
- the know-how to anticipate and exceed the expectations of its clients;
- the know-how to interact in a constructive and evolutionary way with IT professionals and systems analysts;
- the know-how to educate and update its clients in the uses of the enabling technologies;
- the know-how to ride the wave, created by these enabling technologies, with sufficient vision to create the library's continuous programme of development.

Thus, the *digital library of the future* will be: a library staffed by professionals who have the know-how to apply existing enabling technologies in a practical, pragmatic way to exceed the expectations of its clients as well as the know-how to influence and guide development of future technologies in the pursuit of the library's continuous development programme.

There are several other useful *definitions of the digital library* concept where authors variously refer to the electronic library, the virtual library or the library without walls.

The term, *electronic library*, has appeared in literature for several years, having been included in the title of several monographs on the subject, or been the title of serials such as, for instance, the one published by Learned Information or ASLIB's new journal (1997) "Electronic Library Research" from the International Institute for Electronic Library Research, at de Montfort University, in the United Kingdom.

Prof. Mel Collier is Head of Divison of Learning Development and chair of this recently created Institute. He states that the electronic library is:[1] *"a managed environment of multimedia materials in digital form, designed for the benefit of its user population, structured to facilitate access to its contents and equipped with aids to navigation of the global network."*

The *virtual library*, on the other hand, postulates a society in which the library concept does not presuppose the existence of a physical building, since the whole of its contents has been digitalized. This situation will naturally take some time to evolve, since it requires a radical change in the practice of the main actors in today's library world, namely authors, publishers/booksellers, companies supplying subscription services, document supply centres and of course, users.

Whatever terminology is used, the *library world is changing* rapidly as a consequence of the emergence of new tools for storage, searching, processing, creating, retrieving, displaying and assessing information, in networked environments.

The enabling technologies allow the digital library to acquire additional functions in publishing/creating/recreating information which in themselves stimulate the conditions for a forum where clients can look forward to a fruitful exchange of ideas, points of view and experiences, thereby contributing towards the rapid advance of knowledge and know-how. Such a forum can also provide training in the new technologies and their interfaces with the Information Highway.

Broering gives an excellent breakdown of the essential components that will make up the virtual or digital library of the future.[2]

THE LIBRARY OF THE FUTURE

As professionals, students, researchers and academics become more sophisticated in their search methods, the conventional links between information and its delivery will no longer be relevant. Librarians will need to exercise their know-how in the development of knowledge management techniques and human-computer interfaces.

At the same time, the characteristics of the user population will change; they will become increasingly diverse and more geographically dispersed. The digital library must address the communications issues as part of their continuous development programme if they are going to reach this wider market. Intelligent customers are not going to be satisfied with fax and e-mail; the issues of universal access, distance learning, collaborative working and document delivery cannot be avoided for long.

The library as a knowledge management system

In the value-adding process, organized data becomes information and processed information becomes knowledge. The knowledge cycle obeys the g-t-r heuristic, that is generate, test, regenerate.[3] In other words, existing knowledge is used to develop a hypothesis; additional data is collected by experimentation and ordered into information; this information is applied to the hypothesis, which is then accepted or rejected; the new knowledge thus created or regenerated completes the cycle.

This process can be seen to have a response time associated with the time from discovery or generation, through dissemination to use and then on to regeneration. If it is accepted that the intrinsic value of the knowledge resource lies in its timeliness, relevance and accuracy, then knowledge management must concern itself with optimising these components of value, as follows:

Timeliness - the timescale of the knowledge cycle has been drastically reduced by use of networks and the enabling technologies. It is this aspect which has had the most dramatic effect on information generating, disseminating, seeking and using behaviour. The limitations of hard-copy publishing processes are self-evident. Their long timescales and rising costs can no longer be subsidised in today's climate of budgetary constraints and competitive pressures.

Relevance - this is just as important in this new scheme of things as it ever was, except that the choice is so much wider. The management task is therefore to present these choices in such a way as to constructively narrow the field for the end user, while making the final selection as comprehensive as possible. It requires a multidisciplinary knowledge management team, which includes academics, scientists, librarians and information technologists.

Accuracy - the knowledge management team must accept the responsibility for advising on the quality and reliability of information accessed. It will need to put in place some form of rating measure; the skills of the management team must be such as to enable them to do this.

KNOWLEDGE MANAGEMENT

Lucier [4,5] is of the opinion that Knowledge Management has four components,
- collaboration
- knowledge base
- knowledge management processes
- knowledge products and services.

To become the focus of a Knowledge Management System, the library must move away from a static storage and retrieval mode of operation towards one which is more aligned with the dynamics and response time of the contemporary knowledge cycle and its contributors.

NATO/AGARD - International Aerospace Information Network (IAIN) Initiative

As a practical example of a geographically dispersed community, the aerospace industry worldwide is experiencing significant changes. The research, development and manufacturing activities have become ever more international in scope and conduct.

To busy researchers, more information does not necessarily mean better information. In the interests of cost-effective R&D, it makes sense to provide an information service which is targeted at this particular community, the International Aerospace Community.

Considering the advances that have been made in Information and Communication Technologies, the increased international participation in the aerospace field and the realities of scarce resources for every nation, the impetus for international cooperation and resource sharing is readily apparent.

The IAIN Working Group was set up by the Technical Information Committee of NATO/AGARD, the Advisory Group for Aerospace Research and Development, in 1995 and will operate for two years. This Working Group is concerned with the development of IAIN - International Aerospace Information Network - initiative [6]. I am a founder member of this NATO/AGARD Working Group. Its work is directly relevant to the digital library concept as it relates to the management of a diverse and distributed knowledge base for the benefit of the aerospace community.

IAIN's mission is: "To facilitate access to, use and understanding of aerospace and aerospace related information, worldwide."

IAIN is developing a prototype organizational and technical infrastructure that will serve the community of aerospace research scientists and engineers and the broader community of policy analysts, resource managers, educators and to some extent, the general public.

IAIN's objectives are:
- to identify major collections of data relevant to aerospace R&D;
- to provide mechanisms to access these data and information resources;
- to create a vehicle to stimulate the integration and access of multidisciplinary data related to aerospace R&D;
- to achieve a self-sustaining, worldwide network of partner organisations committed to sharing their data and information resources.

The IAIN prototype Homepage URL is (September 1996): **http://web.dtic.mil/iain**.

The developing Information Society in Portugal

In Portugal, it is possible to discern a growing interest in and awareness of Information Society issues, as they concern Public and Private Bodies, the Media and the general public.

By the publication of the Lei nº 10-A/96 (Law)[7] which approved the Planning Options for 1996, the Government has demonstrated its commitment to a policy of developing the Information Society in Portugal; several initiatives are already underway.

The government strategy for the creation and development of Portugal's Information Society was welcomed by all sectors of the community (business, industry, researchers, educators and citizens at large). It will enable Portugal to take its rightful place in the development of a successful and prosperous European Union.

It is my belief that these actions, towards the creation of a Global Information Society, strongly indicate the need for a National Programme for the Development of Digital Libraries in Portugal.

National Programme for the Development of Digital Libraries in Portugal

GOALS OF THE NATIONAL PROGRAMME

As an information manager professional and researcher my thoughts regarding the goals of such a programme should be:

- to highlight Portugal's presence in the Global Information Society arena, by making available our Knowledge base, Culture and National Heritage;
- to promote knowledge transfer within the Portuguese R&D environment, encouraging the formation of multidisciplinary and transnational teams;
- to improve Portuguese competitiveness in the global marketplace;
- to create "electronic archives" of National Heritage material to allow ease of access for researchers and citizens alike;

ACTION LINES OF THE NATIONAL PROGRAMME

This National Programme must provide for the following action lines, among others:

- To develop Specialisation Diplomas/PostGraduate Degrees, in the area of Digital Library / Electronic Publishing;
- To promote Lifelong Learning Professional Programmes to enable existing librarians and other Information Management staff to update their education by continuous Personal Development Programmes;
- To ensure that all students acquire modern information skills in order to encourage a vibrant information culture in future generations;
- To provide resources for University Libraries to enable them to make available independent learning materials to be used not only by University students but also by external users (for Personal Development, distance learning, Business, etc.);
- To develop the required physical infrastructure of networks, servers and terminals;
- To review and update the required legal framework to take into account information in digital format (e.g. copyright and related rights, personal data protection, access to government information)
- To launch a National Research Agenda for the development of Digital Libraries in Portugal; this must take into account the continuous emergence of new

technologies, the demand for more sophisticated services and high quality products. The research programme should promote projects developed through national and international cooperation, which will aim at focusing on best practice and enable Portugal to "leap-frog" the competition in this important economic sector;

Conclusions

This paper offers a basis for consideration and outlines some courses of action regarding the Development of Digital Libraries in Portugal. The scale of action proposed is significant. There is a strong and urgent need for an integrated effort towards cohesive development of Digital Libraries to support and nurture a healthy Information Society in Portugal.

References

[1] Collier M. Defining the electronic library. In: Electronic Library and Visual Information Research - Elvira 1. London: Aslib, 1995, p. 1-5
[2] Broering NC. Changing focus: tomorrow's virtual library. Serials Librarian, 1995;24(3/4):73-94
[3] Plotkin H. The nature of knowledge: concerning adaptations, instinct and the evolution of intelligence. London: Penguin Books, 1994, p. 84.
[4] Lucier RE. Embedding the library into scientific and scholarly communication through knowledge management. Proc Clinic on Library Applications of Data Processing, 1992;(April):5-18
[5] Lucier RE. Building a digital library for the health sciences: information space complementing information place. Bull Med Libr Assoc 1995;83:346-350
[6] IAIN Concept and Proposal, 24 May 1995. Includes Series of Reference of the IAIN working group. IAIN WD-05.
[7] Portugal. Assembleia da República. Lei no. 10-A/96: Aprova as Grandes Opções do Plano para 1996. Diário da República, I Série-A, no. 71/96, 23 de Março de 1996, p. 584-(2)

HIGHLIGHTS OF HEALTH SCIENCES INFORMATION IN AMERICA LATINA AND CARIBBEAN

Celia Ribeiro Zaher, BIREME/PAHA/WHO, São Paulo, Brazil

Abstract

To counteract the problems of retrieval of scientific medical information and availability of journals in Latin America, the Pan American Health Organization decided, in agreement with the Brazilian Government and support of U.S. National Library of Medicine, to create a Center to operate as a reference center and clearing house for health science researchers and professionals. BIREME today acts as coordinator of the Latin American and Caribbean Health Sciences Information System, assembling 37 countries and 602 medical libraries within its network. The System promotes introduction of modern means of communication and information technology and organizez training of professionals and users developing its capacity in applying the most update concepts of information systems management and computerized information handling.

Description of its goals and future developments towards a virtual library network were considered, as well as the accomplishments and setbacks were described, including statistical data for the period in review for the counterpart countries.

Future outlooks of BIREME itself and of the network have been highlighted in view of the needs of the scientific community.

S. Bakker (ed.), Health Information Management: What Strategies?, 31.

INFORMATION MARKET SYNERGY: WILL EUROPEAN CONTENTS BECOME EUROPEAN PRODUCTS?

Maria Joaquina Barrulas, INETI/CITI, Portugal

Introduction

Information market synergy is a topic of general interest, since what happens in the information market has consequences in the overall management of any library.

My recent work at the Centre for Technical Information for Industry of INETI, the National Institute of Engineering and Industrial Technology, is related to information market issues and, in particular, with the actions undertaken by the European Commission under the IMPACT2 and INFO2000 Programmes. The concepts of information industry and information market will be dealt with from two perspectives: from a wider view of an industry with various identifiable segments, towards a converging sector showing a trend for cross-merging.

Major work being carried out at the European level to develop and strengthen the information industry and information services market in Europe is referred to and finally I refer some thoughts on the roles of librarians and information managers.

Information industry: sectors and dimensions

The well-known matrix produced by researchers at Harvard University's Centre for Information Policy Research in the beginning of the eighties, is referred to as the first description of the "total range of business entities in the USA's information industry".[1] In McLaughin and Birinyi's map (Fig. 1), about 80 entities are placed alongside the axes content and conduit and products and services of the matrix, according to the extent to which each represents one dimension, or another.

This matrix shows a very broad spectrum of entities and activities considered to be part of the information industry. It includes traditional products and services, such as books and libraries, printing and publishing as well as the technology-based services and products such as on-line directories and professional databases and videotex. It covers also the wide range of telecommunications services and products, audiovisual and film.

Defining information industry with such a wide scope stresses the importance of information within society, and produces figures confirming that information workers are the majority of the work force in modern societies. It also provides the basis to consider information a major economic sector. However, segmentation is necessary to understand how the market works and to identify major actors in it.

S. Bakker (ed.), Health Information Management: What Strategies?, 33-40.

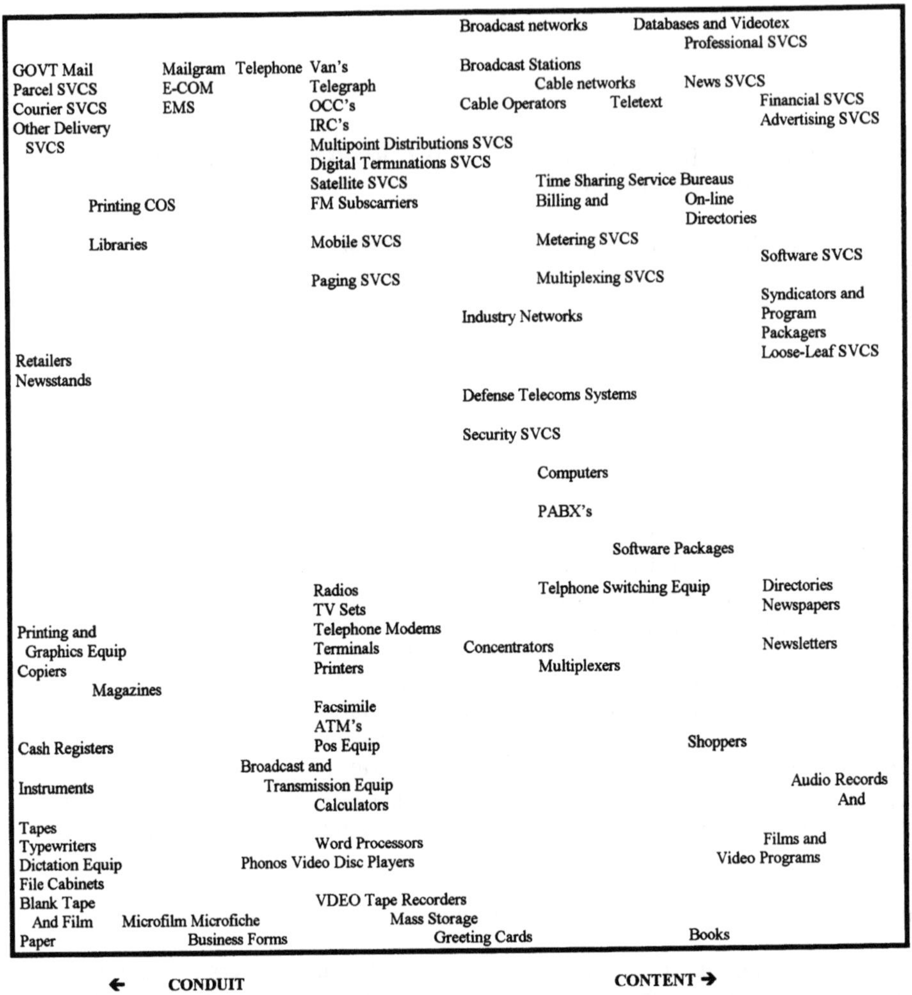

ATM-Automated Teller Machine; E-COM-Electronic Computer Originated Mall; EMS-Electronic Message Service; IRC-International Record Carrier; OCC-Other Common Carrier; PABX-Private Automatic Branch Exchange; POS-Point-of-State; VAN-Value Added Network.

For example, "Electronic information services" is one of the traditional designations used to frame the boundaries of an industry that includes the providers of information services and the organisations involved in providing the means of distribution and processing such services. The major stakeholders being the on-line database providers and vendors, the real-time information service providers and CD-ROM publishers. This segment of the information industry was seen as fast-growing and innovative, but rather small if compared to the cluster formed by telecommunications or hardware and software manufacturers and producers, sectors of the information industry that are often considered completely independent. Also, well defined and previously seen as very distinct sectors are the audio-visual and film industries.

Technological development within a decade has been made several of the products and services of the matrix, obsolete, as for instance, the telegraph or videotex services, while others such as mobile phones or electronic mail were just emerging and are now mass-produced and/or used. At present the information industry is facing a "convergence phenomenon".

CONVERGENCE

The convergence phenomenon in the information industry results from technology integration. At the lowest level, the ability to digitalize all kinds of data provides the basis for incorporating different elements, such as sound, video, text, image into a single product. The time is near that all these elements, incorporated into a single device including television and film, will be accessible locally or remotely, via broadband networks and through an "information machine".

Convergence in the information industry leads to recognition of the importance of information content. Companies operating in the equipment, infrastructure and distribution/delivery of information services and products, do realise that the information contents is their primary raw material, and begin to look for strategic alliances with content owners.

The advent of multimedia and the total range of interactive electronic information and entertainment services, are opening new, mass consumer markets sufficiently attractive to interest the giants of film, television and telecommunication industries.

A study by the Policy Research Institute, UK, commissioned by the EC not only compiles the main events and developments, but divides the information sector into three broad groups: information content, information delivery and information processing:[2]

"*Information content*: the intellectual property which forms the basis of an information service, whether it be a piece of text, a collection of photographs, a film or a piece of music;

Information delivery: electronic communication channels (such as telecommunications, cable and satellite) or off-line distribution channels which are used by information content providers to distribute their services, and by users to access these services;

Information processing: the hardware, software and communications equipment required by users in order to view and process information and entertainment services and by information content producers in order to develop and design their services."

Within these three major groups a great variety of industries can be found, with different structures, scales and revenues, but increasingly interrelated and with a growing co-operation (see Table 1).

As pointed out in the Report, "without alliances and, in some cases, investments in channels of delivery and viewing/receiving equipment, information content producers have little hope of getting their services to the users. Equally, the hardware manufacturers are finding that their products will not sell unless their potential customers have a range of suitable applications from which to choose."

Table 1: The Composition of the Wider Information Industry

Information Content	Information Delivery	Information Processing
Primary Producers	**Primary Infrastructure**	**Primary Equipment**
Print, electronic and multimedia publishing Film, video and TV programme production / publishing Audio production / publishing	Public telecommunications (PSTN) Fibre optic networks Cable networks Satellite networks Radiowave, cellular and mobile networks	Computer & peripherals manuf. Processor manufacturing Consumer electronics Telecoms / satellite receiving equipment Operating software Applications software
Secondary Agents & Services	**Secondary Infrastructure**	**Secondary Products / Services**
Trade, retail and specialist distribution Design, specialist production and replication Rights brokerage and clearance	TV / radio broadcast channels Value-added network services Intelligent 'superhighways'	Distribution, bundling and replication Specialist programming / interface design Software production tools

Source: Policy Studies Institute / IMO Annual Report 1993 - 1994

To scope and to define the Information Industry is difficult as increasingly more organisations are moving beyond their traditional areas of activity and operating across the full range of "information-related" industries. Examples are the growing number of cross-industry mergers, acquisitions and strategic alliances, and the extent to which companies make investments in related industry sectors. Companies recently involved in such transactions in the USA and Europe are, among others:[3]

- VIACOM (US) buying Paramount Communications: Cable operator buying content
- US West buying 25% of Time Warner Entertainment: buying content
- Time Warner (US) Buying American television & Communications: content owners expanding into delivery channels.
- Paramount communications buying Macmillan Inc. (US), print publishing: constructing media group
- Microsoft (US) buying 50% of Continuum Inc. (US): company that has rights in images in St. Petersburg Museum and London National Gallery.
- Reuters (UK) acquiring Quotron (US), real-time finance services: buying into the US market share
- Pearson (UK) buying Software Toolworks (US): multimedia software/ videogrammes.
- Reed/Elsevier (UK/NL) buying Official Airline Guide (US): extending market share.

A global information market in a global information society

The interdependency of economies in an open market environment is a phenomenon that economists have identified, businessmen are experiencing and some politicians are still learning on how to cope with. Global is a term that now qualifies economy as well as society. "Global Information Infrastructure" also emerged and according to Leer there are three visions of this expression:[4]

- the predominant one is the *political vision* which transmits the emphasis given by Al Gore (who supposedly has coined the phrase), considering it as the "electronic nervous system for government, education, health care, culture and commerce", therefore the key for the development and prosperity of a society, globally networked;
- the *commercial vision*, mainly shared by the major players of the information industry sectors of entertainment and communications, which envisages the global information infrastructure as a global marketplace.
- the *social vision* that sees global information infrastructure as the basis for the establishment of the global village anticipated by MacLuhan long time before. This vision is shared by many Internet users who accepted this medium as a "place to access free information and to learn, a place for scientists and academics to exchange and develop knowledge".

These three visions encompass different concerns but are not mutually exclusive, and should therefor be accommodated in all development strategies.[4]

A global information society is still to be reached, and many wonder if the infrastructure being built will allow equal access for all or will enlarge the gap between information rich and information poor nations and individuals.

GLOBAL INFORMATION MARKET

A Global Information Market is emerging from the infrastructure of digital networks now seen as a condition for nations development. Acording to Leer[4] the various activities related to information industries within the Global Information Market, can be grouped simply into two main blocks: content and technology.

Content. This block includes network service providers, government and public services such as health care and education and the wide range of value added information services, on-line services providers within various sectors:

- banking and financial services
- health care
- libraries and archives
- on-line information: business and professional research
- on-line information: education and academic research
- on-line information: home market and mass-consumers
- entertainment and culture

Technology. This block starts with the physical communication network (Telephony, satellite, cable, broadcasting-companies), followed by network security, control and performance (manufacturers of microchips, security technology and network control systems). Computer and software manufacturers and consumer electronics producers complete the technology block.

Globalization in the information industries is on its way and the battle field is moving more and more towards the content that ultimately will be the differentiating element offered to consumers. In this respect Europe has a strong role to play: its rich and diverse cultural heritage is an immense and invaluable asset, the basic raw material for value added information services providers.

The European perspective

The level and pace of the Information Society development in Europe are of a rather recent concern to politicians. The European Commission's White Paper of December 1993 "Growth, Competitiveness and Employment" brought to the public discussion the potential for new jobs that is associated with the information and leisure activities. The White Paper paved the way for further actions aiming to define "an European way to the Information Society".[5,6]

However, the "comercial vision" arrived first. By the late 1980s the European Commission had already realised that the European information industry needed a push to become competive and to reduce the gap between its American and Japanese counterparts. The IMPACT (Information Market Policy Action) Programme launched in 1989 is the first co-ordinated action from the European Commission oriented towards information contents, first understood as advanced electronic information services and products, basically on-line databases and CD-ROM's.

Phase one of the IMPACT Programme ran from 1989 to 1990 with three main goals:

- creating the internal market of information services
- improving competitiveness of European information services
- contributing to internal cohesion

The second and most important phase, IMPACT2 was in place from 1991 to 1995 and had a strategy to stimulate the market from both the supply side and the demand side, according to four actions lines:

A. Improving understanding of the market
B. Overcoming legal barriers
C. Increasing user-friendliness and improving information literacy
D. Supporting strategic information initiatives

ROLE OF THE INFORMATION MARKET OBSERVATORY

The Information Market Observatory (IMO - established in 1988 and later incorporated under IMPACT), was one of the first initiatives to shape the information market and industry in Europe.

The results of IMO market research (identification of market actors, market segmentation, market dimension, forecasting and trends) have been published in a series of Working Papers covering a variety of topics. The single enumeration of the titles of these Working Papers gives a perspective of the evolution of advances in technology and product innovation during the last decade.

A full account of the major developments throughout the year is given in IMO Annual Reports. Also, the studies of a more qualitative nature on various aspects related to information use, are valuable tools for new entrants in this very fuzzy industrial sector.

WORK OF THE LEGAL ADVISORY BODY

Under action line two of IMPACT2, the contribution of the Legal Advisory Body in areas dealing with legal and regulatory barriers to the free-flow and use of information is relevant. Experts of all EU member states have addressed key-issues such as data protection, intellectual property, computer crime, etc.

STRATEGIC INFORMATION INITIATIVES

The stimulus to the supply side given under IMPACT2 was mainly through action line 4. Three calls for proposals for pilot projects in Interactive Multimedia, Geographical Information and Information for Business and Industry were launched.

The support given to innovative information products was intended to push European producers to respond to specific needs of European users and gradually improving competitiveness of the European information industry.

The IMPACT programme, with a relatively small budget, if compared with larger technology research oriented European Programmes, helped to stimulate European firms and entities working in information-related areas and to create synergies as a result of joint projects carried out by consortia of different EU countries.

IMPORTANCE OF CONTENT: INFO2000 PROGRAM

The content industry is seen as "one of the key dimensions of the information society" and Europe, in spite of its weaknesses, also possesses many strengths such as the overall market size and population, the presence of world-ranking information and conglomerates, a long-established publishing tradition and a rich content base and linguistic diversity.

INFO2000 is the European Commission contribution to help European content industry to strengthen its competitiveness. This programme was adopted by the EC in May this year and has three long term strategic objectives:

- facilitating the development of the European content industry
- optimising the contribution of the new information services to growth, competitiveness and employment in Europe
- maximising the contribution of advanced information services to the professional, social and cultural development of the citizens of Europe

and will develop under three Action Lines:[7]

- stimulating and raising awareness
- exploiting Europe's public sector information
- triggering European multimedia potential

INFO200 is described as a programme aiming at "the development of a European information content industry capable of competing on a global scale and able to satisfy the needs of Europe's enterprises and citizens for information content" (Work Programme 1996-1999).

Conclusion: Changing roles of the Information Manager

The changing roles of librarians and information managers in the digital era, is a core topic in almost every professional meeting and it is also the topic of some papers in this conference. Two main aspects are particularly relevant in the context of the information industry development: quality assurance and assessment of user needs.

QUALITY ASSURANCE

As in any other industrial sector, the availability of a wide range of products and services enlarges the possibility of choice, but also increases the need for making "qualified choices". This means that a librarian or information manager has to develop his/her ability to distinguish quality products and services from simply "consumer oriented gadgets".

In the health libraries sector, this ability is crucial, and will have to be exercised whenever the librarian or information manager has to decide which products/services in what formats should be acquired to best match their user needs.

Quality assurance of free information sources, e.g. available in the INTERNET, becomes more and more relevant. Librarians cannot leave this new and important role to others.

USER NEEDS

Knowing the users and their information needs and requirements is high priority in order to fully accomplish any library's mission. The vast literature shows that this subject has been intensively addressed and studied by librarians and information scientists.

As the information industry expands and a diversity of products and services are released to the market, user needs and usability aspects also have acquired greater relevance. User-centred approaches become imperative in the design of new information products, and specific methodologies have been developed for information engineering projects.[8] User involvement in every stage is a requirement for any project to be supported under the Telematics Applications Programme.[9] In the libraries sector, two groups of users are specifically mentioned: the libraries and the librarians themselves and the users of library services.

Another very important role for which librarians are most capable, is therefore, to contribute their knowledge of user information seeking behaviour into the design of new innovative "usable" information products, services and systems.

References

[1] Horton Jr FW, Burk CF. InfoMap: a complete guide to discovering corporate information resources. New Jersey: Prentice Hall, 1988

[2] The Main events and developments in the Information Market 1993-1994. IMO, European Commission, 1995

[3] IMO Working Paper. Mergers & Acquisitions in the electronic information industry. European Commission, 1994

[4] Leer AC. Information Transaction in the Global Information Market. ELPUB 102. European Commission, 1995

[5] Europe's way to the Information Society. An action plan. Communication from the Commission to the Council and the European Parliament and the ESC and CR, 1994

[6] Europe and the global Information society: recommendations to the European Council. European Commission, 1994

[7] Communication to the European Parliament and the Council concerning a multi-annual Community programme to stimulate the development of a European multimedia content industry and to encourage the use of multimedia content in the emerging information society (INFO2000), 1995

[8] ELPUB 105: Usability study. Handbook for practical usability engineering in Information Engineering projects. European Commission, 1995

[9] Telematics Applications Programme. IV R&D Framework Programme. European Commission, 1994

NEW TOOLS IN BIOMEDICAL RESEARCH: DYNAMIC FULL TEXT COLLECTIONS

Bette S. Brunelle and Dana Johnson, Ovid Technologies

Introduction

For at least fifteen years various models for full text searching, browsing and presentation have been widely discussed in the information industry, but it is only in the past few years that significant bodies of electronic full text have begun to be available. Predictably enough, the explosion of full text activity has resulted in a variety of forms, or models, for full text delivery.

PUBLISHERS MODEL

On the Web, one can find many publishers offering full text with a variety of search engines and features. A conspicuous feature of publisher-provided full text is that only a small amount of text, usually either abstracts or selected articles from recent issues, is actually available. Although that may change, the biggest drawback to single-publisher sites is a conceptual one: too many different "stops" on the information superhighway to get all the information needed -- and at each stop there is a different software, data structure and interface. It's as if each library in a system only held the ten or twelve subscriptions from a single publisher, and patrons had to go from library to library to find all of the journals of interest, learning each time how and where a particular library shelved the issues. Further, although many of these offerings are on the Web, the linking capabilities -- and linking is the raison d'être of the Web -- are severely restricted by the limited scope of the offerings.

VENDORS MODEL

From vendors provide two prominent models for full text: the image-based document delivery system, which may or may not include ASCII text for searching, and ASCII-based full text, which usually does not include images, and thus cannot be a realistic replacement for the original publication. Although ASCII/Image hybrids (systems that allow searching of the text but deliver a page image for viewing) sound promising, the numerous projects of this type have had many problems, mostly to do with the sheer size of a complex full text article, with graphics, rendered into a page image. These images are cumbersome to download, and often beyond the capabilities of a workstation's memory. Furthermore, if you take a user-oriented view of the research

S. Bakker (ed.), Health Information Management: What Strategies?, 41-44.

process, static images, even when supplemented by ASCII text, do not take advantage of the richness and diversity provided by the most elementary Web site: linkages.

DYNAMIC MODEL

A completely new full text model is also beginning to appear -- one that takes advantage of both the richness of "traditional" searching and that of the Web hypertext model of linkages. In this model, collections are designed both with individual document structure and cross-document structure and cross-document linkages in mind. A good way to think of the new full text is in terms of "dynamic full text collections." This model is best approached by looking at the many uses to which full text is put in the research environment.

Browsing Full text

PERUSING AN ISSUE

Browsing -- perusing an **issue** or issues of a journal to see what's there -- is a good way to see what's new in a field, to catch up on "hot topics". Table-of-contents (TOC) features, when available, provide a fast, efficient way to browse. At a minimum, a TOC feature is a "must-have" feature for full text -- otherwise the electronic version will be lacking a major advantage of print. And in fact, with the exception of some image-based document delivery systems, most full text offerings do include this important feature.

MULTIPLE TITLES

Of course, a full text **collection**, as differentiated from an individual full text title, can enhance the utility of browsing by extending the serendipity of browsing one title to the that of browsing multiple, related titles. If the current hot topic in your field is "apolipoprotein and alzheimer's disease", then quickly finding articles on that topic in the British Medical Journal, Lancet, Science, the Journal of the American Medical Association, the New England Journal of Medicine, the Archives of General Psychiatry, etc. is a lot more useful than accessing only the publications of a single publisher.

SEARCH MENU

TOCs are usually made available via a menuing system that leads the user through a title, to an issue, and then to articles. This is a good method if the user already has in mind a particular issue of a particular journal to peruse. At other times a user may not even realize a wish to view a TOC until after an article of interest is located - therefore a good technique for full text is to make TOC browsing evident to the user at several points during the browsing process.

Locating Documents

Another of the common uses of full text is simply to locate a known, or "semi-known" article. A known article is conceptually straightforward -- "Dr. Gloth's article in the March issue of Lancet on "Vitamin D Deficiency." Of course, if Dr. Gloth's article actually appeared in JAMA, then the "known" article is really "semi-known," and searching a collection with multiple publishers will be much more gratifying than searching the works of the single, wrong, publisher.

In addition to mistaken "known" articles, "semi-known" items include such things as "a book review of Humane Medicine" or "a good picture of a transtracheal needle." For these types of items, *fully* searchable full text really shines. Searchable full text should include searching on such document elements as the caption text As an added bonus, full text is often available *before* an indexed and abstracted citation, making it particularly good for searches such as a book review of a new title.

Subject Searching

As is widely known, the majority of searches for any database are subject searches. It is also well-known that a good subject index can generally out-perform "keyword" searching both for precision and recall -- but full text, with very rare exceptions, is not subject-indexed. This is one area where a large, online collection that includes bibliographic and full text databases can improve the retrieval aspects of full text -- by linking the output of bibliographic searching directly to the available full text. In this type of linking, a user searches a database such as Medline, EMBASE, Current Contents, Biosis, Psychological Abstracts, etc. -- using all the searching tools available in these databases.

In Medline, for example, the user's original entry of "ear infection" can be mapped to the controlled vocabulary term "otitis media" and restricted to the treatment and therapeutic subject headings by the mapping process in Ovid. The search is then limited to full text. If any viewed citation corresponds to an available full text article, the citation is marked in such a way that it's clear that full text is available. A simple mouse-click or keystroke links to the full text database and the complete text of the article, with illustrations, is retrieved.

The Ovid system has a particularly rich web of bibliographic-to-full text links. The system not only links to full text from a variety of bibliographic databases, but also knows what full text titles are available to a particular user, and where they are located. Full text from Ovid may be located either on-site or at a remote location such as at an affiliated institution, or on the Ovid Online system. An Ovid user only sees the link capability if a particular full text title is available to him or her, in spite of the fact that different sites may have the same bibliographic databases but different collections of full text.

This linking from bibliographic citations to the corresponding full text essentially brings the full power of an advanced searching system, including automatic mapping of natural language to subject indexing, to full text.

Interacting within a document

One of the great advantages of dynamic, linked full text over page images is the interaction that is possible within a document. Unlike a static page image, dynamic full text allows the user to move from point-of-interest to point-of-interest within the article with ease. Once a full text document is displayed, dynamic full text will give the user a variety of navigational aids, including: 1) a link from the sections in a structured abstracts to the corresponding document section, and back again, or 2) a link from an outline to sections within the full document.

In dynamic full text, figures, tables and illustrations may appear in context within the article, or as links. A good technique for graphics is to show a thumbnail of the item, and the thumbnail itself becomes a link to the fully enlarged graphic. Links to references, right from the place in the citation in which the reference appears, are a basic part of dynamic full text.

Other kinds of inter-document links can be imagined, such as "bookmark" links, which allow a user to make comments on parts of text, and create a personal "trail" through the document.

All these inter-document links make for a convenient and lively interaction with the full text, which mimics the ability to "thumb" through a printed article (e.g. links between sections) and extends the capabilities of print (e.g. bookmark links).

Linking beyond document boundaries

The most exciting instances of linking technology, as shown in the Web, are those linkages which go beyond a document to other items of potential interest. Thus, for example, it's nice to be able to view references in context while reading an article, but it's even nicer if from a reference you can link to an abstracted citation for that reference in another database (and of course, right back again). And even better might be the capability to link from a reference *to its full text*, as is possible with Ovid full text.

The rich web of linkages that can be created within a collection are truly amazing -- in the Ovid Core BioMedical Collection, which contains the full text for 3½ years of 15 journals there are 366,060 reference links to Medline -- and over 14,000 links from a reference to *its* full text in the collection.

There are a number of other imaginative links which go beyond collection boundaries, such as links to email for a primary author or links to other databases on the Web -- for example, a link from an article about a new piece of the DNA map to the GenBank EMBL Data Bank and the citation for this structure.

Linking beyond document boundaries is one of the most exciting features of the new full text, and it is just beginning to be fully developed. An important question to ask of full text software is "how is it architected for links?" If links from a reference back to its citation or full text is available now, will links forward to articles that cite this one be available in the future? How about links to "similar" articles -- something that can be accomplished by certain statistical and clustering techniques.

Summary

Once you begin thinking in terms of linkages beyond the boundaries of a particular database, the possibilities are endless -- and, as is clearly seen on the Web -- not always advantageous when time is of essence. One of the nice things about a dynamic full text collection, is that full text is presented within a coherent context -- with titles selected for compatibility and provenance, and with software features informed by a consistent design philosophy. For full text, this design philosophy should not just mimic the printed page or provide an alternate form of document delivery. Dynamic full text collections should actively support the research process with interesting new functionality.

MAKING YOURSELF INDISPENSABLE: EXPERIENCES FROM 25 YEARS OF NETWORKING

Lotta Haglund and Ulla Ch. Hanson, Spri Library, Stockholm, Sweden

Introduction

In 1993 when Spri celebrated its 25th anniversary, the opportunity to reflect on how Spri Library and Research Report Bank had evolved into the "complete library" presented itself. Compared to other corporate libraries, our library had not only survived but grown into a national resource library for health care, with extensive international contacts. In addition to our high standards concerning quality we are convinced that networking, from both human as well as technical points of view, has had a great impact on the development of the library. And today we can also proudly tell you that we have been nominated, for the second time, to the award "Library of the year", in Sweden.

Spri Library and Research Report Bank

Spri Library and Research Report Bank is an associated national resource library with special responsibility towards health services. Together with the Karolinska Institute, answering for medical literature, and the National Institute for Working Life, answering for occupational health literature, we have a national responsibility for purchasing the Swedish literature in our fields as well as the most important international publications. The library contains Swedish and international literature on health services, including unique research material such as unpublished studies from county councils, health service units and universities.

Collection development of the Research Report Bank

Today we will pay special attention to that unique collection of grey literature called the Research Report Bank, and present the methods we have used to make the acquisition rational and effective.

GREY LITERATURE

According to our instructions from the Swedish Government and the Federation of County Councils, it is our responsibility to collect and disseminate information about

S. Bakker (ed.), Health Information Management: What Strategies?, 45-48.

grey literature in the health care field. In Sweden a great deal of very interesting research and development projects in the health care field are presented as unpublished reports by both the county councils, the nursing colleges and the universities. These documents are virtually impossible to find outside these institutions. The difficulties in finding the documents in normal bookstores have forced us to find new methods of acquisition.

CONTACT PERSONS

We realised early on that our good connections with the staff from the health care field or libraries in the county councils, could be useful to us in order to facilitate the collection of grey literature. The procedure has been to ask people in key-positions to take full responsibility for the delivery of reports from their own institutions. There are usually no problems in convincing people to become a contact person and we can see an increasing interest among researchers to be accessible in reference databases. They serve us voluntarily with information on interesting projects and make sure that the documentation of these projects is distributed to us as soon as possible. Together these contact people create a human network and they are a vital prerequisite for the growth of the Research Report Bank collection.

GROWING NETWORK

The network has developed rapidly and today it also contains staff of the university institutions, nursing colleges, private companies and end-users interested in getting their work registered in the Spriline database. The collaboration with the lecturers in the nursing colleges does also involve articles published in international journals. They deliver their articles and we add them to the holdings of the library and to our database Spriline under a special tag called SUECANA. To nurture this network is an inspiring but time-consuming task, but all sides have strongly benefited from the collaboration since we all share the same objectives, namely to make the literature accessible. That is one of the best ways of making yourself indispensable.

This is one way to obtain grey literature, but we are also using all the traditional methods like scanning journals and literature lists from other health care libraries.

Educational initiatives

As you are no doubt aware, grey literature's presentation can be everything from poor stencils to glossy pieces of art. The latter is seldom a problem but when you get a bunch of paper with very poor bibliographic information and furthermore in an unreadable condition, you can be less than enthusiastic in accepting it.

There must be a mutual interest between libraries and researchers, that publications are accessible in databases, available in libraries, but also professionally written and edited.

To support our colleagues in the company but also our library-customers in writing and editing texts we have produced some guidelines like: "Scientific writing: a short handbook of the process of developing research projects including writing and editing according to international standards".

Another project directly tailored for nursing college students is a guideline about the construction of scientific articles: "What is a scientific article: guidelines and literature".

"How to organise your literature references", is another example.

This kind of support is going to be very important in a future with problem based learning as educational instrument. It is a great chance for us librarians to conquer new fields and in the long run make ourselves indispensable.

The complete library

Unlike other database producers we have since the start of our database Spriline made it our goal to take full responsibility for both database production, hosting the database, and a complete document delivery service. It is our firm belief that there is no use in building a large database if one is not able to order the documents found in the database! The consequences of this philosophy is that we have made it possible for anyone - library or individual - to borrow the documents directly from us. Today it is possible for any individual to call or write to us to receive help with a database search, without any charges. They can then phone, fax, e-mail or write to us and order the documents they want to borrow. Unlike most Swedish libraries we mail documents directly to customers all over Sweden, as well as abroad if required. Our policy is to send the documents from Spri no later than 24 hours after we received the order. Over the years we have continually developed our document delivery service, adding on-line ordering procedures to the databases. The most recent addition to our services is offering SDI-profiles.

Building databases in collaboration

In building our database and library catalogue with the aim of having a complete coverage of Swedish and other relevant material in our field we have found partners for cooperation in database-building. We currently have four partners: Swedish Public Health Institute, the Swedish Handicap Institute, the National Board of Health and Welfare and the Stockholm Gerontology Research Centre. They have special responsibilities for HIV/AIDS, elderly care, care and aids for the disabled and the public health field. They add their references to Spriline and lend their material on the same terms as we do.

UNION CATALOGUES

We also host a union catalogue database called LOKAT for journal holdings in the libraries of the Swedish County Councils. All the libraries annually submit a list of their holdings and a librarian at the Spri Library and Research Report Bank inputs the information and also produces a printed version of the database. To this database we have connected an on-line fax order service that gives the searcher the opportunity to order directly from the library of their choice.

In 1993 we decided to participate in the building of the Swedish national union catalogue LIBRIS by adding our holdings of books not published in Sweden. In consequence our holdings have been opened up for new groups of readers in the university community.

HECLINET

Since 1976 Spri Library and Research Report Bank produces the database Heclinet (Health Care Literature Information Network), together with health care institutions in Denmark, Germany, Austria, Switzerland and Poland. The database is reached via the host DIMDI, and before the end of 1996 also via Spri.

Technical developments

To meet the demands from our customers we aim to be well ahead with technical innovations. We have had our on-line order and autofax services in operation for several years, and in December 1994 we released our first CD-ROM with four databases. The CD has been a success and our loans have increased by 60% over the last 18 months, most likely because it has made the databases easily accessible for students. We also have considered optical storage for the articles indexed in our database Spriline, together with a fax order service. As you can understand copyright is the big issue here. In addition to this we have developed our own home-page on the Internet, with all the information about our library, useful links and e-mail addresses to our staff. The homepage also includes a special search form for free searches in our databases.

Collaborating with Europe

Spri Library and Research Report Bank is the Swedish national *WHO Documentation Centre*. We receive all the publications from WHO Regional Office for Europe in Copenhagen. Since we are the host for the WHO database WHOLIS we also offer to acquire any WHO document not found in any other Swedish library.

We act as the Swedish partner in the international *Cochrane Collaboration* on randomised controlled trials working with the Nordic Cochrane Centre in Copenhagen, Denmark.

Spri Library and Research Report Bank is currently involved in three *European Union projects*, European Clearing House on Health Systems Reforms, European Clearing Houses on Health Outcomes and European Information Network for the Field of Ethics in Medicine.

Conclusion

What has collaboration done for us? The strong emphasis on collaboration in the policy of Spri Library and Research Report Bank, not only with similar institutions in Sweden but in the Nordic countries and in the European Community, has made our library one of the largest health care libraries in the Nordic countries. By offering the package of services that we do, we have made ourselves indispensable to our customers, both individuals and libraries. We have not only survived these 25 years but grown from a small company library to a National resource library!

EUROPEAN CLEARING HOUSES: TWO APPROACHES TO MANAGING INFORMATION

Pat Spoor and Alison Brettle, Nuffield Institute for Health, University of Leeds, UK

Nuffield Institute for Health

There are two European Clearing Houses with information functions based at the Nuffield Institute for Health, University of Leeds, UK:
the *European Clearing House on Health Outcomes* and
the *European Clearing House on Health Systems Reforms*.

Both projects are funded by the European Union under the BIOMED programme and are similar in that they both involve co-operation with other European institutions, and that information and the use of technology such as the Internet play an important part in the project. However, two different approaches have been taken to the collection and management of information, one centralised and the other decentralised.

The poster presented compares and contrasts the different models adopted and evaluates their success.

S. Bakker (ed.), Health Information Management: What Strategies?, 49.

IMPROVING ACCESS TO GREY LITERATURE BY COOPERATION

Caroline Sawers, South Thames Library and Information Services, UK

South Thames Library and Information Services (STLIS) consists of 108 library service points staffed by 270 library staff providing for the needs of over 100,000 healthcare staff serving a population of nearly 7,000,000 people within South East Britain. The mission of STLIS is to help all NHS staff make effective use of the knowledge base of healthcare, and to deliver relevant and accurate information to healthcare staff at the time of need.

The regional library unit, acting on behalf of the Postgraduate Medical Dean, co-ordinates the work of the libraries and monitors the contracts with individual NHS Trusts. This includes: encouraging the development and improvement of library services; advising users, managers and librarians on library matters; and providing central support and professional leadership to librarians.

In order to raise the standards of library cataloguing throughout the region,[1] reduce duplication and make the resources of each library, particularly the grey literature widely available, the database HEALTHBASE has been developed over the last ten years and standard tools for database production have been produced.[2-4] The entry of data has always been closely controlled. In the 1980s output was in the form of catalogue cards, a monthly microfiche, microcomputer diskettes or paper printout. More recently online access via local and wide area networks has been possible. Future plans are to make HEALTHBASE available using World Wide Web technology over the Internet, and within the UK, over the NHSnet.[5]

Collecting grey literature on health related topics produced within their geographical areas is part of the contracting process for the librarians. Questions like "Are there any models for developing services for the home care of elderly people with mental health problems?" can easily be answered from HEALTHBASE. With HEALTHBASE interlibrary loan between the cooperating libraries has increased substantially. Separate figures for grey and conventional literature are not collected, but anecdotal evidence indicates that the grey literature is largely responsible.

References

[1] Lever R. Cataloguing in small medical libraries. Guildford: South West Thames Regional Library Service, 1978

[2] South Thames Library Service. Subject cataloguing guide. 5th ed. Guildford: STLS, 1996

[3] Williams E (ed.). Authority list for corporate headings field. 3rd ed. Guildford: South Thames Library Service, 1996

[4] Holman J (ed.). A quality library service: management manual for health care libraries. Guildford: South West Thames Regional Library Service, 1993

[5] Sawers C. Developing resource sharing tools. In: Carmel M (ed.). Health care librarianship and information work. 2nd ed. London: Library Association Publishing, 1995. pp.197-217

S. Bakker (ed.), Health Information Management: What Strategies?, 50.

RESEAU DIC DOC INSERM: DU TRAVAIL PARTAGE À LA MISE EN COMMUN DES CONNAISSANCES

Nicole Pinhas and Jocelyne Chevalier, Réseau DIC DOC INSERM, http://www.inserm.fr/dicdoc, France

INSERM DIC DOC Network: from groupware to knowledge sharing

In a context in which supply never stops increasing and diversifying, new technologies applied to scientific and technical communication and electronic management of information change the part and functions of various partners. According to these upsetting habits, organization of work may be reconsidered and new managing structures may be expected.

INSERM's documentation (National Institute of Health and Medical Research) has been re-organized in a network built on the shareware of knowledge and ability of not only documentation specialist but also scientists. Members of this network are located all over the country with various specializations and complementary thematics.

This paper reports on: a) - the chronological steps of this experience which began after a requirement survey built out of questionnaires and interviews; b) - the necessary tools of a shared management of work (electronic mail, groupwares); c) - the knowledge data bases collectively built and enriched, then put at the service of the international scientific community on Internet network by means of a Web server; d) - the new applications which have been developed for the best satisfaction of users (bibliographic data synthesis and statistical analysis).

Three years later, we can strike the balance giving the positive points, the difficulties we met and out hopes for the future.

Introduction

l'INSERM, Institut National de la Santé et de la Recherche Médicale organisme public sous la tutelle conjointe des Ministères en charge de la santé et de la recherche a pour missions de contribuer à améliorer la santé de l'homme et de transférer les connaissances produites par les chercheurs vers les acteurs économiques et sociaux. Plus de 10 000 personnes, INSERM ou partenaires associés, travaillent au sein de 270 laboratoires de recherche répartis sur l'ensemble de la France. Conscient de l'importance stratégique que représentait la maîtrise de la gestion des connaissances, le département de l'information et de la communication (DIC) a engagé dès 1993, une réflexion pour déterminer comment les nouvelles technologies de communication qui commençaient alors à s'implanter dans le monde de la recherche pouvaient permettre de mieux organiser les flux d'informations produites et diffusées par les chercheurs en tenant compte d'un contexte technologique et institutionnel en mutation.

S. Bakker (ed.), Health Information Management: What Strategies?, 51-53.

Contexte

Au sein de l'INSERM, la mise en place progressive du câblage et l'accès au réseau Internet ont facilité les échanges et les transferts de données, induit de nouvelles méthodes de travail, et mis en évidence des besoins accrus et ciblés en matière de gestion de l'information scientifique et technique (IST). Parallèlement, on assistait au regroupement fonctionnel de laboratoires travaillant sur une thématique proche et motivés par des perspectives d'évolution communes. Ces différents facteurs: implantation de nouvelles technologies de communication, création de fédérations de recherche thématiques et analyse d' importants fonds bibliographiques ont fait naître, au sein de l'Institut, des demandes d'un nouveau type en matière d'information scientifique. Pour être le plus possible à l'écoute de ces besoins et répondre efficacement aux attentes des utilisateurs, il fut décidé d'adopter un fonctionnement en réseau qui seul permettait, avec des effectifs réduits et dispersés, d'atteindre ces objectifs. Cette structure souple et évolutive met efficacement à profit les nouvelles possibilités offertes par l'informatique et les réseaux de communication.

Le reseau DIC DOC

Le réseau DIC DOC est composé d'un noyau dur comprenant une vingtaine d'ingénieurs en information, quelques chercheurs motivés et un informaticien autour duquel s'articule un second cercle constitué des documentalistes de sites par lesquelles transitent les flux d'informations destinés aux chercheurs. Pour mener à bien un tel projet deux composantes indissociables sont nécessaires:
- la composante humaine basée sur des individus motivés qui doivent apprendre à travailler en groupe et bâtir ensemble de manière interactive des produits à valeur ajoutée.
- la composante informatique qui doit mettre à disposition des outils permettant de travailler à distance selon un processus coopératif.

Les outils informatiques

La mise en place des réseaux de communication a ouvert la voie aux développements de produits informatiques qui rendent opérationnel le travail en commun entre des communautés géograhiquement dispersées.Pour fonctionner, les membres du réseau doivent avoir à disposition:
- une messagerie pour communiquer et faciliter la circulation des documents
- un logiciel de "groupware" à partir duquel seront développées et structurées les bases de travail.

Nous avons choisi le logiciel "Lotus Notes" qui fonctionne selon le mode client/serveur. Un serveur central gère les accès et coordonne les flux d' informations tandis que chaque membre du réseau dispose sur son bureau de la partie "client".

Lotus Notes repose sur l'architecture des trois C: Communication, Collaboration et Coordination. Communications et collaborations sont régies par des règles et des procédures qui permettent le fonctionnement de groupes de travail. Lotus Notes est orienté "documents": chaque document se décompose en des champs aux formats variés (textes, images, chiffres) pouvant faire l'objet de divers traitements.

Chaque participant au réseau travaille en local puis transfert au serveur son apport individualisé. Ces informations sont envoyées au gestionnaire de la base pour validation et acceptation: ce processus appelé "replication" permet la mise à jour partielle ou totale de toutes les copies des bases disponibles. Ainsi chacun peut, soit consulter l'information disponible, soit dans un processus plus actif l'enrichir, la modifier ou la commenter. Mais, seul le gestionnaire déclaré de la base ou de la sous-base, possède le droit de valider les modifications apportées par les autres membres du réseau. Lotus Notes permet de gérer une hiérarchie de la redistribution de l'information. De programmation complexe au niveau informatique, cet outil reste pour l'utilisateur simple et convivial.

Le travail en reseau

Le travail en groupe, favorisant échanges et discussions, permet une plus grande efficacité et une plus grande créativité: il est évident qu'on est plus intelligent à plusieurs que tout seul. Pour apprendre à fonctionner selon un processus collaboratif et pour se familiariser aux outils disponibles tout en les évaluant, nous avons décidé de réaliser une première base de travail sur la documentation et de structurer avec Lotus Notes les flux d'informations qui transitaient déjà par notre réseau informel (informations sur les bases de données, sur les CD-ROM, sur Internet, sur les publications électroniques....). Par la suite, nous avons mis sur pied un système de "veille" nous permettant de repérer et d'évaluer les nouveaux produits: un forum fut créé autour de la base "Panorama de Presse" qui analyse une vingtaine de publications en sciences de l'information pour partager commentaires et analyses.

Chaque membre du réseau n'est plus uniquement consommateur d'information mais devient aussi producteur.

Bilan et perspectives

La mise en place d'un tel projet a nécessité près de trois ans. Actuellement, se développent plusieurs projets thématiques avec une problématique documentaire (oncologie, prions...) Il s'agit maintenant de mettre à disposition de la communauté scientifique les savoir-faire que nous avons acquis dans la gestion électronique des flux d'informations.

Le fonctionnement en réseau est, surtout au début, dévoreur de temps et d'énergie. Mais le partage des ressources et des expériences génère un enrichissement constant et stimulant, véritable source de créativité. La connaissance et la maîtrise d'outils communs tend à uniformiser les compétences des membres du réseau et à créer de ce fait une culture collective.

Le fonctionnement en réseau engendre une véritable révolution culturelle qui conduit à la prise de conscience que le pouvoir n'est plus de posséder une information mais de savoir l'exploiter donc la partager. Comme l'indiquait Hervé Serieyx (1993): "Le défi c'est d'acquérir une organisation en réseau qui permette d'organiser l'information".

Bibliographie

[1] La gestion électronique des informations scientifiques en sciences biomédicales et en santé: expériences à partir de l'exemple du réseau d'informations DICDOC de l'INSERM. Séminaire Obernai 17-18 octobre 1994

[2] INSERM Rapport d'activité 1994

[3] Hawkins DT. The evolving Lotus Notes information industry. Online 1995;(sep/oct):64-73

[4] Bates ML, Allen K. Lotus Notes in action. Database 1994;(aug):27-38

[5] Liberman K , Rich JL. Lotus Notes databases: the foundation of a virtual library. Database 1993;16(june):33-46

[6] Derouet T, Flores J, Vermel C. Le groupware renaît de ses cendres. PC Expert 1996;(févr):149-165

L'INFORMATION SUR LA SANTE: LES DEUX AUTRES DIMENSIONS

Daniel Baudin, Centre International de l'Enfance, Paris, France

Summary

Health information dissemination is characterized by a nearly exclusive production from industrialized countries. Health research and publications in developing countries rarely reach the famous Science Citation Index considered by many as the international bible of scientific journals. Over recent years, the International Children's Centrer (ICC) is engaged in an information exchange program with documentation centers in developing countries. ICC's database on children carries a good proportion of publication references from these partner countries. This is a possible approach to a better and more objective information provided to health personnel worldwide.

L'accès à l'information

Depuis sa création par Robert Debré en 1949, le Centre International de l'Enfance se (CIE) consacre à la santé et au bien être de l'enfant. La santé y est abordée dans un contexte préventif selon trois axes de travail qui sont la formation, l'information et la recherche-action. Deux tiers des activités du CIE sont tournées vers les pays en développement. Dans le domaine de la santé, les auteurs d'articles, de thèses ou d'ouvrages se trouvent au nord comme au sud, dans les pays industrialisés comme dans les pays en développement. On ne peut cependant pas ignorer que les signatures que nous voyons sont beaucoup plus souvent celles des chercheurs du nord que celles des chercheurs du sud. La place faite aux publications du sud, dans notre activité quotidienne, est en fait presque inexistante. De même, l'accès à l'information scientifique est extrêmement difficile au sud alors que la profusion règne au nord. Notre objectif au CIE a été de favoriser l'accès de l'information aux utilisateurs du sud, ainsi que l'échange d'information entre nous et nos partenaires.

L'ACCÈS PAR INTERNET

Lorsque l'on parle d'accès à l'information pour les pays du sud, on se dit généralement qu'il passe par un effort des pays du nord pour mettre l'information à la disposition des utilisateurs du sud. Le schéma consistant à subventionner et à pourvoir le sud en revues scientifiques, ouvrages et bases de données est devenu classique. On va même plus loin depuis quelques années, en s'appuyant sur Internet, et la révolution

S. Bakker (ed.), Health Information Management: What Strategies?, 54-56.

promise dans la circulation de l'information. Certains n'hésitent pas à affirmer, qu' "Internet va sauver l'Afrique "... Revenons plutôt à la réalité.

En France, l'Aupelf-Uref[1] a développé un réseau et installé dans près de 25 pays francophones du sud des "points SYFED"[2], qui permettent la consultation gratuite des bases de données internationales, en ligne ou sur CD-ROM. Il reste ensuite à commander les documents primaires à la source. Ainsi, les médecins et les chercheurs de Yaoundé ou de Cotonou peuvent-ils accéder à Pascal, Medline ou BIRD (Base d'Information Robert Debré). Présent dans les capitales, les points SYFED illustrent l'effort fait par la France pour aider la diffusion de l'information au sud. Des programmes dans ce sens ont été mis également en place par l'UNESCO et l'ONU dans le passé. En dehors de ces initiatives, l'accès à l'information demeure problématique au sud, et l'Internet, "Réseau des autoroutes virtuelles de l'information interplanétaire" ne semble pas être en mesure de jouer le rôle annoncé, en particulier au sud pour au moins deux raisons:

- la gratuité d'Internet est plus que relative, elle coûte par exemple 40 F par heure de connexion à Nairobi et 80 F à Montevideo. Avec un salaire de 500 à 1000 F par mois pour un chercheur, "surfer" sur Internet est un grand luxe que peu peuvent s'offrir;
- de plus, les grandes bases de données internationales ne sont pour ainsi dire pas présentes sur Internet; lorsque ce sera le cas, elles seront payantes, et à des tarifs qui ne permettront pas leur consultation par les utilisateurs des pays en développement.

Il reste donc à Internet à faire le preuve du rôle qu'il pourrait jouer pour les utilisateurs du sud.

L'EXCLUSIVITÉ DE L'INFORMATION DANS LES BASES DE DONNÉES

Une autre caractéristique de l'information aujourd'hui est sa provenance presque exclusive des pays industrialisés. L'article de W. Wayt Gibbs est à ce sujet instructif[3]. On y découvre que dans le Science Citation Index,[4] 78% des articles proviennent de 11 pays! La contribution de ces 11 pays va de 2% d'articles provenant de revues espagnoles à 31% d'articles provenant de revues nord-américaines. Le reste du monde, plus de 170 pays, représente 22% des articles scientifiques "d'importance" au nord. On constate la grande disparité de traitement entre les publications du nord et celles du sud, par les grands diffuseurs. Ce phénomène est d'autant plus frappant que le nombre des revues du sud répertoriées dans le SCI baisse régulièrement. Il était de 80 en 1980. Il n'était plus que de 50 en 1993 sur les 3 300 retenues[3].

L'échange des documents

Le CIE n'a pas l'ambition ni la prétention de vouloir modifier ces données, mais nous considérons que la multiplication des initiatives pourrait contribuer à développer des termes nouveaux dans la diffusion de l'Information. Au cours des dernières années, le CIE s'est rapproché d'un certain nombre de centres de documentation sanitaire et sociale dans les pays en développement. Ceci s'est fait souvent grâce à des contacts directs au cours de réunions ou de stages de formation ayant eu lieu au CIE.

Travaillant principalement dans le domaine de la santé publique, les scientifiques du CIE ont besoin d'informations sur le sud. C'est ainsi que nous avons proposé des accords de coopération et d'échange. Nous demandons à nos partenaires de faire de la veille documentaire pour nous dans leurs pays respectifs et de nous faire connaître les articles, les thèses, les ouvrages, les rapports sur les données sanitaires et sociales et sur la recherche dans leur pays dans le domaine de la mère et de l'enfant. Après un travail de sélection, nous leur demandons de nous envoyer ces documents que nous indexons ensuite sur la base BIRD. Certains d'entre-vous ont sans doute profité de cette information souvent rare au nord. L'INIST, le grand centre d'information du CNRS, fait régulièrement appel au CIE pour ce type d'information, de même que l'Institut Pasteur-Mérieux en France.

En échange, le CIE fournit à ses partenaires du sud les documents répertoriés dans la base BIRD, voire leur fournit un exemplaire du CD-ROM BIRD. Ces prestations mutuelles ne sont bien sûr pas facturées. Nous considérons que ce type de coopération profite à chacun des partenaires et contribue à faire connaître les publications sur le sud aux chercheurs et aux acteurs de la santé du nord. Elle valorise les travaux de recherches réalisés au sud et très souvent négligés ou ignorés au nord.

La base BIRD sur CD-ROM

Notre ambition toute relative ne s'arrête pas là puisque nous essayons de compléter cette politique d'échange par une troisième dimension. Le CIE produit la base BIRD et publie tous les dix huit mois environ un CD-ROM sur l'enfant. La troisième édition du CD-ROM BIRD est sortie en juin dernier avec près de 135 000 références bibliographiques. La diffusion de notre CD-ROM dans de nombreux pays à travers le monde permet donc de faire connaître aussi un nombre non négligeable de publications des pays du sud. Sur les 450 revues que nous dépouillons, 50 proviennent du sud. A cette sélection s'ajoute bien sûr les données qui nous sont fournies par nos partenaires du sud, qu'ils soient documentalistes ou chercheurs. Le CD-ROM BIRD contribue donc à la diffusion au sud de l'information qui provient du Sud. Un chercheur vietnamien peut donc avoir connaissance d'une étude réalisée au Bénin, par des béninois, sur le paludisme. Conscients de l'intérêt pour eux que présente cette expérience, de plus en plus de médecins et de chercheurs partenaires du CIE nous confient leurs articles ou leurs thèses pour les faire figurer dans la base BIRD.

Conclusion

Chacun de nous, soucieux de répondre aux besoins des utilisateurs doit en permanence proposer des informations provenant de sources multiples. La pluralité de l'information contribue à l'objectivité et à la pertinence de notre travail, et surtout à une meilleure information des professionnels de la santé. Les moyens du CIE et sa contribution relative dans la diffusion de l'information au niveau international ne lui permettront pas de changer fondamentalement le cours des choses. Nous voulons toutefois apporter notre contribution à une prise de conscience qui nous semble nécessaire dans le domaine de la diffusion de l'information.

Pour nous, ces trois dimensions, nord/sud, sud/nord et sud/sud doivent être prises en considération pour faire de la diffusion de l'information une activité qui reflète mieux les efforts, les connaissances et les besoins des acteurs de la santé qu'ils soient au nord ou au sud.

Bibliographie

[1] Association des Universités partiellement ou Entièrement de Langue Française

[2] Système Francophone d'Edition et de Diffusion

[3] Gibbs WW. Lost Science in the Third World. Sci Amer 1995;(aug):92-99

[4] Le SCI "cite" 3 300 revues scientifiques internationales sur les 70 000 disponibles dans le monde

QUALITY MANAGEMENT IN THE INFORMATION SERVICE CENTRE OF THE FIOH

Irja Laamanen, Finnish Institute of Occupational Health, Helsinki

Introduction

The Information Service Centre of the FIOH started to develop the quality system about three years ago. First, information and examples were collected. The examples were from industry, where the quality system also covered the libraries and information services. The quality system chosen by the executive committee of the FIOH is based on the principles given in ISO 9004-2 (Quality management for services) and in ISO 9001 (Total Quality Management). The aim is to have a system, which develops and updates itself continuously.

What is quality?

Quality is a vague concept, used in relation to various everyday things. But is it possible to say exactly what is meant when speaking about the quality of the library or the information service? Although quality is not an easy concept, the meaning of it can be agreed upon and there is an accepted way of describing what quality is. IFLA has published indicators of the quality for academic libraries. They are:

1) relevance in collection development
2) degree of satisfaction
3) hours open
4) delay between order and availability on shelves
5) percentage of requested items obtained

These indicators can be measured. The list is short; it could be much longer, but IFLA felt that a short list could be applied in all countries.[1] IFLA also sees that academic libraries are changing, and new indicators might be added in the future. Academic libraries all over the world display great variation in organisational, financial, and technical conditions. Quality is a relative term, related to all these factors.

WHY IS QUALITY SO IMPORTANT?

For years, quality has been important for industry. Quality is now seen also as one of the important means for public organisations, which are not competitive economically, but can compete with the quality of their services and products.

S. Bakker (ed.), Health Information Management: What Strategies?, 57-60.

Quality aims at satisfying the customer, but quality should also be improved in order to find key success factors, to ensure the better availability of resources, etc. Eighty per cent of academic libraries conduct performance measurements, which do not tell anything about the quality (EUSIDIC, spring meeting in Cologne, 1996). The next step should be the combining of both of these.

QUALITY IS LIKE A TWO-SIDED COIN

One side of the coin is the customer with his or her expectations and the other side is the work done in the libraries for producing services and products of high quality. This work done is important, because it entails the promise for quality. But are the expectations of the customer as regards quality and the promise given by the qualitative work process, always met?

Work processes in managing information

The libraries always have taken care of the quality of the very central tasks. The libraries and information services use cataloging guidelines to make uniform catalogs of books and journals, and other materials acquired. This has assured even quality of the catalogs. The catalogs are kept in order according to some rules. The shelf order is based on the classification system that each library uses. So quality is controlled and assured by the guidelines prepared for these workprocesses. But this does not mean that the total quality of some library or information service is managed well.

How to assure the quality of all functions?

Some system is needed for assuring quality. The system must cover all important functions and work processes of the organisation. ISO has produced several standards for the development of a quality system, meant to describe how total quality is managed. Quality management is comprised of three steps:

* planning (what we want to do)
* control (what we are already doing)
* improvement (how to improve what we are doing)

Quality management at the FIOH

Quality management is also an important strategic tool for the Finnish Institute of Occupational Health. The executive committee made a decision concerning the quality system of the FIOH, prepared the quality policy for the Institute and decided on the tools to be used in building the quality system of the FIOH. The application of the quality standards at all levels of the Institute has been under way for several years. At present there is agreement on the structure of the quality handbook of the FIOH.

INSTITUTIONAL LEVEL

The quality handbook at the institutional level describes the quality system as a whole. It gives the quality policy statement, descibes the structure of the system, informs how to carry out documentation. It also gives the principles for purchasing, marketing of services, the control and measuring system, the principles for continuous improvements using internal audits, management reviews, corrective and preventive actions, etc. covering all the elements in ISO 9001.

The handbook also includes the general description and quality objectives for our main activities, which are: a) research, b) services, c) training and education, and d) dissemination of information

DEPARTMENTAL OR FUNCTIONAL UNIT LEVEL

The various departments and some functional units have drafted their own quality handbooks, which describe in detail the procedures and work tasks of the unit.

The Information Service Centre. Our department started building its quality system three years ago. First several crucial questions were posed: Why is quality important? What should be included in the handbook? How is quality defined in the context of our functions, services and products, and how is it created and maintained, and to whom is it targeted? Should quality be divided into internal quality (work processes, etc) and external quality (fulfilment of customer needs)?

In the beginning we also collected information. When collecting examples, we became aware that we had to make the handbook by ourselves. There is no other similar library or information service, nor handbook to be copied. The examples and information only helped us.

In order to create a positive attitude toward quality, it was discussed continuously.

Guidelines. The examples provided the ideas for making and carrying out guidelines:
* Develop and maintain a good way of working or a good workprocess;
* Describe the process on paper;
* Motivate and advise the staff to act as planned and agreed together;
* Describe procedures which makes it possible to show, when needed, that you have done the task as have described in the guideline.

Handbook. The quality handbook is still under preparation but will include:
* the mission of the Information Service Centre;
* user groups and needs of the users;
* general description of the functions, services and products offered;
* goals and objectives;
* quality policy;
* measurement of quality;
* continuous improvement of performance;
* information about personnel;
* continuous education and training of the personnel;
* equipment;
* appendices with descriptions of each of the work processes.

Profits. This enormous task of producing a quality handbook, and of keeping it up-to-date, has been profitable. At its best, it has had positive effects on the work in the centre. The employees can influence the system themselves, and together plan changes, taking into account the available resources and strategies. Some other benefits of this work for the employees:
* the processes are not only mastered by some few persons;
* the processes are not random;

* the processes are not instinctive.
And, customers get more attention and are appreciated as the most important actors.

How to know the opinion of the customer?

Quality is defined by the needs of the customer. Although the library does its best, the clientele of the individual institution defines the quality.

In order to find out the opinion of the clientele, we conducted a user survey, using a questionnaire. When preparing the questionnaire, we had to consider: 1) what are the services that should be included: the quality of the overall performance of the library, or the quality of a specific activity or service, 2) what should be asked, 3) what kind of a scale to use, and 4) how often to repeat the questionnaire..

After collecting the information from the customers the results were analysed. The complaints of the customers, got special handling. Customer complaints were used to make improvements.

The customer is not the only inspector of the library

About once a year there are audits by a group of auditors from inside of the organisation or from outside. Outside auditors are used if the organisation or department is certified. Also in striving for a quality award, the auditors come from outside the institute. The auditors control to make sure that the quality handbook is in operation. If some exception from the handbook is found, mistakes are asked to be corrected, or the processes changed, or guidelines rewritten.

Conclusions

Quality is meant to fulfil the needs of the customers by best possible ways and to help the personnel in everyday work in serving the customers.

References

[1] Poll R, te Boekhorst P. Measuring quality: International Guidelines for Performance Measurement in Academic Libraries. IFLA Section of University Libraries & Other General Research Libraries, 1996. 171 pp. (IFLA Publications 76)

Brockman JR. Just another management fad? The implications of TQM for library and information services. Aslib Proc 1992;44:283-288.

Haines Taylor M, Wilson T. Q.A.--Quality Assurance in libraries: The health care sector. Canadian Library Association, 1990. 158 pp.

Fisher WW, Reel LB. Total quality management (TQM) in a hospital library: identifying service benchmarks. Bull Med Libr Assoc 1992;80:347-352

Line MB. Strategic planning as an instrument of improving library quality. Inspel 1991:1-16

Wormell I. Information quality: definitions and dimensions. Proceedings NORDINFO Seminar. Copenhagen: Royal School of Librarianship, 1989. 139 pp.

ENHANCING THE VALUE OF A HEALTH LIBRARY AND INFORMATION SERVICE TO CLINICIANS

Christine J. Urquhart and John B. Hepworth, University of Wales, UK

Introduction

The Value project examined the effectiveness of UK health library and information services in assisting clinical decision making, and showed how services could be enhanced.[1] Clinicians at 11 hospital sites were asked to assess the value to them of information obtained from inter-library loan requests, mediated searches and end-user searches. A sample of British Medical Association (BMA) Dial-Up MEDLINE users was asked similar questions.

To set the value judgements in context details were obtained of the information-seeking behaviour of both information and library service users and "non-users".

An audit survey of over 30 health libraries provided additional data for the quality assurance toolkit,[2] which helps library and information services to:

1) check their effectiveness (against attainable performance criteria);
2) to target existing services better; or
3) gain evidence for extended or new services.

Evaluation of library services

The quality assurance toolkit is based on the audit cycle comprising: information needs assessment, service provision, and assessment of outcomes. From those assessments of outcomes (benefits to clinical decision making) information needs can be assessed more precisely and services provided to match needs.

Each section of the toolkit is set out in the same way. First, there is an introduction recommending "what to find out". Next come the reasons "why". These reasons are related to the evidence from the Value project research. Lastly, there are suggestions "how" to find out, with details of data to be collected and possible survey methods to be used. As the toolkit is based on actual research and observation of over 40 libraries throughout the UK, the guidelines are certainly "evidence-based".

Libraries should be able to devise local solutions to their own, local problems using the toolkit. There is a strong emphasis on the customer, echoing a TQM philosophy. The Value project has shown that information services can have significant effects upon clinical decisions and that these effects can be quantified.

S. Bakker (ed.), Health Information Management: What Strategies?, 61-63.

However, it has also shown that some information services are not as effective as they might be. For example, some information services are allowing a handful of vigorous users to dominate resources, while neglecting other groups of doctors, (often the most junior doctors). The neglected groups of doctors would actually benefit more from the information than other groups, but they do not receive the services they need.

Using the toolkit

The toolkit is not meant to be prescriptive, and there is no need to complete every section. The recommended starting point is an evaluation of the impact of the library service on clinical decision making. The research suggests that positive findings are likely, and managers are more likely to be convinced that the library is worth funding if the benefits of the library service are related to organisational aims (usually more cost-effective patient care). In the Value project, 89% of the clinician respondents indicated that the information provided would, or did contribute to clinical decision making. The response rate to the survey was very satisfactory (68%, 486/713 questionnaires). Some 88% of the respondents indicated that some of the information was new to them, and 76% said they would share the information with colleagues. Obtaining evidence like this shows that the library service has a positive impact on patient care activities, and that impact is probably dispersed quite widely.

The library service might examine the immediate impact of information on the knowledge of clinicians, by asking questions about gains to knowledge as well as the benefits to clinical decision making. The immediate impact questions used in the Value project were based on those used in the Rochester study.[3] To obtain more details about the clinical decisions affected, the categories of clinical decisions were based on those derived from an NLM study of the impact of MEDLINE on clinical problem solving.[4] As the questionnaires and interview schedules in the toolkit are closely based on those used in the Value project, they are therefore tried and tested methods. Advice on conducting surveys is also included.

Using the findings of an impact survey

One of the interesting findings of the Value project was the demonstration of different clinical decision making priorities of junior doctors and senior doctors. The junior doctors were more likely to be concerned with "improved quality of life for patient and/or family", while the consultants were more concerned with "audit or standards of care". Junior doctors might therefore need information on the psychosocial aspects of care, while the consultants need access to clinical guidelines and clinical audits. Differences in outcomes of information use are reflected in differences in information needs.

Interviews illustrated exactly how the information supported more cost-effective patient care and evidence-based medicine. This case-study evidence helped to check the questionnaire survey findings and provided convincing evidence of how the doctors valued the information provided. Some typical extracts from the transcripts are: "will probably now change medication advice given to pregnant asthmatic patients"; "wanted evidence to critique proposal for (form of expensive emergency care) ... found that there was no medical benefit". The case study details from the interviews do show that information does help to provide more effective patient care, and occasionally real cost savings might be demonstrated.

Monitoring performance

The most junior doctors (senior house officers) and some other medical staff groups do not always use the library services provided. As there was a wide variation among the libraries in the uptake of certain services, performance targets are included in the toolkit to help libraries assess whether their performance is above or below average for their size of library. The better performances did not always come from the better resourced libraries.

Conclusions

The Value project demonstrated how UK health libraries affect clinical decision making, and how health libraries can enhance the value of their services by using the Value toolkit. A complementary project on library services for nurses, midwives and health visitors (EVINCE, Establishing the Value of Information to Nursing Continuing Education) is in progress.[5]

References

[1] Urquhart CJ, Hepworth JB. The value to clinical decision making of information supplied by NHS library and information services (British Library R&D Report no. 6205). Boston Spa, West Yorkshire LS23 7BQ, UK: British Library Document Supply Centre, 1995

[2] Urquhart CJ, Hepworth JB. The value of information services to clinicians: a toolkit for measurement. Aberystwyth, SY23 3AS, UK: Open Learning Unit, Department of Information and Library Studies, University of Wales Aberystwyth, 1995

[3] Marshall JG. The impact of the hospital library on clinical decision making: the Rochester study. Bull Med Libr Assoc 1992;80:169-178

[4] Lindberg DAB, Siegel ER, Rapp BA, Wallingford KT, Wilson SR. Use of MEDLINE by physicians for clinical problem solving. JAMA 1993;269:3124-3129

[5] Davies R, Urquhart CJ, Hepworth JB. EVINCE: Establishing the Value of Information to Nursing Continuing Education. Project funded by BLR&DD, November 1995-October 1996. More details from Christine Urquhart, DILS, University of Wales, Aberystwyth, SY23 3AS, UK; email cju@aber.ac.uk

COSTING LIBRARY SERVICES

Anne-Marie Cawasjee and Maureen Forrest, Cairns Library, Oxford, UK

Introduction

In the current climate of limited funding, it is important to know exactly how the funding is being spent: to identify how much each service costs and to apportion the cost to our funding bodies who now demand that we relate the money we receive to the services we provide. They want to be sure that they are only paying for the services to their own staff and students. The Cairns Library currently receives recurrent funding from a number of sources. We are at present in the process of setting up Service Level Agreements with the funding bodies in which the services to be provided and the funding required to provide them will be specified.

In this situation, we decided that it was essential to set up an on-going exercise to cost our services. The exercise itself carries a cost but there are a number of benefits to be gained:

Benefits of costing

Value: We have a responsibility to our users and our funding bodies to ensure that we provide a cost-effective service.
Allocation: To identify the cost of each service in order to monitor the cost-effectiveness of the expenditure. We must ensure, for example, that we are using the appropriate level of staff for each task.

- Identify where money can be saved.	- Revenue.
- Calculate the cost of new services.	- Income generation.
- Discard expensive, under-used services.	- Self-financing services.

Data: To provide management data on the use of the service and identify areas where more data should be collected. To provide data for funding bodies in support of bids.

The Costing Categories

Direct Costs: These consist of salary costs and materials costs.
Salary costs: The cost of staff time involved in the delivery of each service. Activities involved in delivering the services was compiled. Each member of staff identified the

S. Bakker (ed.), Health Information Management: What Strategies?, 64-65.

activities they carried out and a customised timesheet was prepared for each person to complete daily over a chosen period of time.
Materials costs: These costs represent the expenditure on books, periodicals, databases, equipment and all items needed to deliver the services.
Indirect Costs: These include overheads such as rent for premises, heating, lighting, cleaning etc.

The Costing Process

Identify Direct and Indirect Costs.
Allocation to specific services: Some costs can be allocated to specific services, others such as conference fees, can be apportioned to all services. The different services which are divided into five packages: Core Service, Current Awareness, Document Delivery, Enquiries, User Education. Funding bodies have the option of selecting which packages they wish to purchase.
Apportion to Each Funding Body: Calculate the percentage of the total to apportion to each funding body (contribution required from each funding body).

Our user registration records are coded according to the funding body for each user. We calculated the percentage of users for each funding body and used these percentages to identify the contribution required from each one.
Divide the total amount by Number of Registered Users: To establish the cost per user.
Costing: The calculation consists of direct and indirect costs to which are added an inflation figure, salary increments for staff and a figure covering the depreciation of equipment. Computers and other electronic equipment, in particular, have a short life and a programme for replacement is needed.

A figure for inflation should also be added to the indirect costs.

To raise the funding required to develop the service, a further figure should be added.

Conclusion

We have taken the approach that the cost per user represents the access to the facilities rather than the use of them. To use the analogy of a health club: the club provides a number of facilities such as a swimming pool, a gymnasium, a sauna etc. The basic subscription allows unlimited use to each member although most members will probably not use all the facilities. In addition, the club may provide extra, specialised facilities such as massage and beauty treatments which are not included in the subscription but which are charged for at the time of use. A parallel in libraries for such amenities would be inter-library loans for which the user may pay at the time of making the request.

In our view, retrospective charging based on use over the past year, should be avoided as it is difficult to plan the service and to budget for it under this system. Records of use can be used to support the basic cost calculation and adjustments can be made if necessary.

HOW HEALTHY ARE YOUR HEALTH DATABASES?

C.J. Armstrong, CIQM, Aberystwyth, UK

Information for the end-user

Increased use of local area networks with CD-ROMs as well as the Internet has resulted in information being available to most health professionals. In addition more and more "traditional" online services are targeting information at consumers through one-stop shops such as the Microsoft Network (MSN), CompuServe or Europe Online and databases are being made available to users in subscribing institutions over the World Wide Web; a recent example from Ovid Technologies has mounted a range of databases including PsycINFO and MEDLINE on a server at Stichting Academisch Rekencentrum Amsterdam (SARA).

This means that information professionals are often left out of the research loop - the implication being that the information providers believe end users have both the ability to locate appropriate sources for the material that they want and the experience to use them wisely. Clearly, this offers an exciting challenge in the provision of training and support to information professionals.

This paper, however, is concerned with the implied assumptions made by the information providers and the consequential challenge to end users.

UNMEDIATED ACCESS

If a resource is intended for direct use by "researchers", not only does it have to provide the information needed in a straightforward way but it must also be of a sufficient quality to meet expectations. The direct provision of information - like any other form of publishing - implies that the material is suitable and of sufficient quality to be so transmitted. Conventional print sources often have a self-evident pedigree, possibly they are peer-reviewed; in any event, users can resort to published reviews or - because access is not so immediate - have time to consult peers or information professionals. There are many fewer evaluative reviews available for electronic resources and in many cases such resources are located and used on the fly - users have nothing between them and the data.

A QUESTION OF QUALITY

Experience at the Centre for Information Quality Management (CIQM) makes it very clear that this is a state of affairs which places users at risk. Quality, or the degree to

S. Bakker (ed.), Health Information Management: What Strategies?, 66-68.

which users can trust a database, varies considerably even among the long established, traditional online and CD-ROM databases; many resources on the Internet may have no quality control at all. Without previous experience of information sources, end users may not see a need to question results - we have all heard how information delivered electronically is infused with a fidelity it may not have: coming from a computer it is obviously valid.

If information professionals no longer have the chance to help in the selection of sources or to authenticate results for end users, there is clearly a risk that flawed material may be accepted and find its way into the next level of some research project, gaining a further spurious authentication along the way!

The first online databases could be safely welcomed as they were little more than electronic versions of known and respected print indexes. Certainly, they offered more power and flexibility, but their pedigree was known: scientists had been using their print equivalent for many years - and had been doing so after that print service had been evaluated, refereed and reviewed by many of their peers as well as by their reference librarians and information scientists. Many databases and electronic resources now available are new on the scene and have never had print equivalents. Lacking the review and editorial stages imposed by traditional publishers, such "publications" come with no guarantees as to their merit or value.

The Centre for Information Quality Management

The Centre for Information Quality Management was originally set up by The Library Association and the UK Online User Group to act as a clearing house to which database users could report problems relating to the quality of any aspect of a database being used (search software, data, indexing, documentation, training). CIQM still fulfils this role as a free service to users but, as time has passed, CIQM has begun to take a more proactive role in improving data quality.

ERRORS

Examination of some of the issues reported to CIQM demonstrates clearly that there is a need for such action. Many of the issues reported stem from input errors, but because this affects the indexing, turn into retrieval errors. Records cannot be found because an author has been left out or a publisher mis-spelled. In one case, the producers of a medical database had mistyped the abbreviation for "lymphocyte specific protein tyrosine kinase" as "ick" rather than "lck" throughout one record. While the error probably arose from the fact that the original article was printed in a sans-serif font which did not clearly distinguish between an upper-case "I" and a lower-case "l", the error is quite important because users searching for the concept have to rely on free-text searches for the term "lck" as the thesaurus terms are not sufficiently specific. An important article from a top biomedical journal was lost to searchers - although it is nice to be able to report that this has been corrected now.

CHANGES

Recently there has been a series of complaints about software changes and the lack of warning that customers get when this happens. Not only does this cause problems in searching backfiles (developed for the old software which is no longer supported) but frequently the utility of the software is diminished or so changed that users must be retrained. The proliferation of MEDLINE resources on the Internet with limited search features may be another cause for concern.

In response to such needs, CIQM decided to address the often apparent gap between user expectations of a database and the actuality of searching at the terminal.

Database labels

Now, responsible database producers can produce mini-specifications of their database-as-it-exists and publish these as CIQM Database Labels.[1] Each Label contains a fixed set of parameters and quality assurance statements; all are factual and based on the existing database and its structures and existing production routines so that users know the exact degree to which they can trust a database as well as the exact capabilities of the database. A fuller description can be found in the second issue of *db-Qual*, CIQM's newsletter.[2]

Other bodies have also seen the need for evaluating the quality of data resources. Articles have been published which seek to point up both the need to and the means of evaluating CD-ROMs and networked information sources;[3,4] more recently Web sites have been advertised which contain lists of criteria against which an Internet resource can be judged.[5] Understanding the need to preview, prejudge and direct users, a number of sites have sprung up which offer such guidance, possibly in particular subject areas, to the best and most appropriate sources. The McKinley Internet Directory is a catalogue of evaluated sites while the OMNI Project and Achoo offer a similar approach in the biomedical arena.[6-8]

Where does this leave the prospective user of databases? CIQM's Database Labels and Internet resources such as OMNI and McKinley are two sides of the same coin. Indeed, as CIQM publishes Labels on the Web the similarities become even more marked. At the moment, the Database Labels refer to versions of databases which are available from "conventional" online hosts or on CD-ROM but it is certain that Internet versions of these databases and Internet resources will produce Labels soon. As more and more Database Labels are created for the major databases, it is hoped that users will turn to the resource - either in its Web version or on paper - as a first port of call when they wish to locate a "good" database that meets their needs. Producers will find that the scheme drives quality upwards.

References

1. CIQM Database Labels <URL **http://www.fdgroup.co.uk/labels.htm**>
2. db-Qual: The CIQM Newsletter. <URL **http://www.fdgroup.co.uk/ciqm.htm**>. 1996-. Twice/yr
3. Harry V, Oppenheim C. Evaluations of Electronic Databases, Part I: Criteria for Testing CD-ROM Products and Part II: Testing CD-ROM Products. Online CD-ROM Rev 1993;17(4):211-222 (Part I) and 1993;17(6):339-350 (Part II)
4. Stoker D, Cooke A. Evaluation of Networked Information Sources. In: Helal AH, Weiss JW (eds). Information Superhighway: the Role of Librarians, Information Scientists and Intermediaries. Proceedings 17th International Essen Symposium 1994. Essen: Universitatsbibliothek Essen, 1995. pp.287-312
5. Grassian E. <URL **http://www.ucla.edu/campus/computing/bruinonline/trainers/critical.html**>
6. McKinley Internet Directory. <URL **http://www.mckinley.com**>
7. OMNI <URL **http://omni.ac.uk**>
8. Achoo <URL **http://www.achoo.com**>

RETRENCHMENT AND COST-EFFECTIVENESS IN THE REDUCTION OF SERIALS SUBSCRIPTIONS

*Laura Cavazza and Rita Iori**, *Soprintendenza beni Librari, Bologna;
**Biblioteca Arcispedale S. Maria Nuova, Reggio Emilia, Italy

Introduction

The Library of the Arcispedale Santa Maria Nuova - Azienda Ospedaliera of the City Hospital of Reggio Emilia provides information services to the medical staff of the National Health Service. The Library owns 450 current and 537 ceased journals, the majority focusing on clinical medicine and a smaller proportion on research.

In 1994 the Library was facing a critical situation:
a) users, in order to cover new research subjects, were asking for more new titles, which would have cost Lire 2,090,000 ($ 1300);
b) the Hospital Administration decided to follow the trend of 1992 and 1993 by limiting the 1994-95 journals budget to Lire 195,000,000 ($ 120,594);
c) due to increasing inflation, the subscriptions paid in foreign currency were growing in cost.[1]

Selective criteria based only upon costs were immediately rejected and, following a first analysis, the Library decided to launch a retrenchment plan. The aim was to select journal subscriptions without exhausting the native quality of the collection.[2]

Methodology

The Library shortlisted titles to be discontinued against the following grid:
a) current *frequency of use* (in an open-shelved library, only a questionnaire could indicate the frequency of use and 44% of the users were happy to comply);
b) *lending frequency* in the previous year;
c) threshold size granted for each *NLMC class* represented (at least three subscriptions - American, European, Italian - for each medical discipline, quality tested against relevant sources);
d) *availability*: possibility of finding the same title in the GIDIF,RBM Union Catalogue (a private enterprise devised to supply documents to members);
e) *Impact Factor*;
f) *costs*.

Italian journals were not considered for cancellation as they are locally relevant and cheap. As a result 278 foreign journals were left for consideration. The librarian would take the final decision after discussing the cuts with the directors of the hospital departments.

S. Bakker (ed.), Health Information Management: What Strategies?, 69-70.

Results

Answers to the questionnaire on use frequency showed that 109 journals (40% approximately), were never requested for reading (between 95% and 100% of negative answers). These titles were checked against those never requested for lending and a list was drawn of 12 subscriptions which could be discontinued after considering c), d), e), f) as above and discussion.

Ten subscriptions (3.6%) were cancelled, saving Lire 3,227,000 ($ 1996). Seven new subscriptions were made for an amount of Lire 2,090,000 ($ 1293). The difference was credited forward on the 1996 budget.[3]

Conclusion

The effort made in effectively reshaping the collection, impressed the hospital administrators, who were satisfied to the point of not requiring further cuts in the 1995-96 preliminary budget. In fact, as more resources were made available in the course of the year, a further Lire 15,000,000 ($ 9276) were allocated to the Library. A by-product of the exercise, was that of confirming the quality and relevance of the collection. The retrenchement enhanced the most typical features of the Library by tailoring the collection to the users' needs. Feedback shows that users who specifically suffered from cuts of titles in their field of research were actually satisfied with the new ones they could get. Document delivery service did not suffer from the cuts, i.e. there was no significant increase in the requests for outside documents, because the Library is mainly a supplier.

References

[1] Kronenfeld MR. Update on inflation of journal prices in the Brandon-Hill list of journals. Bull Med Libr Assoc 1996;84:260-3

[2] Revelli C. Quando i tagli riguardano i periodici. Biblioteche Oggi 1993;(1):42-4

[3] Spang L. Reconciling rising serials costs, the serial budget, and reference needs in a medical library serials retrenchment program: a methodology. Med Ref Serv Q 1995;14(1):33-44

IMPROVING ECONOMIC MANAGEMENT OF AN INFORMATION UNIT

Armelle Martin, Sylvie Guillo, Hélène Breul, Bernard Sarrut and Christian Doreau, SIMP, Paris, France

Cost comparison

A cost comparison of databases' access was made for: Medline, Embase, Biosis and Pascal, available through several competitive vendors.[1,2] All parameters involved in pricing tariffs of any online searching were studied.[3] According to a specific database, search cost prices through four hosts (Datastar, Dialog, ESA, Questel) were analysed and compared.[4-6] This comparison dealt with the connect price per hour and the printing price of citations. The objective of this study was (a) to make an objective cost saving choice and (b) automatisation of searching costs and control of the budget.

Results

Results were graphically presented for each database by: Hourly rates, Charges per reference printed (AU,TI,SO,AB) and total search cost with two variables: time (10, 20, 30 min.) and number of references (10, 50, 100, 150).
MEDLINE (Fig. 1). Questel is clearly the most expensive, whatever the connect time and the number of references printed. Datastar and Dialog have similar costs.
EMBASE (Fig. 2). There is no significant cost difference between the two hosts. Datastar is a little bit cheaper if a large number of references are printed.
BIOSIS (Fig. 3). Dialog and Datastar costs are similar (Dialog is slightly cheaper). ESA is more expensive but becomes assimilable to the two other hosts for a long connect time, particularly if the number of references printed is low.
PASCAL (Fig. 4). Dialog and Datastar costs are similar and more expensive than the two other host costs. With regards to a short search duration, Questel is cheaper, particularly if a large number of references are requested. For a longer connect time, ESA becomes more interesting if many references are not requested.

S. Bakker (ed.), Health Information Management: What Strategies?, 71-73.

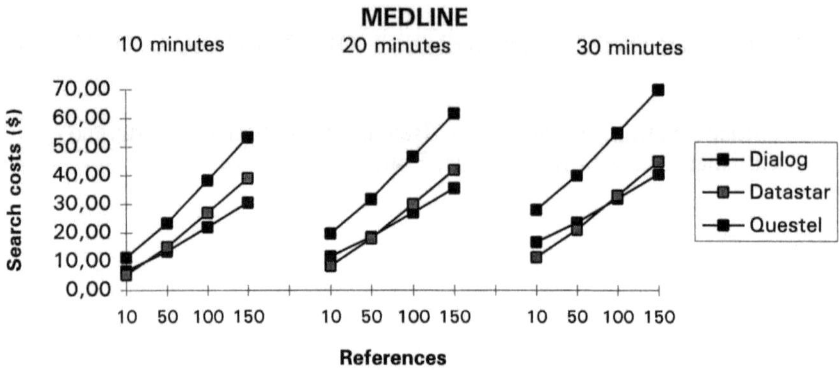

Figure 1. MEDLINE search costs.

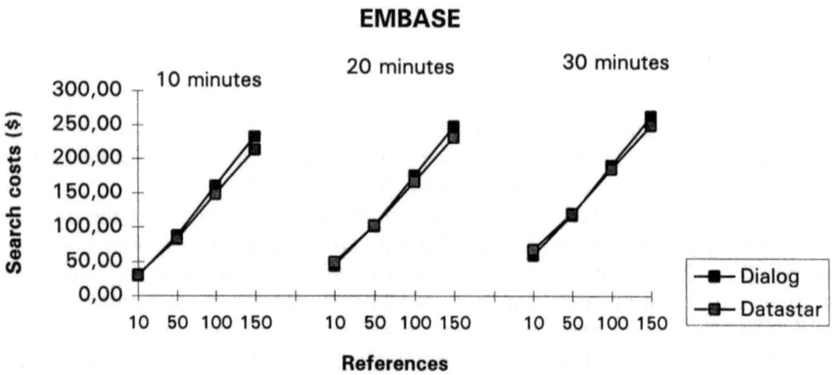

Figure 2. EMBASE search costs.

Conclusion

The choice is not obvious and involves several components. *ESA* is of interest for searches reaching 30 minutes or more, except if the number of citations printed is large. *Questel* is interesting for searching Pascal and a connect time of less than 30 min. It is the only host which allows the search in french language. Otherwise *Dialog* or *Datastar* are prefered, both offer a wide range of databases.

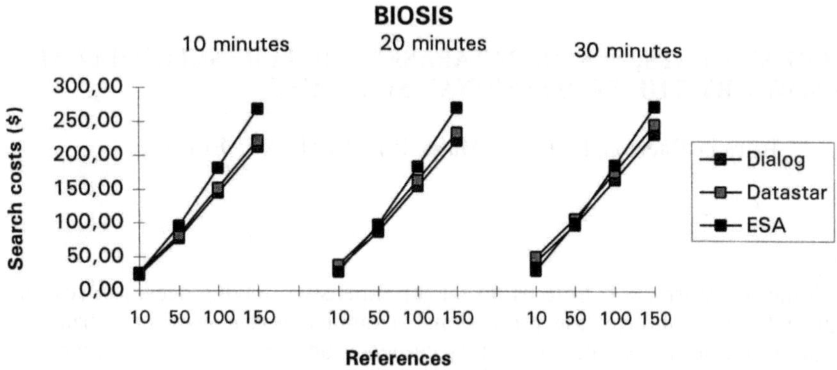

Figure 3. BIOSIS search costs.

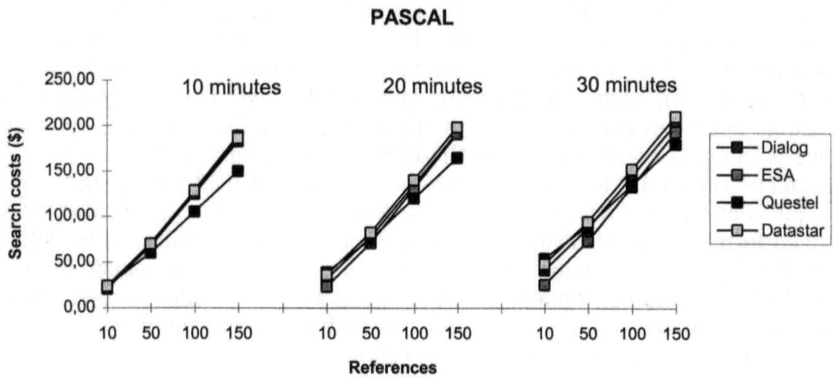

Figure 4. PASCAL search costs.

References

[1] Libmann F. Le prix, élément de concurrence entre les serveurs? Bases 1993;81:1-9

[2] Mariani AM et al. Performances et coût de trois serveurs documentaires à travers des bases biomedicales. Documentaliste 1985;22:201-7

[3] Rowley JE. How much will my online search cost? Online CD-ROM Rev 1993;17:143-8

[4] Feinglos SJ. MEDLINE at BRS, DIALOG, and NLM. Bull Med Libr Assoc 1983;71:6-12

[5] Haynes RB et al. Computer searching of the medical literature. Ann Intern Med 1985;103:812-6

[6] Walker CJ et al. Performance appraisal of online MEDLINE access routes. Proc Annu SCAMC 1992. AMIA, 1993:483-7.

DIFFERENT HOSTS, "SAME DATABASE" : DIFFERENCES THAT MUST BE KNOWN BY THE PROFESSIONAL SEARCHER[1]

Patricia Baert and Vincent Maes, Pfizer Belgium, Bruxelles

Subscribing to information hosts is no longer expensive, having access to several is not unusual for the information professional. Completeness may so be enhanced, with duplicate access to some databases. Host influence on the database is examined for Data-Star, Dialog, Dimdi and Ovid Online on Medline, Embase, Biosis Previews and SciSearch (not available on Ovid Online).

FREQUENCY OF UPDATES differs only for Biosis Previews, the other databases are updated on a weekly basis whichever host is considered.

SEARCH FACILITIES: *Search language comparison* can be quite difficult: even with comparable basic search commands, the policy for each language can be quite different. *Help* can be provided in printed formats, online, or via an Internet homepage. *Specific tools* exist to enhance the search, e.g. specific indexes (Dialog's 413, 414 and 416 files), or multi-database search possibilities (CROS in Data-Star, Superbase in Dimdi). Many hosts recently launched *Graphic User Interfaces* for end-users. Some interfaces can be used partly offline (Probase for Data-Star), another interface is in use for both online and CD-ROM (Ovid Online, Dialog).

PREDEFINED OUTPUT FORMATS for the most often used field arrangement can save time. This is even more interesting when the availability of free information by a predefined format is highlighted. Some hosts offer additional features to be defined by the user (Dialog), or offer a highlight feature. Two formats, bibliographic information only or the full record description, are available in all hosts. Although predefined formats can be combined, some hosts prefer to multiply the range of possibilities

COSTS are one of the most important selection criteria for an experienced searcher, but is a very difficult topic to assess, due to the complexity in pricing structures and variation of currencies. Even if database prices alone are compared on a steady currency basis, significant differences appear. An example was shown here for Medline, with 1995 prices and mean currencies.

Conclusions. The poster showed only some of the most significant findings, but, even for the limited number of criteria studied, we can conclude that accessibility of information from a database certainly varies from one host to another. Professional searchers must be aware that database searching is significantly and at many levels influenced by the hosts. For choosing a host, not only availability of databases and costs should be taken into consideration, but also other criteria depending on the type of search to be performed. Purchasing several hosts can be a strategic issue. This underlines the importance of the role of the host in information delivery: a lot of value can be added by designing the tools for searching efficiently.

[1] Based on the thesis of P. Baert for the degree of Information Specialist (=Bibliothécaire-Documentaliste)

S. Bakker (ed.), Health Information Management: What Strategies?, 74.

QUALITY REQUIREMENTS IN MANAGEMENT OF SUBSCRIPTIONS

*Giovanna F. Miranda and Jeanet Ginestet**, *Sanofi Winthrop, Milano, Italy and **Sanofi Recherche, Montpellier, France

Introduction

Recent years have witnessed many changes in medical information science and corporate librarians must reengineer the library for the new information age. Introduction of end-user oriented products, electronic journals and electronic document delivery systems are only a few examples of the changes. Greater access to information by clients, stemming from the ubiquitous spread of networking within organizations, will have a substantial impact on the traditional activities of librarians and/or information professionals. This concern results in growing pressures "inside" and "outside" the library profession to adopt the tools of management sciences. In this context, management of the library involves providing resources and cost-effective services to anticipate and meet increasing user needs.

For librarians, the optimization of the management of subscriptions and the relationship between the collection's coverage and demand are two of the major problems. Library subscription service manages subscriptions of journals, magazines, CD-Roms, etc, and is designed to facilitate management by the librarians themselves. A published study of a "user rating of library subscription services" takes into account parameters such as the service's reliability and capability, the vendor's integrity and the overall satisfaction of the customers.[1] We have developed a "chart" with more technical parameters or standards for checking the correspondence of the various subscription agencies to these quality requirements.

Methods

The "chart" of quality requirements for subscription agencies was developed and sent to four of the most important subscription agencies in Europe and USA, asking whether they applied these parameters. The quality requirements were divided according to the categories of global support, subscriptions, general services and invoices, and according to their importance: indispensable or optional.

Global support: completeness and adequacy of support to regional offices, language of the country, rapid delivery services (Table 1);

S. Bakker (ed.), Health Information Management: What Strategies?, 75-79.

Table 1.

	Subscription agencies			
GLOBAL SUPPORT	1	2	3	4
Regional offices		Y	Y	Y
Language of the country		Y	Y	Y
Same handling charge for all Divisions of Sanofi Group	Y	Y	Y	

Table 2.

	Subscription agencies			
MANDATORY SERVICES	1	2	3	4
Renewals	Y	Y	Y	Y
Cancellations	Y		Y	?
Changes of address	Y	Y	Y	Y
Claims	Y	Phone/fax within 8 days	Online twice/week	Online
Cost-saving on multiple copies		Y	Y	Y
Memberships		Y	Y	
Single issues		Y	Y	
Back issues service	Y	Y	Y	Y
Missing copies services	Y	Y	Y	Y

Table 3.

	Subscription agencies			
GENERAL SERVICES	1	2	3	4
Specific departments e.g. STM		Y	Y	
Subject catalogs			Y	
Special alert reports			Y	Y
Collection development reports			Y	
New title announcements		Y	Y (serials directory)	Y
WWW Access	Y	?*	Y	Y

*in preparation

Table 4.

	Subscription agencies			
GENERAL SERVICES (CONT.)	1	2	3	4
Bar code journals for check-in	Y	Y	Y	Y
Macro to Gedbib			Y	Y
Routing lists internal circulation	Y	Y		Y
Reprint orders		Y	Y**	
Free samples	Y	Y	Y	

**large experience with other pharmaceutical companies

Mandatory subscription services: renewals, cancellations, change of address, claims, cost-saving on multiple copies, memberships, single issues, back issues service, missing copies service (Table 2);

General services (value-added services): bar code journals, macro to Gedbib (Gedbib is the internal Sanofi library management system and a macro permit an automatic check-in of journals received), routing lists, document delivery, specific departments for technical/medical libraries (STM), subject catalogs, special alert reports, collection development reports, new title announcements, free samples, Internet access (Tables 3,4);

Invoice services: electronic invoices, historical price analyses, advance notice of publisher price increase (Table 5);

Optional services: table of contents, copyright-cleared document, library management software, document delivery management reports, host activities (Table 6).

Results

All the subscription agencies answered our questions.

Quality of answers (Table 7): The delay for answering to our letter ranged between a few weeks and two months. Three agencies answered our questions point by point, the fourth one gave us only details about its business, without considering the questions. One agency gave us an answer at a national level, the others replied from their central European agency. Two of the four agencies organized a visit for presentation of their services.

Global support (Table 1): Two of the four responders have similar quality standards that correspond to our quality requirements. Agency no.1 has no regional office and agency no. 4 can not apply the same handling charge to all the subsidiaries of Sanofi Group.

Mandatory subscription services (Table 2): As expected for the mandatory qualities, all the subscription agencies cover almost all the requirements, such as renewals, time-saving claim systems, missing or back issues services. Agency no. 3 answered all our requirements positively.

General services (Tables 3,4): Unlike mandatory qualities, agencies differ in general services. Only two of the four are able to supply a macro for our library management system Gedbib and have a specific department for technical/ medical libraries, but only agency no. 3 has both. All the agencies have bar-code journals for the check-in, to enable you to enter all the needed information automatically into your system. All the agencies have a Internet access.

Optional services (Table 6): Three of the four agencies have a table of contents service and a document delivery copyright cleared service, but only one is able to supply a document delivery management report to evaluate the relationship between the cost of a journal subscription and the cost of document delivery for us to effectively manage expenditures and resources. A specific library management

Table 5.

INVOICE SERVICES	Subscription agencies 1	2	3	4
Invoices indicating: publisher's price currencies exchange rate handling charges	Y	Y	Y	Y
Electronic invoices	Y		Y	
Historical price analysis		Y	Y	
Advise of publisher's price increase	Y	Y	Y	

Table 6.

OPTIONAL SERVICES	Subscription agencies 1	2	3	4
Table of contents		Y	Y	Y
Document delivery copyright cleared		?*	Y	Y
Document delivery management reports			Y	
Library management software	Y	Y	Y	Y

*in preparation

Table 7

QUALITY OF THE ANSWERS	Subscription agencies 1	2	3	4
Delay of answering to our letter	1 month	2 months	same month	same month
Exact answers to our questions		Y	Y	
International level of the information	Y		Y	Y
Presentation of the services (visit organized)			Y	Y

Table 8.

RESULTS	Subscription agencies 1	2	3	4
Global support	1/3	3/3	3/3	2/3
Mandatory subscription services	6/9	8/9	9/9	6/8
General services	4/11	6/11	10/11	6/11
Invoice services	3/4	3/4	4/4	1/4
Optional services	2/5	3/5	4/5	3/5
TOTAL	**16/32 (50%)**	**23/32 (72%)**	**30/32 (94%)**	**18/32 (56%)**

software was proposed by two agencies, but was not of great interest to us, since we have developed our own system, set up worldwide, to ensure continuity of the service. All the four agencies have a Host activity service, a client/server search and retrieval system for bibliographic data which is accessible on line to the customers through direct electronic transmission or internet.

Invoice services (Table 5): The aim of itemized invoices is to reduce the work of accounting departments. This service is a common quality standard , but only two of the four agencies are able to supply electronic invoices. Agency no. 3 answered all our requirements positively.

Discussion

Table 8 summarizes the results obtained. The correspondence of the various subscription agencies to our quality parameters ranged from fifty to ninety-four per cent. Although the results show that none of the subscription agencies currently apply all the things we asked for, but two of the four responders have similar standards of quality that are very close to our quality requirements, ranging from 72 to 94%. As expected the overlap between quality required and services supplied was better for the mandatory subscription services and the invoice services. Correspondence of global support, general and optional service varies for the different agencies.

Finally, in times of tight budgets, the choice of a subscription agency will depend on which parameters you judge to be the major critical points in your libraries management.

Reference

[1] Cibbarelli P. Cibbarelli's Surveys: user ratings of library subscription services. Computers Libraries 1995;15:29-33

LIAISON PROGRAMME AT A MULTI-FACULTY UNIVERSITY LIBRARY

Felicity Grainger, Glasgow University Library, Scotland, UK

Background

Glasgow University Library is one of the major academic libraries in the UK. In addition to its role of collection it has a tradition of providing services to readers based on subject-divisional structure.[1] Services had concentrated largely on teaching but by the late 1980s the Librarian and newly appointed Head of Reader Services recognised the possibilities of providing support to academic staff.[2] There was increasing pressure to carry out research but a decreasing amount of time to spend in the library which was, due to funding cuts, subscribing to fewer journals.

The move in the 1980s to allocate funding to universities on the basis of the results of a five-yearly Research Assessment Exercise highlighted the need to maximise research performance. Glasgow's research staff do not have the benefits of focused library and information services provided by smaller units[3] and by other medical schools in the UK. Glasgow is unusual in having no medical school library - the medical collection is incorporated into the main multi-faculty University Library.

The design of library services based on feedback from library users using traditional mechanisms of committees, communication at senior management level and questionnaires was thought to be unreliable. After discussions between the Head of Reader Services and Faculty Deans the existing mechanism was replaced in 1991 by an active liaison programme to be carried out by Subject Librarians. At least 20% of their time was to be spent in academic departments.

Their brief was to be the "marketing arm" of the Library, assessing the needs of users, reporting back to Library management and responding, together with the rest of the library staff, to the needs expressed. A task force at Rutgers University later came up with similar recommendations.[4]

Process

From October 1991 Subject Librarians received training in interview techniques and were briefed and provided with documentation on library policy and procedures.

Altogether there were fifteen full-time equivalent Subject Librarians, four in Arts and Humanities, four for Social Sciences, six in Science and one for Medicine. Medical Faculty has approximately 450 academic staff and 950 Honorary Clinical teaching staff. Faculty has special requirements as most departments are off campus,

S. Bakker (ed.), Health Information Management: What Strategies?, 81-83.

information needs are high and staff find it difficult to visit the University Library which is distant from all except one of the eight teaching hospitals.

Subject librarians were given considerable freedom in the way in which they carried out their brief. In Medical Faculty the Heads of Department were visited first and then active research workers. Initially the meetings were with individuals but this has been extended to include groups - members of a department or research laboratory or team. Interviews are structured, "trigger" questions asked and notes taken. The aim is to discover what use is being made of the Library, whether the Library provides for the needs of the user, whether access arrangements and holdings are adequate and what other facilities are required. The library services are described eg. document delivery, current awareness services, some of which are new.

Results

REACTION TO VISITS

The initial response from the academics was one of surprise that library staff were taking a proactive role and initiating visits to them. They clearly find it easier to think of and talk about the information needs relating to their research while they are in their offices or laboratories than when they are in a library environment. They also like to have one named contact in the Library.

INFORMATION NEEDS EXPRESSED BY ACADEMIC STAFF

Feedback from academics has varied depending upon their subject discipline, but is fairly consistent within disciplines. Medical Faculty find opening hours inadequate and journals too few, particularly specialised titles, but they are very positive about services provided. Many requests have been placed for current awareness searches using subject profiles set up on bibliographic databases. Most readers accept that document delivery represents an acceptable alternative to low use journals (provided delivery was fast) especially if there is access to networked bibliographic databases.

Many have taken up offers of demonstrations and hands-on tutorials of bibliographic databases to groups within departments. In addition to appreciating not having to leave the department, people prefer to use their own equipment which is familiar to them although often hair-raising for the Librarian!

RESPONSES FROM THE LIBRARY

Although little can be done (because of funding constraints) to increase opening hours and journal subscriptions, changes have been made to library services in response to the needs expressed. Delivery of photocopied articles has been speeded up, the current awareness service expanded, full-day course on information skills run for research students, letters of introduction and information are sent to new staff who are invited to presentations on the Library and its services.

Mechanisms have been set up for notifying academic staff of changes and new services; initially newsletters but increasingly e-mail and web pages are being used.

OUTCOMES

Image of the library. The Library has achieved a very different image and a closer relationship with academic staff has developed. Subject librarians are perceived as working for the academic departments as much as for the Library and have been invited to join Faculty and departmental committees and working groups.

The closer relationship provides the opportunity for library staff to be involved in discussion of new plans with implications for the Library right at the start. This has extended to teaching, and the appreciation of tutorials to staff has meant that library sessions have now been timetabled into the undergraduate curriculum.

Although more information is now delivered electronically and by post to the science and medical staff than before, subject librarians are actually consulted more - they have established themselves as information experts.

Visits to departments were used as an opportunity to develop closer links with the hospital libraries and this has led to more co-operation.

Impact on subject librarians. As subject librarians have developed closer relationships with their research staff conflicts have sometimes arisen - do their loyalties lie with the Library or their departments? Most have welcomed the change in the style of their work but others would prefer continue to have a more retiring role.

Library structure. The programme has had a considerable impact on the Library and the management structure has been affected by the amount of work generated. The increase in requests, especially for current awareness services, has been far more than subject librarians could service themselves and, as a result, more of the work they carried out previously has been centralised.

Quality assurance

Success of the programme is in no doubt as shown by the report of the 1995 Quinquennial Review in which the subject librarians were singled out for praise. However measurement of achievements is not easy as academics in different subject disciplines have very different requirements.

This is being addressed and now that the needs have been identified, research support is to be formalised by means of Service Level Agreements between the Library and academic departments. These have already been agreed in the area of teaching and are being drawn up for research in order to create realistic and measurable guidelines for services which the Library can provide.

The liaison programme continues and is being constantly updated.

References

[1] MacKenna RO. Subject-Divisional Organization in a Major Scottish Research Library. In: McAdams F (ed.) Of one accord: essays in honour of W B Paton. Glasgow: Scottish Library Association, 1977:99-109

[2] Heaney HJ. Subject-Divisional Organisation: The Standard Still Flies. Libr Rev 1991;40(2/3):21-26

[3] Pratt GF. A health sciences library liaison project to support biotechnology research. Bull Med Libr Assoc 1990;78:302-303

[4] Wu C, Bowman M, Gardner J, Sewell RG, Wilson MC. Effective liaison relationships in an academic library. Coll Res Libr News 1994;55:254+303

TRADITIONAL AND ELECTRONICAL LIBRARY SERVICES

Judit Szabó Szávay, Semmelweis Medical University, Budapest, Hungary

Central Library of the Semmelweis University of Medicine

The Central Library of the Semmelweis University of Medicine, founded in 1828 and operated as an exclusive faculty library, is the largest and oldest medical library in Hungary. The Central Library is an academic library and serves as a medical information centre in Hungary. The present collection of the library consists of more than 250.000 volumes and 550 current journal titles and databases. The library acquires Hungarian and foreign literature mainly in medical and biomedical subjects.

The poster showed the main structure and the activity of all services of the Central Library of the Semmelweis University of Medicine including photos. The different functions of the library such as cataloguing, serials, and circulation, are based on an integrated library system called Dynix Horizon.

THE MAIN LIBRARY SERVICES

Loan during 64 hours a week;
Interlibrary loan attends to other libraries all over the country;
Help desk with reference collection: dictionaries, almanacs, directories, registers, periodical lists; bibliographic and commercial databases; information sheets about the library services;
Card catalogues: author, subject, series, congresses;
OPAC terminals;
Copy service: self service by multifunctional copy card and coins and according to special wishes as enlargement, lessening, colour technique etc. by ordering;
Reading rooms: periodical-, book- reading rooms with video casettes and magnetic tapes collection;
Information center with 5 PC and 5 Macintosh workstations where the CD-ROM databases and all the Internet possibilities can be used;
Internet services: Gopher, WWW, electronic mail system, some word processing and spreadsheets etc.
Closed stacks: Current books and periodicals, old books, closed periodicals.

S. Bakker (ed.), Health Information Management: What Strategies?, 84.

EVALUATION OF MEDICAL LIBRARY COLLECTIONS IN HUNGARY

Lívia Vasas, Semmelweis Medical University, Budapest, Hungary

Introduction

There are four medical universities in Hungary: in Pécs, Szeged, Debrecen and Budapest (Table 1).[1] To these institutes belong the largest libraries (Table 2).[2] The stock amounts to 1,066,304 pieces, 90 full time employées work in the 4 libraries.

The Hungarian language literature can be found in these libraries totally.

The holdings of non-domestic materials are on different levels, as all over the world. However, these collections constitute the main basis of the medical literature in Hungary. It was an important task to know exactly the stock data, qualitatively and quantitatively.[3]

The Conspectus system - the exact method of collection analysis - is extraordinary difficult and takes up very much time. We established an easier, but correct method of analysis, based on common consent of the 4 university libraries.

Evaluation of book-collections 1990-1995

Quantitative and qualitative analyses were carried out relating the book collections according to elected subjects of the medical terminology.[4]

QUALITATIVE ANALYSIS

The whole procedure can be seen in figure 1. We established an ideal, so called basic book-list for qualitative analysis.[5,6] First of all we made the offering lists and we sent them to the leading professsors because the professors as chief users knew the demands best. So we get the basic lists processed in text processor.

We compared the basic lists of books with those in our holding, these are the "available" books. Then we examined the coincidence between the recommanded and available books by subjects, and expressed the coincidence in per cent, then we created 3 groups according to the coincidence percentage:

Between 3-15%: 7 subjects; weak supplied themes. Between 16-50%: 32 subjects; needed better supply. Above 50%: 8 subjects; next to convenient. Half of the most important books we have in these areas.

S. Bakker (ed.), Health Information Management: What Strategies?, 85-89.

Table 1. Medical universities in Hungary[1]

Name	Founded	Staff	Students
University Medical School of Debrecen (DOTE)	1918	751	1163
Medical University of Pécs (POTE)	1923	644	2178
Albert Szent-Györgyi Medical University (SZOTE)	1872	721	2635
Semmelweis University of Medicine (SOTE)	1769	1291	3994

Table 2. Main data of the university libraries[2]

Universities	Library Foundation Year	Holding (volumes)	Non-domestic Current Periodicals (titles)	Staff (FTE)
DOTE	1947	158.756	790	20,00
POTE	1961	212.558	668	20,00
SZOTE	1926	186.461	724	24,50
SOTE	1828	508.304	530	26,25

Table 3. Missing periodicals according to impact factor (IF)

IF GROUPS	TITLES	PRICES $
IF higher than 2	82	30.987
IF between 1-2	104	50.110
IF lower than 1	171	110.837
without IF	170	27.207

QUANTITATIVE ANALYSIS

The four university libraries counted the books acquired in the past 6 years and controlled in the inventory books the prices and the sources of the acquisitions, finally we filled the data in the uniform worksheets.

For analysis, we summarized the data of the 4 universities separately and cumulatively, so we could see, how many books were purchased between 1990 - 1995 by the 4 universities (per university and altogether) and at what cost. The summarization has been performed by subjects, too, for selected subjects.

The final conclusions are: POTE is the best supplied in one topic, SZOTE, DOTE and SOTE in 9, 13, and 25 topics, respectively.

It was a surprise that among the 4 libraries SZOTE preferred the theoretical subjects while DOTE the area of clinical practice. The SOTE has the largest holding, and shows a more balanced collection.

The comprehensive data of the last 6 years for the 4 libraries show, that because of the increasing prices, the quantity of acquisition is somewhat decreasing. The acquired books, however, are invariably the best ones.

We analyzed the language of the acquired books, too: English was the most important language, and after a large gap followed German and French.

We analyzed the purchased and the donated book collections separately. The donated books, mainly in English, are valuable books. We will find very nice numbers, if we compare (per libraries) the value of the purchased books and the value of the total acquisition of the libraries
- to the staff of the universities and
- to the student number.

Regarding the purchase expressed in $/student, DOTE is on the first place with $145/student.

Periodicals

To show which periodicals can be found in these university libraries totally, together with the copy numbers, subscription sums, and the respective impact factors (IF), and to show the gaps as well, we established a list of core periodicals in different subjects in more steps. The process was similar to that applied to books (fig. 2).

The professors of the 4 universities compiled from the different subject lists a single list of core periodicals. The core list contains 1727 different titles in alphabetic order. In this list we indicated the census i.e. the finding-list of the current holdings in the 4 libraries. This gave us the possibility to compare one by one the present holdings with the core list.

From figure 2 we can see, that round half of the necessary periodicals are missing in every library. This is rather insufficient.

On the course of the work we fixed the actual subscription data of periodicals for 1995, and analyzed the costs per student. The numbers indicate that, although the sum spent annually on periodical subscriptions is rather high, the per student values are rather low and the periodical collections are weak (as seen from the IF-s) round 30 per cent of the desired periodicals is missing.

We analyzed the missing periodicals according to the impact factors (IF) and prices. Numerical data shown in Table 3. It would be very important to subscribe to the periodicals with IF-s higher than 2, as well as the recent or new periodicals.

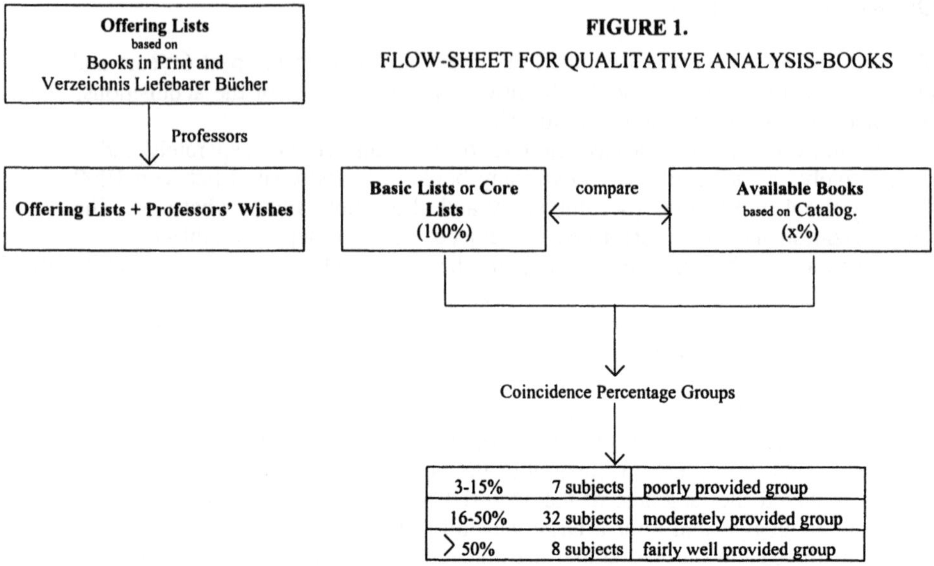

FIGURE 1.

FLOW-SHEET FOR QUALITATIVE ANALYSIS-BOOKS

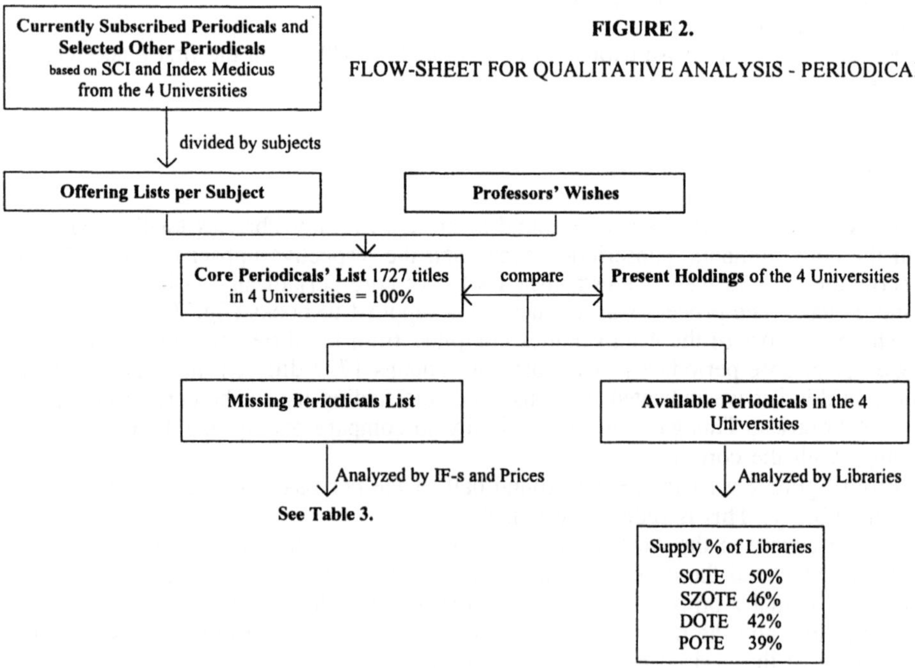

FIGURE 2.

FLOW-SHEET FOR QUALITATIVE ANALYSIS - PERIODICALS

Databases

Of the most important databases, we have some on CD-ROM: MEDLINE, Biological Abstracts, Science Citation Index. The Medline is used everywhere: in POTE (LAN on 4 terminals), SZOTE and DOTE (on 400 terminals). SOTE has a large optical backbone with several local area networks. About 1550 terminals are integrated to one campus-wide network connection. They assure remote accessibility to the databases round the clock, promoting the flow of medical information.

In the budget this is a new, significant and year by year larger expenditure, but everybody is convinced, that neither the libraries nor the universities are able to work without these databases.

Conclusions

A simple method has been worked out to analyze the holdings of 4 Hungarian university libraries and proved to be useful in the evaluation of the collections.

The results of this survey show the necessity of acquiring new books, the gaps of the collections, the exact items of collaboration which must be solved in the near future. We have to adopt a deliberated and coordinated strategy of the acquisition, to maintain a highly reduced locally-held core collection to meet primary needs with rapid and comprehensive access to external sources, backed up by an effective document supply service. From traditional reference and lending libraries we have to move to networked libraries with information services, providing access to local, national and international resources.

Acknowledgement

This work has been done in cooperation with Márta Virágos, Dr Rózsa Földvári and Dr János Marton, respectively head of the library in DOTE, POTE and SZOTE, and their staff.

Reference

[1] The World of Learning 1995. London: Europe Publications, 1994

[2] Semmelweis Orvostudományi Egyetem. A magyarországi egyetemek és foiskolák könyvtári kalauza. Kézirat. Budapest: SOTE, 1995

[3] Vasas L. Az orvosi szakterületet átfogó állományátvilágítási vizsgálat. Tanulmány. Budapest, 1995

[4] National Library of Medicine. Permuted Medical Subject Headings, 1995. Bethesda: NLM, 1994

[5] Books in Print compact disc. London: Bowker, 1995

[6] Verzeichnis Lieferbarer Bücher compact disc. Frankfurt am Main: Buchhändler-Vereinigung, 1995

COPING WITH INADEQUATE RESOURCES IN SOUTH AFRICA

John van Niekerk, Medunsa Library, Medunsa, South Africa

Introduction

The resources, facilities and services of the Library of the Medical University of Southern Africa (Medunsa) will be discussed, including the results of a survey of users carried out in 1995. This evaluation indicated that the Library had difficulty in providing for user needs. A strategy to enable an effective service will be outlined.

The Medical University of Southern Africa Library

Medunsa, situated near Pretoria, is devoted to the health care professions and concentrates on training health professionals to serve the developing sector of the population. There are approximately 3600 undergraduate and post-graduate students in the faculties of medicine, dentistry, veterinary science and basic sciences.

Material of the Medunsa library consists of about 45,000 books, 2,000 audiovisual items and 800 journal titles. An integrated computer system called Erudite is used in the Library for circulation, interlibrary loans, the online catalogue and acquisitions. The South African Bibliographic and Information Network (Sabinet) is used to obtain and download bibliographic information. Literature searches are mostly done on CD-ROM in the Library by users and there is also online access to a wide variety of databases. The library staff of 31 includes 16 professionally qualified personnel.

Problems faced by the Medunsa Library

In recent years funds from the university have been inadequate to maintain and develop the Library's collection and services to satisfy user needs. Several factors have contributed to the problem.

INCREASE IN USERS AND DEMAND FOR SERVICES

There has been a steady increase in library membership each year from 271 in 1978 to 4198 in 1995 with a growing pressure on library facilities and services (Table 1).

S. Bakker (ed.), Health Information Management: What Strategies?, 90-93.

Table 1. Some library statistics:

	1978	1995
Items issued	3,298	55,940
Literature searches	6	709
Photocopies	7,101	1,322,423

HIGHER COSTS

Price increases for publications are often higher than inflation. Aggravating prices in South Africa is the significant decline in the value of the currency, the Rand. Average price rises per annum in South Africa for books and journals often exceed 20%.

INADEQUATE RESOURCES

From 1982 to 1995 the Library's budget increased a little over five times, which has proven inadequate to deal with inflation, the declining currency and more users. Book acquisitions declined dramatically (only 1840 books were acquired in 1995) and many journal subscriptions were cancelled (700/1500 = 47%).

Table 2. Library users and collection development:

	1982	1983	1991	1995
Members	1156			4198
Book acquisitions	2703	5187	893	1840
Journal subscriptions		1500		800

User survey

Informal evidence and statistics suggested that the Library was struggling to adequately satisfy the needs of the users. Consequently, it was decided in 1995 to conduct a detailed survey and a questionnaire was distributed to a sample of 1255 staff, students and outside members. The main part of the questionnaire dealt with library material and services and the service preferences of respondents.

RESULTS

The response percentages, ranging from 20% for undergraduates to 29% for staff, were regarded as satisfactory.

Library material. There was widespread dissatisfaction with books, journals and audio-visual material amongst all user groups. Dissatisfaction with the quantity of books ranged from 58.2% for undergraduates to 68.4% for staff, and with the availability of books from 41.4% for staff to 64.2% for undergraduates. There were similar figures for journals.

Library services. Satisfaction with library services was much higher, e.g. approval for library staff assistance with the loan service, ranged from 80.9% for undergraduates to 94.6% for outsiders.

Information provided by the library. High dissatisfaction with library material seemed to be confirmed by considerable dissatisfaction with the provision of information, e.g. 35% - 45% dissatisfaction for basic information and 55% - 66% for new information.

Service preferences. Substantial numbers of users wanted more personal help from the library staff, especially undergraduates (58.2%) and outsiders (59.5%). Many users wanted an enhanced service with publications being supplied to them from the Medunsa Library or elsewhere, even if fees were to be charged.

CONCLUSION OF SURVEY

In general, users regarded service aspects favourably, while there appeared to be significant shortcomings in library material.

A strategy for the future

It is unlikely that financial provision will change sufficiently to solve the problem. A strategy is required and certain measures have already been implemented.

MAXIMISE FINANCIAL PROVISION

The library has tried to create an awareness amongst its users and key staff in the university administration of its difficult financial situation. The cancellation of large numbers of journal titles had a big impact on users. This awareness may have helped in obtaining budget increases, e.g. 25% in 1996, although such increases were often negated by inflation and the declining currency.

CHARGE FOR SERVICES

To eliminate wastage and increase income only basic services are provided free and other services, such as interlibrary loans, literature searches and photocopying, must be paid for by users, even if in the case of academic staff it is from a library allocation to academic departments.

SELF-SUFFICIENT SERVICES

Photocopying was changed to a self-contained service, with income having to pay for all the costs of the service, excluding staff salaries. This principle of self-sufficiency could conceivably be extended to other activities in the library, or at least there could be greater cost-recovery.

COLLECTION DEVELOPMENT

The Library is now more active in determining aspects of the collection that need improvement and an additional senior staff member has been allocated to collection development to concentrate on this task.

ACCESS TO LIBRARY MATERIAL

To improve access to publications, the Reserve or Short-loan Collection has been substantially expanded. Students can use this material in the library on an hourly basis.

DOCUMENT DELIVERY

The Library does have access to various document delivery services, including interlibrary loans and some full-text databases, e.g. Adonis. It is hoped that more use of such services will improve access to journal articles.

USER GUIDANCE

Guidance is extremely important at Medunsa where many students come from disadvantaged backgrounds. A variety of library guidance programmes are available, but a major task will be to reach more users so that they are able to make effective use of limited material and services.

LIBRARY COOPERATION

The extensive cooperation between libraries in South Africa, e.g. in interlending, networks and consortia, is very important for the Medunsa Library as it can get access to material, services and expertise that it would otherwise not be able to afford.

Conclusion

The strategy of the Medunsa Library thus centres on maximising income and organising services and facilities in such a way that the best possible use is made of available resources. It will be essential to regularly evaluate the library and make adjustments where necessary.

References

Cronin B (ed.) The marketing of library and information services 2. London: Aslib, 1992
D'Andraia FA. The business of libraries is staying in business. J Lib Admin 1994;20:81-91
Williams TL, Lemkau HL, Burrows S. The economics of academic health sciences libraries: Cost recovery in the era of big science. Bull Med Libr Assoc 1988;76:317-321
Wood EJ, Young VL. Strategic marketing for libraries: A handbook. New York: Greenwood Press, 1988

MULTIMEDIA IN AN ACADEMIC MEDICAL LIBRARY

Lubomira Soltesova, P.J. Safarik University, Kosice, Slovak Republic

Introduction

The library as a provider of information should present development in information technology, new information media and communication methods. Though it isn't easy in a period of severe budget cuts, unappropriate status of the library within the university or broader social systems, lack of qualified librarians, the University Library of P.J. Safarik University tries to introduce results both to its users and staff. It was the first place where university faculty and students have had access to INTERNET, to hypertext documents, and to CD-ROM databases.

After getting acquainted with the new document type on CD-ROM we started to think about implementing multimedia to our library services. What seemed to be important for our final positive decision? We considered multimedia to be:

- ideal information media for medical education by merging text, graphics, animation or other information forms in mutual different level relations;
- progressive information media showing users in a practical way the latest developments in information technology and supporting their information skills.

The possibilities of end-users in using the library equipment are limited because of an unsufficient number of public workstations. Due to weaker technical equipment and related reasons patrons in our library are still more passive recipients than active users. Democratic access to information and documents from various sources for different patron categories in many foreign libraries sustained our effort to give end-users a more active role. One of the ways to reach this aim was to offer them the new attractive media:

- ○ for playing and learning;
- ○ for improving their information, retrieval and general computer skils supported by consultations and training program;
- ○ for visiting library on a regular basis and focussing their attention to other library and information services.

Of course, we had to consider also our financial possibilities for:
a) appropriate equipment; b) databases; c) experienced staff. It almost seems too courageous to buy multimedia products, when the library budget is not sufficient even

S. Bakker (ed.), Health Information Management: What Strategies?, 94-97.

for journal subscriptions and when the books are acquired thanks to grants and gifts. We realized however that if we didn't try to keep-up and apply some of the new technologies, further development could be beyond our reach for a long time. In 1994 some extra money was used for buying the first multimedia titles and PC.

Definition

There are various definitions for multimedia. Generally, it is an information product combining on one medium at least 3 of following forms of information presentation:
- text
- data (statistics, tables, graphs, etc.)
- audio (human voice, music, sound effects, etc.)
- graphics (both classic and computer)
- photographs
- animation
- videorecord

By taking advantage of more forms of information multimedia could be a very effective communication platform and retrieval tool.

Besides on content, hardware facilities, interface, etc. the quality of multimedia depends primarily on the quality of graphics. What regard to animation it could be two-dimensional (window animation) or three-dimensional which enables the reproduction of objects in their 3 dimensions (virtual reality).

Because sound, video and all above mentioned applications require large memory and storage capacity, CD-ROM became the most universal medium with its capacity of 650 MB.

Standardisation was necessary to reach compatibility from technical and software point of view. Leading platforms are Macintosh and IBM compatible PC. A few years ago the standard for multimedia PC was introduced which lists minimal requirements for any product or system able to read multimedia document:
MPC, level 2:

PC 486 SX, 4MB RAM (recommended 8MB), 160MB HDD

CD-ROM unit with double speed min. 300KB/s, 16-bit digital sound card and speakers,

VGA 256 colours, min.13" monitor

Windows 3.1 or higher, MS-DOS 5.0 or higher, MS CD-ROM Extension 2.1 or higher.

We were able to buy a Pentium, 60 Mhz, 540MB HDD, 15"colour monitor, video, sound and network card, etc.

Benefits for medicine

Multimedia products have found their practical application in various fields: in learning languages, in geography and touristics presentations, in history, in public information systems, in entertainment industry, in video conferences within network environment and also in medicine and medical education thanks to their specific functions.

Multimedia databases and programs in medical education support in recipients logical and systematic thinking and learning
- by navigation between logical relations

- by incorporation of different information forms.
If the multimedia title can provide a student or other user with a large amount of information for a specific problem in the form of graphics, text, video, audio, etc. it enables him/her to see and understand the problem in a broader context and mutual relations.

There is also another crucial attribute of multimedia - interactivity, which enables the user to be active during browsing and learning. Interactivity is that feature which differenciates multimedia from TV or video. Multimedia allow the user to interact with the content through the use of menus, icons and hyperlink. They enable to personalise information by using annotation tools, electronic bookmarks, to create presentations by exporting the images or text to a presentation program. They are ideal for self-testing and knowledge refreshment.
Besides, they allow to:

- search large collections of references, full texts, images, sounds and other information very quickly and user friendly using graphical user interface
- create and label own images using samples from the database
- print text linformation in different formats and styles or to export them to the text file.

Multimedia medical atlases, electronic libraries or teaching programs enable to explore and learn medicine in new, dynamic and modern way.
According to survey published by the Slovak National Library in 1995, the University Library of P.J. Safarik in Kosice owns the largest number of CD-ROM databases in Slovakia, among which also some general and medical multimedia are provided in the Medical Library:

I. MEDICAL SPECIALIZED

1. Springer's The Comprehensive Classification of Fractures. Part 1: Long Bones. With Radiographic Examples and Proposed Treatment.
2. Elsevier's Interactive Anatomy. Atlas of Continuos Cross-sections on full motion CD-I. Volume I. The Head and Neck. Paranasal Sinuses and Anterior Skull Base.
3. Mayo Clinic: The Total Heart.
4. Albertina Icome's MultiMedica Thorax. X-ray Images and Data. Children's Lung Diseases.

II. MEDICAL GENERAL

1. Mayo Clinic: Family Health Book
2. Dorling Kindersley's The Ultimate Human Body. A Multimedia Guide to the Body and how it works.

III. GENERAL ENCYCLOPEDIAS

1. Encarta
2. The New Grolier Multimedia Encyclopedia

Example: The first listed database provides comprehensive classification of fractures of long bones (Humerus, Radius and Ulna, Femur, Tibia and Fibula). Fractures are devided into 3 types according to the bone segment (proximal, diaphyseal and distal) and further into groups and subgroups in an ascending order of severity according to the morphological complexity of the fracture. Treatment recommendation with possible problems is easy to attach, such as X-rays with possibility to magnify the desired part. A complete dictionary and glossary is also included to explain terms and concepts. Fracture code with all related information can be added to the individual patient record (name and ID, sex, date of birth, date of surgery and evaluation, etc.). The information could be retrieved from the database by saving results to a text file or printing them directly to the printer. While generating a report the data can be sorted alphabetically by the patient's name or chronologically by the date of surgery. In this way the multimedia database can be used not only for learning, but directly in clinical practice during diagnosis, and treatment documentation is a basis for further multi-aspect analysis or research.

Perspectives

Though the teacher is one of the basic parts in medical education he can improve a standard lecture by presenting information in various forms and relations using LCD panel or other presentation equipment even in a big lecture hall. Multimedia make teaching and learning more interesting and enable control and verification of subject understanding. The students can use the interactive features of multimedia titles during their home studying and learning. In this respect, like for printed documents, the medical library should collect and provide users with a wide range of multimedia documents. The library can also show and train faculty and clinical doctors how to use these databases in their clinical practice and professional development.

Another possible perspective is to make one step further and to start creating one's own multimedia documents both for library prsentation and specific medical education.

This paper summarized just a few experiences of using multimedia documents in a medical library. We do try to learn more and find other applications of more professional and specialized titles to include in library services. Serious consideration of all related aspects, requirements, conditions, e.g. analysis of current services and user needs, which new services, to whom, in what form, space facilities, financial sources, acquisitions plan, technical equipment, training, etc., should result in deep conception of using multimedia in the medical library.

References

Holsinger E. Jak pracuji multimedia. Brno: UNIS Publishing, 1995. 198p.
Hlavaty E. Multimedia a PC. Bratislava: Tecpron, 1995. 161p.
Janovska D. Prehlad titulov CD-ROM na Slovensku. Kniz Inform 1995;27(10):398-404
Informace na dlani. Katalog CD-ROM a dalsich informacnich zdroju. Praha: Alberina Icome, 1994. 176p.
Sokolowsky P, Sediva Z. Multimedia. Praha: Grada, 1994. 208p.
User's manuals of above listed multimedia
Information Sheets and Brochures (Mosby, SilverPlatter, Springer)

USE OF CD-ROM IN THE MEDICAL LIBRARY: 8 YEAR FOLLOW-UP

Françoise Pasleau, Martine Evraud, Philippe Jacquet, Nicole Quinaux and Anne-Marie Severyns, Faculty of Medicine, University of Liège, Belgium

Besides Medline, the local library network contains different databases chosen to enlarge the coverage of specific fields: Biology (LSC: Compact Cambridge Life Sciences), Oncology (PDQ: Physician Data Query), Pediatrics (Base d'Information Robert Debré) and Pharmacy (IPA: International Pharmaceutical Abstracts). Current Contents-Life Sciences (CC) provides a day to day follow-up.

A four months audit of the CD-ROM network was conducted in parallel with a user survey in order to draw a picture of the library network and its use.

Searched databases. Medline is the most frequently used database to conduct 80% of all searches. Within Medline 79% of the queries are made in the 1992-1996 segment. The frequency of access decreases with the publication age. Only 16% of the users consult several databases, most often Medline and CC. The other databases are only occasionally consulted. IPA and LSC are mostly selected by the library staff to answer questions in the field of environmental safety, toxicology, physiology and biochemistry.

Frequency of use. Through the audit, a mean number of 23 daily connections was measured. Access by modem is actually restricted to the University members.

Connection time. Many (55%) users seem satisfied with brief connection times (mean= 21 min). The remainder requires long lasting searches (mean= 93 min).

Users' profile and priorities. The majority (60%) are students, mostly premedical and doctoral students. Major concerns are: the preparation of dissertations or Ph.D. theses, the keeping-up in their fields as well as occasional searches. Another 21% are clinicians, who access Medline, for several reasons including support for clinical decision making. Research scientists (10%) have multiple concerns and a particular interest for the regular follow-up of the most recent publications. Members from the Faculties of Veterinary Medicine, Psychology and Sciences, paramedical workers and private physicians constitute the external users' group (9%). The most striking observation is that all types of users preferentially turn to Medline.

Guidelines to help users in a more efficient approach of the CD-ROM network must rely on improved exchange of information and advice between users and library staff on database selection, retrieval systems and subsequent citation management.

S. Bakker (ed.), Health Information Management: What Strategies?, 98.

INFORMATION NEEDS AND A COUNTRY OF SCIENTIFIC PERIPHERY

Anamarija Bekavac and Jelka Petrak, School of Medicine, Zagreb University, Croatia

Setting and Study

Characteristics of the science in a scientifically peripheral country as opposed to the mainstream science are: smallness - scientific community is small in number compared to the number of the subject fields of its current research, and consequently there are not enough qualified scientists to take part in the peer review process; non-equilibrium within the scientific community and between it and the society as a whole meaning the lacking of self-regulatory mechanisms for quality selection; communication barriers towards world science (local language = lost science). Health researchers and professionals depend on information import and are not members of the "invisible colleges". Libraries play the key-role in information acquisition and dissemination. The use of libraries and their services, thus, reflects not only the importance and quality of a library, but information needs and use generally.

Aims. To identify the reasons for the presupposed unsatisfactory use of the Zagreb School of Medicine Central Medical Library (CML) and to examine whether they are related to library itself or library environment.
Methods. The study was conducted on two levels:

A. There are 154 professors on the official teaching staff list. Only 81 actually used CML in a year's period. The survey was carried out on that group.
B. According to the results on the A level, 10 most frequent users were selected. A group of 10 professors non-users was randomly selected from the official teaching staff list. Both groups were interviewed on the reasons of library use or non-use.

Results. The library is the most important information source for 75% of reporting users. Features inherent to social context are the main reasons for minimal library use for 90% of surveyed users. The group of 10 non-users also reported the use/non-use of CML not to be library related.

Conclusions

The social impetus (competitive behavior, evaluation of professional and scientific ability by the international standards, etc.) is not strong enough to generate systematic information needs and, consequently, to stimulate better use of biomedical information sources.

S. Bakker (ed.), Health Information Management: What Strategies?, 99.

MEDICAL INFORMATION IN TARTU UNIVERSITY CLINICUM

Keiu Saarniit, Tartu University Clinicum, Estonia

Medical Information Centre

Estonia has a fast-developing information environment, its national medical information resources are scattered. Radical changes in medical information services (and in social, political and economic conditions) started at the beginning of the 90s, thus experience of 5 years has been gained from the functioning of the new system. Considering the information demands of the largest medical institution in Estonia - Tartu University Clinicum - the Board of the Clinicum established in 1994 a medical information centre (MIC), to develop an up-to-date technical infrastructure providing facilities to:

- create an electronic medical information centre,
- have access to CD-ROM databases,
- organize training in software usage and retrieval of electronic information,
- have access through INTERNET to the databases of foreign companies and libraries.

The project was supported by the Open Estonia (SOROS) Foundation and the first stage is completed in cooperation with the Tartu University Library, Institute of Computer Science, Computing Centre and with the Estonian National Library. Nine computers are connected to the local network and 20 to the network of the Clinicum. Databases on CD-ROM (Comprehensive Medline from 1966, CCIS a.o.) are in current use. A computer practice unit is set up for training database searching and using computer programs. Regular courses for medical staff, as well as advanced courses in medical informatics (ca 100 persons per year) are arranged. There is an agreement with the Karolinska Institute-MIC to retrieve information from their databases and to order copies. A comprehensive medical information system reaching every hospital of the country, is to be achieved.

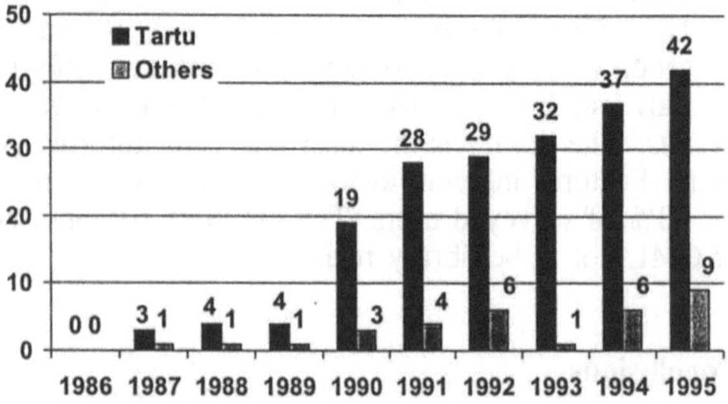

Figure 1. Publications in Medline of Estonian doctors.

S. Bakker (ed.), Health Information Management: What Strategies?, 100-101.

TASKS

The task of information centres includes analysis of both incoming and new generated information. *Evaluation* of the activities of the Estonian medical staff is based on the number of publications in the journals of Medline. About 250 articles per year are issued in Estonian magazines, e.g. "Eesti Arst" (Estonian Doctor), in journals of the former Soviet Union and -increasingly- in international publications (fig. 1).

To achieve a national information system that meets the needs of the medical profession, it would be necessary:
(1) to create an electronic *database of Estonian medical literature*, which would allow fast information exchange in special fields both at home and abroad;
(2) to carry out *bibliometric and scientometric research* on the basis of special literature, which would allow to estimate the distribution and impact of Estonian thought in world medicine.

The Estonian Science Foundation has approved the project. It is to be hoped that combined efforts will result in a system of medical information shared with other European countries.

NEW SERVICES AGAINST OLD MENTALITIES

Ioana Robu and Sally Wood-Lamont, University of Medicine and Pharmacy, Cluj, Romania

Abstract of poster presentation

AIM AND OBJECTIVES

The aim of this study is to obtain accurate data regarding the information gathering behaviours of academic staff and students of the Cluj University of Medicine and Pharmacy. The study is prompted by the present stage of development of the library service, and will mark an important step in decision and medium to long term planning. The introduction briefly describes the development of the library service since 1990. Though the number of library users and visits have increased significantly as compared to 1989, a fairly high number of patrons, most of them with intense scientific activity, stay away from the library.

USER SURVEY

Analysis of a survey by questionnaires show that old mentalities persist despite efforts to improve access to health information: introduction of automated library system, new databases and subscriptions to foreign journals, open access shelves, marketing etc.

FUTURE OF LIBRARY SERVICES

The situation is emblematic for the whole of the Romanian medical community, being one of the sequelae of the communist era. Effects on library service planning are discussed, plus the possible solutions, including better marketing, user education integrated with the university curricula, information delivery to hospital sites.

S. Bakker (ed.), Health Information Management: What Strategies?, 102.

VETERINARY MEDICAL LIBRARY SERVICES IN AUSTRIA

Doris Reinitzer, University of Veterinary Medicine, Vienna, Austria

Introduction

Opened in 1995 the new campus of the Veterinary University in Vienna is an impact for veterinarians in Austria (**http://www.vu-wien.ac.at**). I will present the experience of the first year in the new library building. The underlying concept of the library is to serve as an information center to hospital, students and academic staff and to become an interdisciplinary connection of biomedical disciplines.

The Vienna University of Veterinary Medicine, second oldest school for veterinarians in the world, has now completed its first move to a new 3.1 billion schilling campus on the north shore of the Danube. Forthy seven individual buildings are located on a 143000 square meter area and gives home for clinics, institutes and the library. The university employs about 560 academic and support staff and 2700 students. Compared to other universities our university is a real big project for Austria. We are not only looking back because this year we celebrate the millennium of Austria, the dimensions of this University will suit for the future. This year the university starts the new semester celebrating an open day presenting all its institutions. The library offers a "day of discovery", where we show a special selection for each user group: for pet owners, the academics, private practitioners and veterinarians employed by the government. Last year we conducted an anonymous user survey to find out what the readers want.

Budget constraints

Like other countries Austria has budgetary problems, which means that more and more services should be provided with less money. A reduction of some social services for students and the new contracts for university lecturers and assistant professors evoked a wave of protest at all universities. The process of budget consolidation has raised a number of structural problems that force to change the university and library policies. A new federal legislation provides the basis for the establishment, maintenance and operation of Austrian libraries, called the "University Organisation Act" (Universitäts-Organisationsgesetz 1993, UOG). This law promotes decentralisation and increasing university autonomy. Now we have to discuss both budgetary and personnel affairs with the dean, who is confronted, on one hand, with saving in the university sector and, on the other hand, with increasing operating costs.

S. Bakker (ed.), Health Information Management: What Strategies?, 103-105.

Library cooperation

The recent development of information technology has provided a broad basis for highly-integrated library networks with central and local components. In the area of academic and research libraries, the library organisation system, BIBOS, has been implemented step by step since 1987. The advantages of this cooperation result in coordinated descriptive cataloguing and search procedures, providing efficient and time-saving access to literature to the users. A framework of cooperative cataloguing has been successfully introduced including local and foreign data bases. Today 22 Austrian libraries, including all 18 universities, participate in BIBOS and offer this union catalogue. In the biomedical area useful data also come from other members such as the university of agriculture and the central library of medicine, which is located in the most important hospital of Austria.

Networks

The future is closely tied to digital information, and the Veterinary University promotes changes in information technology by establishing and maintaining a local area network provided by the university computing center. The library offers the most frequently needed medical bibliographic databases on CD-ROM via the LAN: VET-CD, BEAST-CD and Medline. To use our other databases on CD-ROM the visitors can book a terminal in the library. The increasing importance of databases as an information resource for better access to animal health information transforms the role of library into a general knowledge server open to all interested persons in biomedicine. The information center IVetS is headed by an veterinarian who not only provides bibliographic citations, but also gives answers to scientific questions by the help of the library holdings, both electronic and printed media. In addition, the library serves the needs of rural practitioners who are often geographically isolated, to participate in continuing education and research and to stay in contact with their alma mater.

There is a great disparity in telematics infrastructure accessible to our users. Universities and research institutions are interconnected to the Austrian Academic Research Network (ACONET) and there are practitoners using Internet via a special workstation or via modem. But many veterinarians do not have computers yet, but also want to perform data base searches on CD-ROM or online. In this case we answer telephone inquiries and send prints. Continuing courses help our users to become familiar with new technologies. Now a "library course" is a part of the curriculum for doctoral studies. Students working on their theses are our most frequent retrievers of information on CD-ROM databases.

Catalogue

Our input in the online catalogue BIBOS includes all library acquisitions starting from 1990. Unlike other Austrian university libraries we catalogue not only monographs, but also current journals. It is possible for the users to find out online if the last recent issue of the journal is avaiable for them. Furthermore the catalogue BIBOS includes all Austrian veterinary theses and that from our partner universities in Europe. BIBOS, which is not only an OPAC but also a library administration system supporting acquisition and cataloguing, now covers much well over one million titels.

It includes about 25000 monographs and 3700 serials from the complete stock of 153000 items held in our library.

ONLINE CATALOGUE

You can enter this online catalogue by two ways. A telnet connection allows you to access the catalogue directly. To get all the special characters printed correctly on the screen you have to emulate a special IBM terminal. By most of the common net software this is done by a 3270 terminal emulation (e.g. qws 3270 which is a public domain software avaiable on many ftp-servers). The domain name address is **opac.univie.ac.at**. To avoid the inconveniance of this IBM emulation a WWW-gateway has been established by the computing center of the universitiy of Vienna. Using popular interfaces like Netscape or Mosaic you can access this WWW-gateway with the address **http://bibopac.univie.ac.at**.

CATALOGUES ON CD-ROM

A CD-ROM version of the catalogue, covering titles and holdings of all academic libraries in Austria, has been published recently. Also available on CD-ROM is the Austrian Periodicals Data Base ÖZDB (Österreichische Zeitschriften Datenbank) with a similar user interface. In the near future BIBOS will be replaced by a new system. Because library loan is not well supported by BIBOS, we use for this purpose a system called aLF based on the data base system allegro C.

Future developments

With our library services we want to offer new trends in the dissemination of current medical information to practicing veterinarians. Future developments in library automation will proceed in the homogenization of different library systems towards standardized architecture as basis for integrated national and cross-border library services within the European Veterinary Libraries Group (EVLG).

References

Kooperationen: Higher Education, Science and Research in Austria. Wien: Austrian Academic Exchange Service (ÖAD), 1996;3(1&2). **http://www.bmwf.gv.at**

Olensky G. Der Neubau der Universitätsbibliothek der Veterinärmedizinischen Universität Wien auf dem Donaufeld. In: Oberhauser, Otto (Hrsg.): Österreichischer Bibliotheksbau in den neunziger Jahren. Wien: Prachner, 1991. pp. 39-45. (Biblos-Schriften 155)

Bureau for International Research and Technology Cooperation. Telematics Profile Austria. Wien: Bureau for International Research and Technology Cooperation (BIT), 1995. **http://www.bit.ac.at/bit/telemat/studie/**

NORWEGIAN COLLEGE OF VETERINARY MEDICINE: NEW LIBRARY

Anne Cathrine Munthe, Norwegian College of Veterinary Medicine, Oslo

Veterinary medicine in Norway

The Norwegian College of Veterinary Medicine (Norges veterinærhøgskole) is the only veterinary college in Norway, and its library the only one covering the subject of veterinary medicine. The library dates back to 1891, and was atttached to the National Animal Health Institute (Det veterinær-pathologiske laboratorium). After the college was established in 1935 it was transferred to it.

The library serves the staff and the students at the college and the staff at the Central Veterinary Laboratory (Veterinærinstituttet) which is situated at the campus. As a national resource library it serves all veterinarians and the general public who need its literature and services. The collection comprises approximately 75 000 volumes, 480 current periodicals and 350 videos and slide programmes. The staff consists of 3.5 librarians and 1 library assistant.

THE OLD LIBRARY BUILDING

In 1963 the library moved into new premises which at that time were very modern and spacious. They were expected to be adequate for the next 25 years. In the second half of the 1980's it became more and more overcrowded in spite of an active discarding of duplicates and outdated literature. The number of staff members and the amount of technical equipment had increased, and it became impossible to find room for everything. Another factor which contributed to the needs for new facilities was the raising demands to social working conditions and environment in Norway. As a new building seemed to be out of the question, we had to concentrate on making use of the existing ones on the campus. Some alternatives were suggested, but none of them were satisfactory.

PLANNING A NEW LIBRARY BUILDING

In the summer 1991 it was decided that the Norwegian Food Control Authority (Statens næringsmiddeltilsyn) should be transferred to the campus and that a new office building and laboratories had to be constructed. At the same time it was clear that our library was to be extended by taking over a laboratory on the storey above. Later it became obvious to the architects who were engaged that it would be unsuccessful both from a technical and an architectural point of view. They suggested

S. Bakker (ed.), Health Information Management: What Strategies?, 106-108.

that the new building should provide room for the library as well.

By the time we became involved in the planning, the size and the outline of the library were decided. What we have got is a library in two storeys of totally 660 sq.m. and with new stackrooms in the basement. Of course we would have wanted the library even bigger, but it was impossible on the rather limited site for the building. Our great challenge was to make the most of the square meters.

FURNITURE AND EQUIPMENT

The architect's vision was to create spacious and bright rooms and it is achieved by large windows which make most of the daylight. It is also reflected in our choice of furniture and the colours of the textiles used, which are white, clear blue and green and a little black. All the furniture is made of birch and the shelves are of birch and light grey steel.

Information desk. The ground floor with the entrance, has the information/circulation desk, catalogues , indexes and abstracs and PC's for searching our online catalogue and CD-roms. We have also about 300 current journals on display.

Monographs. On the first floor the monographs and the bound volumes are shelved. We have chosen to keep only the literature from 1980 and onwards on open access. Here we have the staff facilities such as offices, a lunchroom with kitchen and a meeting room. Unlike most Norwegian university and college libraries, we do not have a separate reading room, as reading space is available for students elsewhere in the college.

Study and reading rooms. The outline of the library is rather stringent, but we have tried to soften it by the shape of the reference desk and the arrangement of the shelves which are placed so they form shielded corners with tables and chairs. They are very popular for students colloquiums. There are also ten separate desks along the wall for users who want a more quiet area.

Library systems

CLASSIFICATION AND SHELVING

Classification. Since 1965 we have used the «Barnard's Classification for Medical and Veterinary Libraries» for indexing and shelving the monographs. Unfortunately no revisions or extensions have ever been published. We have updated it ourselves within certain subjects, but the call numbers became long and complicated for the users who got difficulties in retrieving the books. The moving was therefore a welcome chance for us to take a decision concerning the shelving system. We wanted it less complicated by organizing the collection in larger subject groups. The Danish Veterinary and Agricultural Library had in connection with their own moving in 1994, and the change from closed to open access evolved a system which was just something we had wanted and imagined. Fortunately our Danish colleagues were pleased we liked their system so much, and we were allowed to use it and make the necessary adjustments.

Shelving. We have divided our subject field in 11 groups designed alphabetically from A to K. Each of the 11 groups have about 10 subgroups which are designed by numbers. The call number for a book consists of one letter and a double figure. We started by using every tenth number in each group so we easily could fit in new subjects. In order to further facilitate, especially the shelving, all the main groups have got their own colour. Every book spine is marked with the colour code and the call number (the letter/figure combination and the four first letters of the title). All the books in each subgroup are shelved according to the title. We have kept the classification system for indexing the books. It means that all the books are classified according to Barnard's and get a call number according to our new system.

CATALOGUE

In 1990 we ended our card catalogue and joined the online catalogue BIBSYS which is a system for all the Norwegian university and college libraries. While we are putting new call numbers on all the books from 1980 and onwards we also convert the catalogue for the period 1980-89. In this way there will be correspondance between the book on open access, the online catalogue and the call numbers.

Results

BUDGET

As we became actively involved in the planning after the decision on building a new library was made, we had no influence on the budgeting of the building and its fixtures. But when it came to the interior the responsibility was entirely ours. We knew that we had to be very modest in our demands, and the grant turned out to be the absolute minimum of what was needed. Due to some unforeseen problems we exceeded the budget quite a lot. Fortunately this exceeding got no consequences to us the following fiscal year.

LIBRARY AS MEETING POINT

After half a year in the new library, we are very pleased with its situation on the campus, its interior and furniture. The reactions from our users are entirely positive. They enjoy coming, not only to find the literature they need, but they spend more time here. Because there are no staff restaurant or other informal meeting place on the campus, the library has become the centre where they encounter colleagues both from the college and the Central Veterinary Laboratory.

INFORMATION RETRIEVAL SKILLS FOR PROBLEM BASED LEARNING

Valerie Ferguson, Sheila Padden, Sigrid Rutishauser and Michael Hollingsworth, University of Manchester, UK

Introduction

Problem Based Learning (PBL) was introduced into the Manchester curriculum for 250 medical and 80 dental undergraduates in 1994/95 in response to the need for tomorrow's doctors and dentists to develop life-long learning skills.[1,2] Working in tutorial groups of fourteen, they study a different clinical case or normal situation each week, setting their own learning objectives to derive a plausible explanation for the case. The need for students to develop skills in finding, retrieving and using information from the library was identified early in the planning process.

Library Skills Programme

Experiences of the first year's provision of a Library Skills Programme (LSP) have been reported elsewhere.[3] This paper reviews progress after two years' experience of the course to show how the delivery methods of the LSP have developed in response to evaluation by students and staff.

AIMS AND OBJECTIVES

The general aims of the undergraduate curriculum in Years 1 and 2 include the development of skills in using technical resources, such as the library, effectively. The overall aim of the Library Skills Programme (LSP), was to introduce the students to library resources and facilities in a timely and appropriate manner. The specific objectives of the LSP were that students should be able to locate books, periodicals and sources of help, understand the range, status and use of library resources, know how to search for information on a specific topic, cite references appropriately and correctly and evaluate scientific literature.

METHODS AND EVALUATION

Methods used to deliver the LSP took account of the large numbers of students involved, limitations on library staff resources and the constantly evolving nature of the course. They included large lecture theatre events for the whole group and 'cascade' learning via tutorial group representatives.

S. Bakker (ed.), Health Information Management: What Strategies?, 109-112.

Questionnaires designed by the Course Director and the Medical Librarian were administered at lecture theatre meetings for the whole group of students. Confidence/success/helpfulness was rated from 1 (low) to 5(high) as appropriate.

Semester One

WELCOME

In 1994, a 20 minute illustrated welcome talk to all 300 students was given on the first day of the course, followed immediately by informal orientation to the undergraduate facilities of the Medical Faculty Library. In 1996 this will move to the third day directly preceding the introduction to PBL learning methods and a much longer period of up to two hours will be allowed for an integrated introduction to different learning resources including those of the library.

ORIENTATION

Orientation tours of the Main Library were given about six weeks into the first Semester during 'Reading Week'in order to build confidence in using the additional book resources and make students aware of the medical periodical collections. A graphic "slide show" customised for medicine and dentistry and demonstration of how to use the library catalogue (TALIS), was followed by a tour of the relevant areas of the library guided by 2nd year students.

Relatively few first year students attended the tours and questionnaire results showed that 30% felt that they did not need such a tour. In 1995/96 the tours were given by Library staff and students found this at least as satisfactory as the use of senior students (Table 1).

For 1996/97 further changes within the PBL course have redesignated the "Reading Week" (designed as a breathing space with no PBL case studies) as "Review Week". Tutorial groups will be invited to send representatives to an "Open Forum" to discuss their library experiences before taking a library tour based on identified needs.

Semester Two

USING LIBRARY RESOURCES

"Using the Library Effectively" seminars on finding and using different types of material in the Main Library were timetabled at the beginning of the second semester using tutorial group representatives to cascade learning. Finding pre-selected items such as major reference works, research monographs, and periodical articles of different types in the library using TALIS and library guides was followed by examination and analysis of the items, and using printed resources (eg Index Medicus and MeSH terms) for a subject search.

Strategically placed posters and leaflets help to maintain a high profile when these events are repeated for other students. A register of attendees has made it possible to target tutors and groups where attendance has been poor. From 1996/97 communication with students by e-mail will be possible.

MEDLINE SKILLS

A Medline demonstration to the whole student group in a lecture theatre was followed, a week later, by practical classes in the Medical School Microlab working through the *Medline: Step by Step Guide* devised by a course teacher in conjunction with library staff.

The demonstration was not well received in 1994/95 by many of the students mainly because the visual quality of the live searches in a lecture theatre seating 300 was unacceptable for about half the audience and it was difficult to gauge how much information could be conveyed when the majority of students had not yet done the practical work in the library seminars. In 1995/96 the technical presentation was improved by using a Liquid Crystal Display tablet. Instead of starting with a subject search an attempt was made to show how scientific papers arrived in the Medline database. Overhead projector transparencies of the contents page of *New England Journal of Medicine* were used to identify an article which was then retrieved and displayed in Medline format. The students' rating of this session showed a slight improvement. (Table 1)

Mean Scores (Medical & Dental combined)	1994/5	1995/6
Helpfulness of library tour	3.44 n=59	3.88 n=18
Helpfulness of "Using the Library Effectively" Seminars (combined score 6 queries)	3.00 n=83	3.37 n=33
Helpfulness of Medline demo	2.51 n=189	2.59 n=157
Confidence in finding articles after M'lab Medline	3.817 n=169	3.99 n=147
Full marks in simple Medline search (skills exam)	n/a	57% n=316
Success of SSM in developing library skills	3.94 n=146 (Med only)	4.05 n=191 (Med & Dent)

Table 1. Evaluation of Library Skills Programme by 1st year undergraduates
1 = least successful/helpful/confident 5 = most successful/helpful/confident

The Microlab Medline sessions, as part of the Informatics course run by a Senior Lecturer enabled blocks of 80 students to work through the *Medline Step by Step Guide* in 1994/95. Library staff experienced in using and teaching Medline attended these classes to assist students with problems. This was a necessary preliminary to the Special Study Modules(SSM) - mainly literature reviews supervised and marked by academic members of staff - undertaken just before the Easter break.

By 1995 the number of workstations available in the Microlab had increased so that 160 students at a time could work through the *Guide* in pairs. Doubling the student numbers and a shortage of supervisors with a good knowledge of Medline increased the likelihood of inadequate searching strategies. Not all students attended their timetabled session and some clearly made only a superficial attempt to work through the exercise, although their self-reported confidence in using basic skills increased slightly from 3.817 in to 3.99. The students' capabilities for Medline searching were tested in Semester 2 in a regular skills examination. They were asked to retrieve, download and print a simple piece of information from Medline. Fifty-seven percent scored full marks in 1995/96.

SPECIAL STUDY MODULES

Emphasis was laid on the importance of the literature review, even for laboratory-based SSMs. Clearly, only the supervisor who had offered the topic could make a judgement on the adequacy of the review. Library staff, however, were able to make an objective assessment of how successful students had been in citing references in the text and preparing a bibliography.

The only guidance the students received was the rules given in the *British Medical Journal*. The SSMs written in 1994/95 revealed, in general, a poor grasp of how to list a bibliography and how to cite references.

For 1995/96 library staff made available for reference and photocopying a two page document on citation methods. Sampling by library staff of the 1995/6 SSMs showed much improvement in citation methods. Students rated the success of the SSMs in developing their library and information skills more highly 1995/6. (Table 1)

Discussion and conclusions

The questionnaires were designed as a working tool to indicate the students' own perceptions of i) their confidence or success in retrieving information and ii) the helpfulness of the LSP in achieving that level of confidence or success. A mean score of less than three signalled the need to make some adjustment to the course.

Did the LSP make any contribution to the undergraduates' actual information retrieval skills? To make statistically valid claims for the figures will require further analysis. With a more structured evaluation tool it will be possible to build on the Medline skills examination and thereby test the ability of these undergraduates to construct effective searching strategies as they progress through the clinical course.

References

[1] General Medical Council. Tomorrow's Doctors. Recommendations on undergraduate medical education. London: General Medical Council, 1993

[2] General Dental Council. Recommendations concerning the dental curriculum. London: General Dental Council, 1993

[3] Ferguson VA. Planning and providing a course of problem-based library skills for medical and dental undergraduates: the first year. Health Libraries Review 1996;13:43-47

INFORMATION SKILLS IN THE CURRICULUM

Huibrecht Christiana Lombard, Frik Scott Medical Library, Bloemfontein, South Africa

Educational changes

Medical education in South Africa is on the threshold of extensive and radical changes. The call for change in the training of physicians received international acclaim with some world- and regional congresses initiated by the World Health Organisation. Certain paradigm shifts have already taken place and these changes will undoubtedly have an influence on medical education and practice. Some of the changes are:[1]

Community orientated learning. There must be a shift from lecture hall education and training hospitals to community orientated learning. The aims, objectives and basic principles of an institution must be defined by the needs of the community.

Professional thinking. Students must be trained in professional thinking that can be applied over a wide spectrum rather than concentrate on the superficial learning of a large amount of detail which is soon forgotten.

Problem-solving and lifelong learning skills. The student must be able to apply from the start that which he has learned, in the context of handling of patients and health care problems.

Usage of information sources. It is much better to learn how to use information resources and to find information yourself than to receive knowledge from somebody else and try to memorize it. Medical students must be exposed early in their training to the vast profusion of electronic resources. They have to acquire sophisticated skills and manage their own lifelong learning, to be able to respond to the rapidly expanding knowledge base of the biomedical sciences.

Problem-based learning

The Medical Faculty of the University of the Free State has investigated the possibility of changing from a traditional curriculum to a community orientated, problem- based learning curriculum.

S. Bakker (ed.), Health Information Management: What Strategies?, 113-116.

NURSING STUDENTS

From 1997 the Department of Nursing is implementing problem-based learning for all the first year students.

Phase 1: During October 1996 the facilitators for each group, as well as the lecturers and the information officer for the Department of Nursing will meet to plan and design the curriculum that will be used for the first year nursing students. With first hand involvement, the information officer will have a clear vision of the goals of the department. This will also help to ensure that applicable resources would be available for students to use. Because the information officer is also responsible for the information needs of other departments, information retrieval skills will be taught to the facilitator of each group in order for them to assist the information officer in training the students.

Phase 2: Beginning in January 1997, the first year nursing students will be involved in an orientation week at the university. During this time, they will be given a general introduction to the library. The 100 students will then be divided into 10 groups and be placed in the community where they will compile community profiles. Twice a week, these groups will return to the university where they will follow a problem-based learning curriculum.

Because problem-based learning is a new concept for the library and also because the library was not built with the problem-based learning concept in mind, separate discussion rooms for each group are not available in the library. The students will therefore have their introductory sessions at the Nursing Department lecture rooms. They will divide into small groups to discuss the case they have to study. They will identify facts about the case as well as learning issues or areas for further investigation. They will then visit the library to retrieve information about the case.

Phase 3: The third phase is a period of self-directed learning during which the students, independent of the facilitator or lecturer, consult resources in the library. The extent and depth of the issues that has to be persued will determine the time that will be spent on information gathering.

Phase 4: On completion of phase three, the students will convene in their respective groups in the library to discuss what they have learned and refine their knowledge and understanding of the problem and its management. Information material for each specific case will be put into a special reserve collection. A time limit will be set to enable every student to use the material. As the students get more proficient in finding their own information material, these collections will be reduced to include only the core material necessary. Facilitators will be given bibliographies so that they can ensure that the basic resources are identified by the students. Advanced techniques for retrieving references from databases such as Medline will be given on request. The last step will be for the students to assess themselves individually with regard to problem-solving skills, knowledge acquisition, self- directed learning and support of the group. Their peers as well as the facilitators and lecturers will also comment on each self-assessment.

MEDICAL STUDENTS

Because the Medical Faculty has not yet changed to a problem-based learning curriculum, a different approach will be followed to teach information seeking skills to medical students. The training will take place over all four of their study years. As they will not be given a case to study, formal lectures will be given to small groups of students to teach them to:

- analyse a topic and identify relevant key words;
- identify terminology relevant to a topic by using thessauri of databases and Library of Congress Subject Headings;
- use Index Medicus or other printed indexes to find references to information;
- use Medline and other relevant CD-ROM databases;
- interpret bibliographic citations;
- use the Internet to find information; and
- know how to locate books, journals and other information resources in the library.

The formal lectures will be supplemented with practical, hands-on training.

Impact on the library

Labour intensive. Because large group lectures are not very effective, information retrieving skills have to be taught to small groups of students. The UOFS library will therefore make extensive use of videos as educational aids.

Limited space. Additional rooms and areas close to the library will have to be identified for small group discussions. Adequate seating has to be available in the library or nearby tutorial rooms for students using the reserved materials.

Bibliographies will have to be compiled by the information officers.

Collection development will be influenced because adequate and applicable resources must be made available.

Additional computers have to be made available. The Faculty will share this responsibility with the library.

Cultural differences. Many of the students have different cultural backgrounds. It is therefore necessary for the information officer to understand other cultures and the information seeking patterns of the diverse groups.

Language barriers. English is the second language for many of the students. Insufficient English proficiency and lack of adequate English vocabulary make it difficult for them to understand library terminology. This makes it difficult for them to understand the information officer and places a heavy burden on the information officer.

Copyright clearance has to be obtained for all materials placed in the reserve collection.

Conclusion

To meet the challenges of a rapidly growing medical knowledge base and a demanding health care consumer population, medical education will have to change. Each medical practitioner and educator must become part of the process of change and must keep pace with innovations. The health sciences information officer must be acknowledged as an equal member of the medical education team. As a recognised information expert, the information officer can teach medical students knowledge and skills that can be used efficiently and effectively in practice. Their role will undoubtedly shift from intermediary to educator.

Reference

[1] Nel CJC. Die handhawing van norme, waardes en standaarde in geneeskunde onderwys in Suid-Afrika. Geneeskunde 1996; Mei/Jun:31-37.

-.-.-.-.-.-

Figure 1 of: LE CENTRE DE DOCUMENTATION ET LA FORMATION DES PSYCHIATRES ET DES PSYCHOLOGUES. Giuliana Schmid, Claudia Nesa et al.

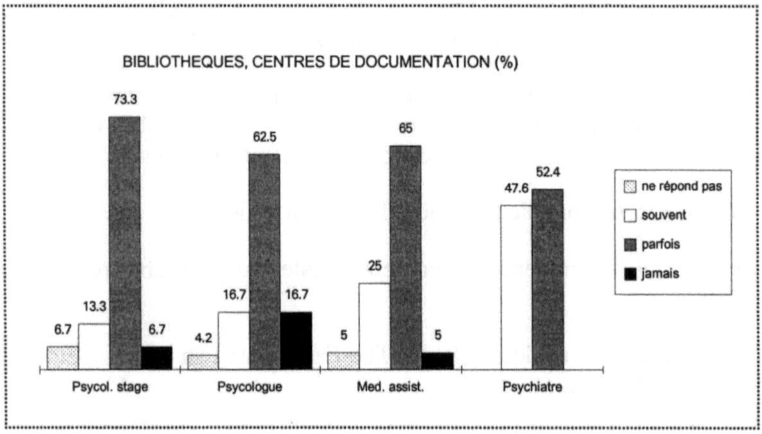

Table 1. of: LE CENTRE DE DOCUMENTATION ET LA FORMATION DES PSYCHIATRES ET DES PSYCHOLOGUES. Giuliana Schmid and Claudia Nesa et al.

	Psych. stage	Psych.	Méd. assist.	Psychiatres
Consultation/prêt de livres	73.3	70.8	60.0	85.7
Commandes d'articles	20.0	75.0	60.0	90.5
Consultation de revues	40.0	50.0	60.0	80.9
Index des revues	20.0	45.8	45.0	81.0
Recherches bibliographiques	33.3	37.5	20.0	66.6
Total	37.3	55.8	49.0	80.0

LE CENTRE DE DOCUMENTATION ET LA FORMATION DES PSYCHIATRES ET DES PSYCHOLOGUES

Giuliana Schmid, Claudia Nesa et al., Centre de documentation et recherche de l'Organisation Sociopsychiatrique Cantonale (OSC), Mendrisio, Suisse

Buts: en s'adressant aux psychiatres, aux médecins assistants, aux psychologues et aux psychologues en stage:
° identifier les sources d'information et les types de documents les plus utilisés;
° vérifier le degré de connaissance et la fréquence d'utilisation des services du centre.
Méthode: questionnaires mi-structurés; tous les interviewés ont été contactés personnellement; population: Totale N=80: 20 médecins assistants et 15 psychologues en formation; 21 psychiatres et 24 psychologues formés.
Résultats:
(1) Sources d'information les plus utilisées: rélations interpersonnelles (souvent 62.5%), cours de formation (souvent 50%); les moins utilisées: les congrès (parfois 67.5%), les bibliothèques (parfois 62.5%). Les psychiatres utilisent plus les bibliothèques (souvent 47.6%). [Table 1, page 116]
(2) Les documents primaires les plus utilisés sont les livres, les revues et les articles; les documents secondaires (bibliographies sur papier, banques de données ON-LINE et CD-ROM) sont moins utilisés: ce sont les psychiatres qui les utilisent le plus (moyenne 39.9%).
(3) Connaissance des services du Centre (moyenne %): psychiatres (96.8%), psychologues (87.9%), médecins assistants (73.8%), psychologues en stage (69.9%).
(4) Les services plus utilisés auprès du Centre sont le prêt de livres, la commande d'articles et la consultation de revues.
Conclusions:
Les différents profils se différencient par leurs comportement envers les services du Centre, soit au niveau de la fréquence que de l'utilisitation des services offerts. Actuellement les psychiatres profitent le plus de ces services (moyenne 80.9%). Ils recourent plus régulièrement aux livres, aux revues et aux articles. Les psychologues y recourent moins fréquemment (moyenne: les psychiatres 66.6%, ainsi que les psychologues en stage, les médecins assistants 60% et les psychologues 41.6%). Les nouvelles technologies se montrent timidement à l'horizon, encore peu connues par cette génération.
Pour atteindre la totalité des usagers potentiels et avoir un rôle de support plus important en rapport à la formation professionnelle, le Centre devra améliorer, à travers une information spécifique, ses différents services à fin de mieux cibler ses destinataires, en particulier les psychologues en stage et les médecins assistants.
Bibliographie:
Perucchi M et al. Biblioteche mediche, utenti potenziali e bisogni. Bollettino AIB 1995;35(1):65-74

S. Bakker (ed.), Health Information Management: What Strategies?, 117.

WHICH LITERATURE RETRIEVAL METHOD IS MOST EFFECTIVE?

Anita Verhoeven, Edzard Boerma and Betty Meyboom-de Jong, Medical Faculty, University of Groningen, the Netherlands

Introduction

Decision making in general practice needs to be supported by evidence-based conclusions published in the literature. However, which method for retrieving citations from these publications is most effective for general practitioners has not been determined.

Objective

Therefore, we studied which method, the printed Index Medicus or Medline on CD-ROM, is most effective for general practitioners to retrieve citations from the literature.

Methods

To answer this question, we developed a post-graduate course for each retrieval method, tailored to the needs of general practitioners. In these courses, 73 general practitioners completed the same four assignments linked to daily practice, using one of the two methods. As outcome measures we used precision, recall and personal score. In an expert group of three, we composed a gold standard to which we related the participants' selected citations. The interjudge agreement was high: 86% of the citations were judged similarly (as relevant or non-relevant). Precision, or efficiency, is defined as the proportion of citations retrieved by the Index Medicus or Medline that is actually relevant for the subject. Recall, or sensitivity, is defined as the proportion of the total number of known citations in the Index Medicus or Medline identified by the search. Finally, the personal score indicates the quality of the search based on the relevance of the citations for general practitioners, the publication type, and the place of the journal in the Science Citation Index, or its Dutch counterpart the KNAW list.

Results

Preliminary results showed that the mean of all three outcome measures of the four assignments were higher in the Index Medicus group. The difference between the

S. Bakker (ed.), Health Information Management: What Strategies?, 118-119.

Index Medicus and Medline on CD-ROM in both recall and personal score were statistical significant with a p-value < 0.05 (see Table 1).

Conclusion

Thus, out of two methods, the printed Index Medicus is more effective for general practitioners to retrieve citations from the literature.

Table 1: Results of 4 assignments in the Index Medicus and Medline on CD-ROM group.

	Precision	Recall	Personal Score
Index Medicus (n=33)	56%	24%	-30
Medline on CD-ROM (n=40)	51%	17%	-36
P-value	0.26	0.002	0.05

SCIENTIFIC LIBRARY: TRAINING FOR EVERYONE

Elisabetta Marinoni, Pierangela Mazzon and Donata Pieri, Universita' degli Studi di Padova, Italy

Vallisneri Library, established in 1990, through the fusion of the libraries of 7 biomedical departments, possesses 100.000 volumes and 800 scientific journals. The staff wants this library to be available not only to academics and university students, but also to other people interested in biomedicine (teachers, medical doctors, etc.).

SPECIAL COURSES The project is aimed at establishing specific courses on the use of bibliographic tools and network facilities, which will be tuned to the different expertises of undergraduate and graduate students. Furthermore, meetings among university librarians will be regularly organized, in order to discuss the specific problems of a large biomedical library.

In 1996 we have initiated, as a pilot experiment, a short course for *young students* of Padua. This very successful course, supported also by the "Assessorato all'Istruzione del Comune di Padova", will be extended and repeated.

In the first stage of the project, the staff of the Library and one of the Interdepartment computer scientists will organize courses addressed to *secondary school teachers*: the "new frontiers" of the reference and information services, as well as selection criteria for Internet resources will be examined in detail (about 20 h.).

In the second stage, the same staff will organize courses addressed to *secondary school-leaving students* (about 15 h.), giving information and instruction on library organization, how to access and use the library material, how to manage and consult at best bibliographic material, how to draw up a bibliography in order to set up a scientific work correctly (e.g. degree thesis).

SPECIAL TOOLS At the and of each course there will be a kind of *"treasure hunt"*: every student will receive a research subject, and the winner will be the one who will succeeded in citing and listing references to published literature, and finding the best way to obtain the required material.

The library staff created *special tools* (quick references, guidelines, etc.) to help attenders and end users to understand and use the library and its resources.

LIBRARY SERVICES During this programme this scientific library operated effectively in its own municipal district, the library staff programmed to extend the opening hours one evening a week: this means, not only increasing numbers of end users, on but also the opportunity to meet all the students-workers and connoisseurs on the subject requirements. During the evening opening hours the library staff will be fully engaged with reference and information service, in order to promote effectively easy library resources access. This opening is tentatively scheduled for February 1997.

S. Bakker (ed.), Health Information Management: What Strategies?, 120.

A PERMANENT ROLE OF UNIVERSITY LIBRARIES IN INFORMATION LITERACY TRAINING: ELECTRONIC MEDIA AND COMPUTER NETWORKING

František Choc and Milan R. Špála, First Faculty of Medicine, Charles University, Prague, Czech Republic

This paper exploits the results of a previous project.[1] Education and training in traditional information literacy for librarians, teachers and students, is no longer adequate to current demands, even if well established and not oversophisticated. In the present electronic era, the information media and technology are still not fully accepted by all their users, although the high efficiency in learning, teaching, and research is acknowledged.

First was determined: the *goals*, the *networking* and the *resource sharing*, and the *electronic information services practical comments*. The electronic information services policy for the university library was defined and based on this analysis and on publications[2] and material from similar libraries.[3]

Second this project was tested and resulted in:

Since 1993/4: Courses for pregraduate medical students (group A) and for postgraduates in biomedicine (from 3 medical faculties, the Faculty of Sciences and the research departments of the Czech Academy of Sciences and the Ministry of Health - group B) were prepared during the last three years by members of the Institute of Scientific Information (ISI) qualified in librarianship and medicine.

Since 1995/6: A course was established for bachelor students (group C) and special courses or demonstrations corresponding to the demands of the users, for teachers (group D) and for members of the ISI (group E); hands-out material was available.

The 4 hour course MEDICAL INFORMATICS for Group A (30 stud/yr) consists of theoretical and practical training in the principles of bibliography and searching in MEDLINE, Current Contents, or Czechoslovak Medical Bibliography (BMČ). CRAFT OF RESEARCH is a training course for Group B (60-80 stud/yr, 24-28 hrs/yr) in the principles of scientific communication and research data presentation including intensive workshops with databases. The 30-hour course SCIENTIFIC INFORMATION for Group C (50 stud/yr) is similar with a more practical approach. Groups D (40 pers/yr, 20 hrs/yr) and E (15 pers/yr, 30 hrs/yr) proposed their topics themselves (multimedia, new databases, research efficiency evaluation, interlibrary loan, document delivery). All the groups received intense training in Internet access.

The constant feed-back contact with the majority of the participants of the above courses, mainly with researchers and postgraduate students, has confirmed the advantages of the electronic information services policy stated at the beginning of this study and the usefulness of these library (ISI) activities. The participants of these courses appreciated the friendly role of the Library staff facilitating to master new electronic trends in information services.

References on page 122

S. Bakker (ed.), Health Information Management: What Strategies?, 121-122.

SOME EXPERIENCE WITH REFERENCE MANAGER

L. Hrcková and F. Mateicka, Research Institute of Rheumatic Diseases, Piestany, Slovak Republic

Personal bibliographies

Reference Manager is a personal bibliographic research system (Research Information System, Inc. USA), which enables to create personal bibliographical databases from the most common literary sources concerning biomedicine area (books, book chapters, manuscripts, magazine articles, notes, unpublished reviews, etc.). records are compatible with international formats (e.g. Medline) and the program enables importing records from other databases as well.

In our institute (the this system is used by individual researchers to create their own databases. This enables quick orientation in their own literature information files.

The program facilitates comfortable searching of desired references, based on defined key words. An advantage of the program is easy export of selected literature citations into a prepared manuscript under current text editors. It is extraordinary effective in reports with numerous literature data, since it manages them comfortably and safely.

-.-.-.-.-.-

References:
of: Chok F, Špála MR. A permanent role in information literacy training. p. 121+122

[1] Špála MR, Choc F. Participation of the medical faculty library in graduate and postgraduate medical education. *In:* McSeán T, van Loo J, Coutinho E (eds). Health information - new possibilities. Dordrecht: Kluwer Acad Publ, 1995. p. 246-8

[2] Fagan LW, Perreault LE. The future of computer applications in health care. *In:* Shortliffe E.H., Perreault LE (eds). Medical informatics. Computer applications in health care. Addison-Wesley: Reading MA, 1990. p.620-44

[3] Lane Medical Library, Stanford University Medical Center, 1994-6 (by courtesy of J.L.Morrison)

S. Bakker (ed.), Health Information Management: What Strategies?, 122.

FINDING SOLUTIONS IN THE LIBRARY

Maria Nardelli and Luisa Vercellesi, ZENECA S.P.A., Basiglio, Italy

Introduction

Pharmaceutical companies nowadays are increasingly evaluating the importance of bringing R&D scientists constantly up to date in their specific fields of interest. Such a continuing education is achieved through a series of different interventions, for example attendance to scientific conferences, periodical workshops on products and indications organised by headquarters, and training programs developed by local companies.

Aims

A local biomedical library can effectively support these programs and favour internal customers' personal updating through a rational use of both traditional sources and advanced information technologies.

In our library are already available sophisticated end-users' workstations, equipped with the most consulted international databases which are tailored to physicians and pharmaceutical researchers. In spite of this, we have realised that our main customers still refer more willingly to traditional sources like books and journals. Otherwise they require direct support from library staff, either due to their limited confidence with advanced information technologies or to the short time they can devote to improve their computer literacy.

As a support to internal training programs, my colleague Luisa Vercellesi and I have developed and started a long term project, mainly addressed to the members of the medical function, which was aimed to improve internal customers' knowledge and use of advanced information resources available and to encourage their confidence in solving their information problems without intermediate interventions.

Materials and Methods

The project entitled "The library as a solution" has been based on an eight-month calendar starting from July 1995 and involving several different initiatives such as:
- production and distribution of informative material on the library activities, products, resources, and services;

S. Bakker (ed.), Health Information Management: What Strategies?, 123-125.

- periodical meetings with the customers involving all the medical department and part of the commercial staff;
- distribution of two questionnaires, the first at the beginning of the project and the second after the last scheduled meeting, to assess the impact of the project itself on the customers involved.

The strategic planning of the project has been carefully carried out to define the organisation of the scheduled meetings and to prepare the informative material to be distributed. Although several new working commitments occurred unexpectedly throughout the project, we have been able to complete the training program to medical and commercial staff by the end of the expected period.

After two months from the last meeting a second questionnaire has been distributed, in order to collect all necessary data to provide a final evaluation of the impact of the project on the customers involved.

One of the first initiatives taken at the beginning of the training period was a widespread distribution of an "orientation map" of the library hall, conceived as a logistic guide and aimed to improve users' confidence in locating primary and secondary sources available.

Throughout the project we have alternated training meetings to the distribution of the informative material previously prepared (see Table 1), including traditional tools as the annual journals' holdings list as well as new products like a series of monographic cards describing the contents of the "top ten" books on the shelf.

The majority of the customers contacted have confirmed their interest in the project, especially those who attended all the scheduled meetings despite their many working commitments.

Results

At the end of the eight-month training program we have observed that more than fifty per cent of the customers contacted took part in the project on a regular basis. As a practical result of the efforts we devoted to this achievement, our subjective impression is that our internal users show to have changed their habits in using information resources available; their self-confidence in approaching advanced information technologies and their computer literacy have improved as well as their awareness of the many resources they have at their disposal in the library.

Conclusions

From our point of view the achievement of these encouraging results required a great commitment as regards the amount of time devoted to the project, which has been considered a priority objective on the top of routine activities. Ww have been able to involve a large number of participants by duplicating some of the scheduled training sessions, despite the experience of a remarkable turnover that caused fifteen per cent of staff in training to leave the Company.

Nevertheless we expect long-term benefits from the completion of the project, therefore we have planned to offer our customers further assistance by inviting them to spend one hour twice a month improving their knowledge of biomedical and commercial databases available in our library; each of this "customer hours", as we called these training sessions, will be devoted to a close examination of a different database and to the solution of real information queries suggested by the users themselves.

The value of the library's image, as a valid solution to any information queries, is undoubtedly increasing among customers. Therefore we are determined to maintain a high quality commitment towards our internal users, in order to be always prepared to face the constant changes that characterise the activities in a pharmaceutical company.

Table 1. The Project: "The library as a solution"

materials	amount		customers involved	
	PLANNED	ACTUAL	PLANNED	ACTUAL
GENERAL GUIDE to the library's activities - products - resources - services	40	40	40 MD	23
MONOGRAPHIC CARDS on the 10 most consulted books available (e.g. Goodman & Gilman's)	40	23	40 MD	23
QUICK GUIDES on main literature databases available	5	3[1]	40 MD	23
GENERAL AND "THERAPEUTIC AREA" PRESENTATIONS	6	2	60 MD+CD	23
"ORIENTATION MAP" of the library hall[2]	60	60	60 MD+CD	60
MAIN LITERATURE DATABASES PRESENTATIONS	3	3	60 MD+CD	23
LIBRARY PERIODICALS HOLDINGS LIST edition 1996[2]	60	60	60 MD+CD	60
QUESTIONNAIRES	2	2	40	30

[1] The databases manuals were self-explicatory
[2] Widespread distribution

CD = Commercial Department
MD = Medical Department

PLANTS TOXIC TO ANIMALS: A CURRICULUM-INTEGRATED HOME PAGE

Mitsuko Williams, University of Illinois at Urbana-Champaign, USA

Introduction

The growth of the activities on the Internet, especially the World Wide Web, is causing a revolution in the way information is delivered in education, commerce, and government. Sophisticated Internet resources, which began appearing early in this decade, are now commonplace. Librarians, long regarded as information specialists, are suddenly finding many other players in their field. This new phenomenon challenges the role of the librarians from one who acquires and organizes printed materials to that of managing dynamic communication mechanisms.

The hype of this new development does not go unchallenged. Critics of the Internet quickly point out that the new resources lack content.[1] As information specialists, librarians are in the best position to seize the opportunity to make the Internet viable and an integral part of the educational process. This paper represents one example of Internet resource development at the University of Illinois at Urbana-Champaign (UIUC) Veterinary Medicine Library.

The Project Background

Plants Toxic to Animals is intended for students in their third year of veterinary school at UIUC where Toxicology (Vet. Bioscience 320) is one of the required courses. Associated with this course are: a) a course syllabus containing over 800 pages, b) a collection of about 2,000 slides with brief descriptions, c) dried specimens of nearly 70 plants, and d) the Poisonous Plant Garden located at the back of the College of Veterinary Medicine building.

Unfortunately, the plant specimens are in poor condition. The slides are discolored, lack adequate explanations, and must be viewed through archaic viewing equipment, Singer Caramate 4,000. Even though the Poisonous Plant Garden, which was established in 1990, contains real plants, the students generally miss most of the growing season as they are not on campus from mid- May to early September.

Under these circumstances, the announcement of a university-wide grant opportunity in the autumn of 1992 was a timely event. The purpose of the program was to encourage faculty members to try technological enhancements in their teaching. The proposal to create a database of poisonous plants received funding from

S. Bakker (ed.), Health Information Management: What Strategies?, 126-128.

the university, and together with additional funds from the Library, eventually led to the creation of the site "**http://www.grainger.uiuc.edu/vex/toxic/toxic.htm.**"

Technical Notes

After reviewing some of the existing slides, a decision was made to use only originally produced images. By doing so, the identify of the plant is assured and the copyright concerns are eliminated. Beginning spring 1995, the plants were photographed using a Canon AV1 35mm camera and Kodakrome slide film. A digital camera was considered but not used due to poor image quality. The developed slides were scanned at 150 to 300 dpi using a high performance Kodak image processor which stored images on a Photo CD.

A most representative image of the plant is shown in 2/3 to full screen size while any additional images are first shown in thumnail with links to their full size counterparts. These plants are either commonly found in the wild in the Midwestern United States, or are common ornamental species. Typically, four different growth stages are represented.

Care was taken to maintain accuracy, overall cohesiveness and consistency. Following the university guidelines, an e-mail link to the author was added at every stage of the entry. Links to external sources are minimally used.One of them is an extensive, text-based information database developed by a researcher in Canada (**http://res.agr.ca/brd/poisonpl/**). Lacking appropriate images, the Canadian database now links to some of the images in our database. A reciprocal linking from our database to the Canadian site is planned in the future, thus making a dynamic exchange of information. The other site is located at Cornell University (**http://www.ansci.cornell.edu/plants.html**). The National Animal Poison Control Center (**http://www.cvm.uiuc.edu/napcc/napcc/html**), which is located at UIUC, is also represented.

Database

The database is made accessible by either the common name or the scientific name of the plants. Other elements of the database include description of the garden, bibliography of books used, structure of the database, and links to related sites.

Each plant entry is shown with its representative image, immediately followed by a descriptive text. At the bottom of the description are links to other images, as well as to five additional pieces of text describing distribution, condition of poisoning, control, toxic principles, and clinical signs. Treatment information is purposefully excluded to discourage animal owners from providing treatment without seeking veterinary help.

Description and distribution information is gathered from various books found in the library. The course syllabus serves as the key source of information for condition of poisoning, toxic principles, and clinical signs. The length of the text varies from plant to plant, while most entries have 3 to 4 additional images representing different growth stages.

The database made its debut in December 1995 with only four entries, each with a single plant image. Today, it contains about 50 entries. Twelve of them are complete with text information and multiple images, while many other entries are at various stages of completion. Through this database, the students have access to the basic facts about poisonous plants and what they look like at various growing stages, long after they leave the school environment. Using the database, the veterinarians can show their clients what the fruits of Japanese yew look like, compare the flowers of poison hemlock and water hemlock, and view the roots of these deadly plants which are sometimes mistaken for a parsnip. Common plants such as tulip or hyacinth are easily recognizable when in flower, but how about the bulbs of these plants?

Impact

As expected, veterinary students, at Illinois and elsewhere, found the database very useful. However, judging from the number of e-mail questions received, the impact of this database is much more widespread than anticipated. Some of these questions bring new challenges in terms of entries that need to be included. Many others are unrelated to animal poisoning but show evidence of general lack of information about poisonous plants.

Conclusion

For an experimental project, this database became much more challenging, time consuming, and interesting than ever imagined. Even though the number of entries are now nearing the goal of 60, we expect the work to continue for a while.

The diversity inherent in the subject of veterinary medicine lends itself to creating new learning materials for their clientele. Additional work in progress at UIUC Veterinary Medicine Library include: a) abbreviations and acronyms database, b) a list of currently acquired journals and other serial publications with dynamic links to content pages or full text, and c) a community-based pet information database.

At the regional level, UIUC is combining efforts with other schools in a multi-state, multi-institutional initiative called Committee on Institutional Cooperation (CIC). Among many projects is Healthweb, which addresses all aspects of medical information including veterinary medicine. The amazing ease of file transfers and home page production challenge veterinary librarians to push the present level of international cooperation to the next level, i.e., to create mutually useful reference sources. With the increasing cooperation among veterinary librarians through VETLIB-L, members of European Veterinary Libraries Group and those of Medical Library Association/Veterinary Medical Libraries Section can indeed combine efforts to make tangible contributions to the field. Such effort will, in turn, strengthen and nurture us in our profession as animal health information specialists.

Reference

[1] Stoll C. Silicon snake oil: second thoughts on the information highway. New York: Anchor Books, 1995

THE AIDA PROJECT AND DOCUMENT DELIVERY IN ITALY

Valentina Comba, Biblioteca Centralizzata di Medicine, Torino, Italy

The AIDA Project

AIDA (Alternatives for International Document Availability) is an EC Project in the framework of the Second Action Plan for Libraries: its aim is to overcome organizational and financial difficulties related to interlibrary loans (ILL) and document delivery in the participating countries, Italy and Portugal. Many libraries in Italy are buying documents and asking for ILLs abroad but have difficulties in lending, providing document delivery and invoicing their services. The partners of the project are: the University of Turin, the University of Bologna, the State Library of Triest, the National Central Library of Florence, the State Library of Milan ("Braidense"), the State Library of Venice ("Marciana"), in Italy; the University of Coimbra and the National Library of Portugal, in Portugal. The INIST in France is an associate partner.

The project started in February 1994 and was concluded in May 1996.

Technical aspects

Most partners are more likely to be considered document supply centres rather than small libraries providing services to end-users. However the Project deals with both sides of the lending process, providing a software which serves the library ("Point Of Sale") asking for a ILL, and the supplying library ("Document Supply Centre"). The software adopts a client/server architecture: the computer used as server, located at the Bologna University, is an Alpha DEC 3000 and the software is a RDBMS package (Oracle 7); client requirements are a IBM or compatible PC (processor minimum INTEL 486, memory 8 Mbyte RAM, hard disk 150 MB free space, network card) and the client software is based on a combination of MS/Windows 3.1, SQL*Net and TCP/IP emulators for Windows.

The AIDA Project uses IP as a layer protocol. This means that all the layers (e.g. ILL/OSI) are transmitted on the network over IP which is the transport protocol to be used by the upper layers such as ISO 10160/1 (InterLibrary Loan standard).

The actual software prototype in use among some Italian and Portuguese libraries allows to exchange messages (ILLs) and to monitor ILLs. The cost of the services, based on a list of fees, can be calculated.

S. Bakker (ed.), Health Information Management: What Strategies?, 129-131.

What ought to be done...

Since the Project was first conceived, there have been major advances in telecommunications, software and services. In the meantime, there have been other EC Projects, some of which connected with AIDA, such as COPIN. Electronic documents, electronic journals are becoming widely available and therefore it is particularly important to define strategies and set fees for electronic document delivery. The Universities of Turin and Bologna are making a joint effort to upgrade library services in order to provide electronic documents as well as paper ones.

Our joint work in the project has been useful when discussing fee-based services with the National Libraries. In Italy Universities have become self managed bodies: they can sell services and invoice users or other Institutions. State Libraries still depend upon the Ministry of Culture which controls incoming revenues and general expenditures. As a result, Universities can bill their end-users and pay any document supplier but State Libraries cannot bill the ILL services they provide.

Medical Libraries and current needs

Nearly all Italian Medical Libraries (IML) are not State run nor they operate under the Government's administration. Moreover, IMLs can benefit from the AIDA network model, based upon the exchange of services between large and small libraries and not a central (or National) Document Supply Centre.

A short questionnaire (annexe 1) was sent to some active IMLs to analyse current needs improving document delivery to their end-users and to other medical libraries. The questionnaire was faxed to 26 libraries, selected among 798 listed in Italian Biomedical Libraries Directory and the List of Libraries of GIDIF, RBM Union Catalog. All of them provide document delivery service to other libraries or Institutions. Seventeen filled in the questionnaire: 5 from Pharmaceutical Companies, 6 from Hospitals, 5 from Universities, 1 from a Research Institute. Most of them had requested more than 1,000 articles from other Document Supply Centres in 1995. Ranking the Suppliers, the first was considered the Union Catalog and its shared services, the Universities Libraries were the second provider; the British Library, Hospital Libraries and other sources, such as the headquarters of pharmaceutical companies, ranked third. Articles accounted for a large part of expenditure, most declaring 1 to 25 million It. Lire a year. Most IMLs requested fees. Delivery of documents and the requests balanced out and 13 libraries delivered more than 500 articles a year. Some respondents suggested making an effort to upgrade the Italian Union Catalog for a higher quality Italian Union Catalog; others felt copyright problems had to be solved.

Clearly the document delivery service is a very important feature of the IMLs. I believe the flow is increasing despite the fee-charging trend. This is why the AIDA software would be very useful to send the requests and control the processing of the ILL or document delivery. AIDA would also be appreciated by medical libraries having to manage their finances and an invoicing system to cash fees such as cash, postal orders, bank cheques, UNESCO coupons, STAMPS! etc.. One of AIDA's possible developments could be to manage the delivery of electronic documents: this is why it may be very useful to medical libraries in the future.

Beyond paper journals. Conclusions

One of the most important trends of the current literature is the increased circulation of electronic journals. Most biomedical publishers are still offering the subscribers to the paper edition free access to their electronic version. The discussion on copyright is very lively, "free Medline" being a good example. However the current opinion is that the "free access" to documents and databases is just a passing phase of the "Internet explosion" and publishers will soon close access to valuable documents and information or, more probably, they will provide access to both information and documents as a combined service, accessible to subscribers on the Net.

We therefore expect document delivery to change: medical libraries will not only organize the retrieval services of copies, be they electronic, paper or other, but also the delivery of electronic journals on the LANs of Institutions, Hospitals, University Campuses and so forth. Electronic "back" issues and storage of full text electronic journals will have to be organized as well. An appealing challenge awaits us: to be in the network and to provide networked document delivery service.

Annexe 1

QUESTIONNAIRE

1. How many articles did you request from other libraries or DSC in the 1995?

2. Rank your most important Suppliers:
   - British Library
   - INIST
   - Libraries cooperating in a Union Catalog
   - Universities
   - Hospitals
   - Pharmaceutical Companies
   - Research Institutes
   - Others ____________________

3. Indicate your 1995 article requests expenditure.

4. Is your library/information centre supplying documents to other libraries/centres?

5. How many articles did you send?

6. Are you charging a fee?

7. If so, please send us your price list.

8. Please, list what you consider to be the main problems.

L'IMPORTANCE DU PROJET AIDA DANS LE TRANSFERT DE L'INFORMATION MEDICALE

Lúcia Veloso, Biblioteca Geral da Universidade de Coimbra, Portugal

Le projet AIDA et les difficultés de la participation Portugaise

La présentation de l'AIDA (Alternatives for International Documents Availability) au Portugal n'as pas obtenu un grand succès auprès des bibliothèques, parce qu'il ne présentait pas un besoin prioritaire pour les bibliothèques portugaises

Au moment où le projet a été présenté, le Catalogue Collectif National - PORBASE - n'était disponible en ligne que dans très peu de bibliothèques; le réseau académique - RCCN - qui devrait lier toutes les institutions scientifiques nationales, n'avait pas inclus, dans sa première phase, la plupart des bibliothèques universitaires qui n'ont pas, encore aujourd'hui, des infrastructures de communication!

L'automatisation des bibliothèques portugaises a commencé en 1986, avec un projet de la Bibliothèque Nationale qui a développé un programme de gestion bibliographique sur Mini-Micro CDS/ISIS (on prépare à ce moment la version 5.0 pour windows). Les raisons de son succès resident dans son utilisation facile par les petites bibliothèques isolées (un équipement très simple a été distribué aux premiers participants), dans la formation intensive faite au personnel des bibliothèques et dans la collaboration de toutes les institutions, même celles qui avaient d'autres projets en cours.

La PORBASE est disponible en ligne, par le protocole X.25 du réseau public (Télépac) et récemment par le protocole TCP/IP qui permet l'accès à l'Internet. De toute façon les bibliothèques ne communiquent pas entre elles: le programme CDS/ISIS n'est pas intégré et ne permet pas de cataloguer en ligne. Les liaisons pour la recherche en ligne sont très coûteuses pour les budgets de la plupart des bibliothèques.

Heureusement, la situation des bibliothèques commence à changer au Portugal, et il faut que les ressources financières et humaines soient appliquées à ces priorités.

L'intégration du Projet AIDA dans un projet national de prêts interbibliothèques, était une bonne manière d'attire les bibliothèques portugaises, surtout les bibliothèques universitaires, pour leur participation à l'AIDA. En effet, il répondait à une préoccupation qui était à solutionner, même sans les sources informatiques que l'AIDA pourrait apporter: la possibilité de donner un apport informatique au travail de prêts interbibliothèques qui pèse sur les services sans structures. Afin d'engager la participation d'autres bibliothèques, les contacts devraient tenir compte aussi de la Bibliothèque Nationale, responsable du Catalogue Collectif National (le seul moyen informatisé de localisation des documents, surtout de la bibliographie nationale), et,

S. Bakker (ed.), Health Information Management: What Strategies?, 132-137.

par imposition légale, centre national de prêt pour la bibliographie nationale. La participation d'autres partenaires qui puissent apporter au projet d'autres fonds documentaires, surtout de la bibliographie spécialisée étrangère, support de la recherche scientifique et technique, était un objectif qui, malheureusement, n'a pas obtenu de succès.

La participation des Services de Documentation et Publications de l'Université de Lisbonne et de la Bibliothèque Universitaire João Paulo II de l'Université Catholique de Lisbonne, comme partenaires associés, a quand même élargi nos frontières dans le domaine de la documentation étrangère des sciences économiques et sociales.

C'est pourquoi le projet AIDA a besoin de vous pour être utile aux sciences médicales où l'importance d'obtenir les documents rapidement et au meileur prix est parfois vitale dans le "strictu sensus" du terme!

Etat du projet au Portugal

LE DÉVELOPPEMENT DU TRAVAIL

L'AIDA est le résultat d'un travail planifié en plusieurs étapes, commencé par une analyse de la situation du prêts dans les pays participants: cette analyse prétendait à travers la lecture des données statistiques rendre plus évident le rôle que les prêts interbibliothèques jouent dans l'activité du travail des bibliothèques de chaque pays et dans le plan national d'accès aux documents.

L'absence d'un système centralisé et d'une politique concertée entre les divers acteurs du prêt interbibliothèques, ayant comme conséquence une grande variété des procédés, une mauvaise qualité des services en ce qui concerne le délai de fourniture et la localisation des documents, par manque de personnel et d'ouvrages de référence, ont créé une dépendance aux services internationaux dont les coûts commencent à être trop lourds. D'un autre côté, la documentation disponible dans chaque bibliothèque n'est utilisée que par quelques dizaines d'utilisateurs ne justifiant pas, la plupart du temps, son coût. Cette situation, semblable dans les deux pays, a été une des meilleures justifications du projet et qui devrait être suffisante pour créer les motivations qui manquaient au début. Cette analyse a eu aussi une très grande importance dans la prévision future de la valorisation du service de prêts interbibliothèques en volume de transactions et de type de services à rendre, en résultats du produit obtenu.

Le questionnaire sur le besoins du marché de l'IDS (Interlibrary Document Supply) et la valorisation que le Projet pourrait apporter aux utilisateurs potentiels, a présenté le prêt interbibliothèque comme une activité secondaire par rapport à la majorité des services de bibliothèques, bien qu'elle ait tendance à augmenter. N'ayant pas de statistiques fiables relatives au mouvement national des fournitures de documents sous la forme de photocopies ou autres, nous avons été forcés à tirer des conclusions de l'analyse de croissance de ce service chez les quatre partenaires portugais.

On a estimé une croissance relative à la fourniture de documentation de 34% à l'intérieur du pays et de 80% pour l'étrange. Les demandes de documentation pourraient présenter une croissance de 23% dans le pays et de 80% pour l'étranger. Pour que le développement du projet soit valorisé, on avait aussi une claire notion des difficultés qu'il faudrait résoudre:

Le développement des services existants:
- un accès meileur et plus rapide aux bases de données
- la réorganisation des services locaux (planification et rationalisation)
- l'activation de nouveaux supports et moyens de tranfert de l'information
- la promotion d'échanges avec d'autres pays
- l'amélioration du type d'utilisateur en ce qui concerne ses exigences et ses besoins en information
- la disponibilité de l'information sur la bibliographie portugaise

Le développement eventuel de nouvelles structures d'information et de services de prêts:
- les services de reférence
- la planification nationale du prêt interbibliothèques
- la connaissance des ressources nationales existantes
- le partage d'une politique d'acquisitions.

En effet, au Portugal, le développement de l'accès à l'information n'est pas accompagné par la facilité de localisation et l'accès aux documents, malgré la contribution importante que la Base Nationale de Donnés Bibliographiques - PORBASE - a apporté à la recherche des documents existants au pays. Les investissements effectués dans le domaine du transfert de documents et dans la production de bases de données en texte intégral ne sont pas encore à la portée de toutes les bibliothèques, ils ne couvrent pas tous les besoins existants et ne s'adaptent pas à tous les documents. Obtenir le document dont on a besoin n'est pas une tâche facile si la source d'information utilisée ne donne pas la localisation du document, ce qui arrive dans la plupart des bases de données commerciales. Donc, la recherche des documents doit être une des fonctions primordiales d'un service de prêt interbibliothèques, exigeant la connaissance des sources de références pour identifier et localiser les divers types de documents. Les services de références peuvent fonctionner dans les bibliothèques ou s'organiser en unités centralisées qui aient l'objectif de prêter leur appui aux bibliothèques qui n'ont pas les moyens nécessaires pour remplir ce rôle.

Il y a, cependant, des conditions préalables pour améliorer l'accès aux documents au niveau national:
1) l'investissement dans une politique d'acquisitions partagée qui ait comme objectif de remplir les besoins d'information nationaux dans tous les domaines;
2) promouvoir les services de références existants, élargissant leurs objectifs, bénéficiant de leurs collections de référence importantes et de l'expérience de leur personnel;
3) être attentifs aux besoins des infrastructures de communication entre services bibliographiques dans les priorités d'acquisitions de services.

Ces conditions sont indispensables au point de vue de la gestion des sources bibliographiques nationales et au point de vue de la promotion de nouvelles structures de développement regional et local, comme les universités.

L'idée d'associer la culture et l'information à un produit qui doit attirer des clients, justifie cette préocupation, surtout dans les pays qui, comme le nôtre, est plutôt client que vendeur, adoptant des solutions coopératives entre des bibliothèques d'un même pays, et même des bibliothèques de pays différents, pour faire face aux grands producteurs. Les prêts interbibliothèques sont des services qui pourraient remplir ce rôle important de coopération.

La définition des fonctions et des sujets de l'IDS. On définit clairement les fonctions, les sujets, les conditions, les produits à fournir, les soutiens, les emprunteurs, les fournisseurs, les utilisateurs de chacun des deux pays, les normes d'enregistrement et de communication de données et finalement les liaisons qu'il fallait établir entre ces divers intervenants.

A partir de cette definition on a construit une structure qui a abouti à l'architecture du système (le rôle fonctionnel de chaque unité, la définition des routines - séquence de fonctions à accomplir dans chaque phase, le réseau de communications à établir entre partenaires, les conditions commerciales de chacun d'eux, etc).

L'objectif était de créer un software de gestion télématique du prêt qui puisse servir de modèle à d'autres réseaux, donc d'utiliser des solutions simples et normalisées, appliquées à un groupe de participants de structure très complexe avec des solutions informatiques très variées.

LE PRODUIT OBTENU

Les tests effectués pour vérifier le fonctionnement du software de l'AIDA ont dû être faits dans un contexte fictif.

Lors des premièrs tests du software effectués de Bologne (vu les difficultés existantes au Portugal et la date finale du projet) les communications aves les partenaires portugais et étrangers ne marchaient pas. Donc, nous avons dû exiger, d'une manière ferme que le software du Centre Service - installé seulement à Bologne - puisse être aussi disponible au Centre Informatique de l'Université de Coimbra, comme c'était d'ailleurs prévu dans le projet, pour définir le réseau portugais, et effectuer les tests avec succès.

Les tests ont été effectués, pendant une semaine, d'une manière intensive. Les quatre partenaires portugais de la base centrale, leurs conditions de prêt et leurs opérateurs ont été définis à Coimbra. Quand ce travail a été effectué et les liaisons testées, on a élaboré un plan d'exécution où les transactions considérées indispensables ont été prévues pour tester le réseau et le software, ayant pris en considération les fonctions de chaque partenaire et leurs possibilités d'exécution, adoptant les produits disponibles, les types de supports et d'envoi.

On a alors établi un schéma pour définir la politique de prêt entre plusieurs sujets de différentes dépendances administratives et ayant différentes conceptions de la politique de prêt. On les a groupés en Groupes d'Affinité ou Groupes Génériques selon que les conditions de prêt (politiques et commerciales) étaient spéciales ou génerales. Dans le schéma prototype on a distingué deux groupes avec des conditions privilégies: les Universités Portugaises (Coimbra, Lisbonne) qui échangeront leurs documents gratuitement. Les participants au projet (Bibliothèque Nationale et les autres partenaires italiens) auront des conditions plus avantageuses que les autres, les clients, partagés entre clients nationaux et clients étrangers avec différentes conditions de prêt et commerciales.

Le résultat des tests nous a permis observer que les communications étaient actives, bien que limitées par les conditions du réseau, entre les bases clients et la base centrale et que le software, malgré certaines contraintes, était facile à installer et à manipuler.

Le futur de l'AIDA

LES POTENTIALITÉS EXISTANTES

Le fournisseur versus client. Un des grands avantages de l'AIDA est la possibilité de chaque partennaire de pouvoir remplir dans le système soit le rôle de Fournisseur soit celui de Client, faisant directement ses demandes, sans avoir besoin de recourir à un intermédiaire. La gestion du prêt est faite à partir du Centre de Service qui peut être situé de l'autre côté du pays. La participation au réseau peut être autorisée sous des conditions établies par le Centre de Service qui doit définir le nom du nouveau participant, son rôle à l'intérieur du système, les produits qu'il peut ajouter, les conditions de fourniture, les moyens de paiement, etc.

Les demandes en liste publique. La demande peut être envoyée à un fournisseur hors du réseau, en choisissant l'option «mettre dans la liste publique» C'est cet aspect qui apporte une nouveauté au produit relatif aux modules intégrés dans un système propriétaire. La communication peut être ainsi établie avec tout ceux qui utilisent les mêmes protocoles.

Le système AIDA/CLIENT est très peu exigent au point de vu de l'équipement informatique

Les besoins d'équipement informatique sont:
- IBM PC ou compatible, doué d'un processeur 80486
- 8 Mb de Ram
- 150 Mb de disc
- disque souple de 3,5" haute densité
- plaque de réseau et le correspondant software
- système opératif MS/Windows 3.1
- SQL net
- émulateur TCP/IP pour Windows

Choisir le fournisseur dans la liste des fournisseurs disponibles. Cependant, l'introduction dans la liste publique exige une décision du demandeur. Cette décision est importante pour permettre la recherche dans le pays par des moyens traditionnels (catalogues imprimés, catalogues non disponibles en ligne, etc.) pour profiter des sources existantes dans chaque pays et simultanément, tester et exercer la capacité de réponse des petits centres et bibliothèques moins encombrés de demandes que les grands centres de prêts! Le participant au réseau AIDA peut aussi suggérer son entrée dans la liste des fournisseurs s'il considère qu'il a une documentation spécialisée qui peut être consultée localement et offerte aux autres participants.

LES DÉVELOPPEMENTS FUTURS

Pendant la présentation et discussion du software de gestion del'AIDA, le Centro Interfacultá per le Biblioteche della Universitá di Bologna et la Biblioteca Centralizzata di Medicina e Chirurgia della Universitá di Torino, ont présenté plusieurs suggestions pour améliorer leur capacité d'intégration et communication avec d'autres systèmes. Ces suggestions ont figuré dans le document final du projet (d.6. Wp4.3, 10 Oct 1994) «Synthesis of approuved system and network specifications»:

Au point de vue de la *fonctionalité*:
a) Intégration dans les OPACs des bases nationaux de chacun des pays (SBN en Italie, PORBASE au Portugal);
b) Intégration de l'AIDA dans les solutions locales;

c) Intégration dans l'AIDA des fonctionalités du «server» WWW afin de permettre l'utilisation de leurs potentialités, comme la recherche de l'information en ligne et le transfer electronique des documents;
d) Intégration du prêt ILL avec le prêt interne de chaque service afin d'éviter l'utilisation de deux systèmes séparés.

Au point de vue des *solutions informatiques*:
a) Prévoir une architecture moins centralisée, ayant la possibilité d'installer des unités plus petites et autonomes du système central;
b) Permettre l'accès à partir d'un terminal, permettant à l'utilisateur final le dialogue direct avec le système;
c) Permettre une meilleure compatibilité du software avec d'autres systèmes (MS/Windows, Unix, Macintosh).

Ces développements exigent de la part du Consortium un investissement qui, pour le moment, doit être séparé en Italie et au Portugal. Ainsi, on a considéré que l'exploitation du produit et les développements devraient faire objet d'un projet indépendent de celui-ci et sous la responsabilité de chacun des pays.

Les développements du software et l'exploitation du produit obtenu ont été définis dans le document «Disseminations and exploitation plan of AIDA Project in Portugal: some proposals». Dans ce document on présente deux plans de développement futur:

1- Le groupe de la PORBASE, constitué par la Bibliothèque Nationale et les bibliothèques nommées «Participants de la PORBASE» qui font la gestion de leurs fonds documentaires à partir du programme PORBASE sur Mini-Micro CDS/ISIS. Pour ce groupe la Bibliothèque Nationale développera quelques adaptations de l'AIDA au module de prêt du programme et fera son exploitation dans ce groupe;

2- Le groupe des bibliothèques universitaires qui intégrera l'AIDA dans les OPACs et dans les modules de prêt des systèmes locaux. Ce développement pourra être objet d'un projet coopératif entre les bibliothèques qui ont le même système. Le produit sera disponible aux autres bibliothèques.

Ces deux solutions prétendent être complémentaires, ayant de fortes possibilités de couvrir un vaste nombre de bibliothèques dans tout le pays.

Ceci pourra être réalisées lorsque les conditions s'utilisation de l'AIDA seront atteintes. Il faut attendre que la situation des bibliothèques évolue dans les prochaines années et que le produit soit amélioré pour que le projet puisse avoir une diffusion et une utilisation généralisée. Je pense qu'il faut avant tout croire au produit et surtout promovoir sa propagation parmi les bibliothécaires et signaler ses réelles possibilités d'adaptation aux différents degrés de développement des bibliothèques portugaises.

Bibliographie

Commission of European Communities. DGXIII, Telecommunications, information market and exploitation of research. Telematic systems in areas of general interest. Area 5: libraries programm. Project: LIB-AIDA/3-2036: Alternatives for International Document Availability (AIDA) - Contract. Luxembourg, 15.XII.1993

LIB-AIDA/3-2036- Alternatives for International Document Availability. D.5.4.2 - AIDA e World-Wilde Web / osservazioni CIB e Torino. Roma, Sept, 1994

LIB- AIDA/3-2036- Alternatives for International Document Availability. D.6.WP4.3 Synthesis of approuved system and network specifications: version: final. prepared by STUDIO STAFF. Rome, 10 October 1994

LE SERVICE FOURNITURE DE DOCUMENTS À LA BIBLIOTHÈQUE DE L'INSTITUT PASTEUR DE PARIS

Emmanuelle Jannès-Ober, Institut Pasteur, Paris, France

Abstract

The document delivery division of the library of Paris Institut Pasteur has first been established in answer to the needs of its scientists. Progessively, the division has turned to other french research institutions working in microbiology and related fields. Since 1994, the management of the division has been thoroughly reorganised in order to fulfill its new commitments: automatization with Excel and Word softwares, specialization of the staff, use of new tools for information searching, diversification of our suppliers and ways of order. To face the development of its actions, the document delivery division is now working on new projects: a Web server will be put into service on the internet network (access to the catalogue and to the document delivery function for all our clients). In the next future, we could editing order forms directly from the databases management software and also adding full text to our databases network.

Introduction

Le service fourniture de documents de la bibliothèque de l'Institut Pasteur de Paris a été conçu pour répondre aux besoins des chercheurs de l'institut. Progressivement, la bibliothèque est devenue un fournisseur du réseau national de prêt entre bibliothèques. Sur les 1000 traitements mensuels du service fourniture de documents, la moitié correspondent à des demandes des chercheurs de l'Institut Pasteur et l'autre moitié à des commandes de clients extérieurs. Pour faire face à ses nouvelles missions et à l'accroissement du volume de ses activités, le service fourniture de documents a été entièrement réorganisé; passant d'une gestion manuelle à une gestion informatisée.

Organisation actuelle du service: ressources humaines et équipement

Huit personnes sur seize participent aux activités du service mais aucune ne consacre la totalité de son temps à la fourniture de documents. Depuis 1994, le personnel a suivi une formation interne en micro-informatique (initiation au traitement de texte et au tableur), à l'interrogation des bases de données sur CD-ROM et aux commandes en ligne par internet. Les logiciels utilisés sont actuellement Microsoft Excel et Word

S. Bakker (ed.), Health Information Management: What Strategies?, 138-140.

pour la saisie des commandes et l'édition des bons de commandes auprès des fournisseurs extérieurs. Parmi les apports de cette organisation nous noterons: un meilleur suivi des commandes passées auprès des fournisseurs, une gestion rationnelle des commandes de nos clients extérieurs, ainsi que la réalisation de statistiques permettant de mesurer les activités du service et donc de les faire évoluer. Par contre, les limites d'un tel système peuvent être pénalisantes: la saisie des données est peu fiable (champs non contrôlés), ce qui limite les possibilités de développement des statistiques. En outre, il n'existe pas de lien direct avec les autres applications informatiques de la bibliothèque. Pour ces raisons, la gestion actuelle à l'aide d'Excel et de Word ne représente qu'une simple étape de l'automatisation du service fourniture de documents.

Par ailleurs, le service dispose, pour la recherche d'information, des outils suivants: 9 répertoires sur CD-ROM, de nombreuses bases de données bibliographiques dont trois sont diffusées en interne à travers le réseau informatique de l'Institut Pasteur (Medline, Current Contents et Biosis), les autres sont consultables en monoposte ou en ligne (abonnement à 4 serveurs commerciaux).

Aperçu des activités du service

Le potentiel de fournisseurs est énorme: l'ensemble des membres du réseau français du Catalogue Collectif National, soit environ 3000 bibliothèques et centres de documentation. Mais les fournisseurs réguliers sont peu nombreux: 6 fournisseurs principaux (dont 5 à Paris et 1 à l'étranger) traitent les trois quarts des demandes. Concernant la nature des documents demandés, 99% correspondent à des photocopies de périodiques. Si l'on regarde le nombre d'articles commandés à des fournisseurs extérieurs, par titre de périodique, on constate que chaque titre correspond au maximum à 2 demandes par an: seuls 3% des titres ont donné lieu à un nombre plus élevé de demandes et ont abouti à une proposition d'abonnement pour les années à venir.

Le profil des nos clients extérieurs est très particulier puisque l'essentiel appartient au réseau I.P. (les Instituts Pasteur d'Outre-mer et instituts associés, les autres Instituts Pasteur et Instituts Mérieux de France). Parmi les clients extérieurs hors réseau, l'Institut National de l'Information Scientifique et Technique représente près de la moitié.

La transmission des commandes auprès de nos fournisseurs s'effectue encore essentiellement par télécopie ou par courrier; les commandes en ligne étant réservées aux fournisseurs occasionnels (afin d'éviter la double saisie). Nos clients extérieurs envoient leurs commandes par courrier ou par fax, seuls les chercheurs de l'Institut Pasteur peuvent passer leurs commandes en intranet via le serveur Web (**http://www.pasteur.fr**). Le mode de livraison des photocopies reste majoritairement le courrier.

Le délais de traitement des commandes de notre clientèle extérieure est de 24 heures (non compris les délais postaux). La plupart des commandes qui ne sont pas honorées (42%) correspondent à des demandes relatives à des collections que la bibliothèque ne possède pas; 38% concernent des numéros récents, non encore reçus, de nos collections.

Perspectives d'évolution. Depuis 1996, la bibliothèque de l'Institut Pasteur est pôle associé de la Bibliothèque Nationale de France; depuis septembre, notre catalogue est diffusé sur internet. Cette ouverture vers l'extérieur devrait aboutir à un accroissement important des demandes au cours des prochaines années. Pour faire face à l'augmentation prévisible de ses activités, la bibliothèque est en train de mettre en place de nouveaux outils de gestion informatique et développe de nouveaux produits et services. D'une part, les clients extérieurs pourront prochainement passer leurs commandes de documents par internet. Pour les lecteurs internes, le système de gestion des bases de données bibliographiques en réseau (Ovid) permettra, dans l'avenir, d'intégrer un module de commandes de documents auprès de la bibliothèque (version futures d'OvidWeb Gateway). Pour la gestion interne du service, le développement d'une nouvelle application est en cours: à partir de 1997, un module spécifique pour les opérations de traitement du service sera intégré au logiciel de gestion de bibliothèque Doris/Loris, utilisé depuis 1994 dans notre bibliothèque. Cette dernière application permettra une saisie contrôlée des commandes, l'édition automatique des bons de commandes (fournisseurs) et des factures pro forma (clients extérieurs), ainsi qu'un suivi systématique des relances et des litiges.

Par ailleurs, de nouveaux services sont en cours de mise en place: accès par internet aux revues pour la fourniture d'articles avant parution, de résumés ou de sommaires; reproduction d'articles à partir de nos revues disponibles sur CD-ROM (2 titres actuellement), ce qui servira de test en vue de l'introduction possible du texte intégral à notre réseau de bases de données bibliographiques.

Conclusion

Les perspectives d'accroissement des activités du service fourniture de documents de la bibliothèque de l'Institut Pasteur nécessitent une constante adaptation des outils de gestion et du personnel. Les solutions informatiques choisies sont donc déterminées par un triple objectif: la nécessaire complémentarité avec les solutions existantes, le développement de l'intranet très apprécié par les chercheurs de notre Institut, tout en ouvrant plus largement nos services au public extérieur.

INTERLIBRARY LENDING AND ELECTRONIC COMMUNICATION

Friedhelm Rump, Veterinary School of Hannover, Germany

Introduction

The Library of the Veterinary School of Hannover has all library functions automated and is part of a major regional library network. With the access to Internet and especially the World Wide Web it has become easy to locate holdings not only on the national but even the international level.

Consequently time is saved in the placing of ILL-requests. But in many cases the process is being slowed down again by making use of electronic transmission. ILL-requests submitted by e-mail or fax reach executives' desks and get delayed there, simply because the person may be on a business trip or a meeting etc. Also it is not always clear, whether electronic transmission is chosen, because requests are urgent or just because a convenient link from the holdings interface was inviting. Requests to discussion lists, such as **VETLIB-L**, will in the majority of cases be served in reasonable or very short time. There are cases, however, where holdings are few, and where no statement concerning the coverage of costs is made by the requesting library. In these cases it may happen that the request gets delayed considerably or is even neglected, if the library, which would be able to fill it, is not in the position to deliver for example photocopies free of charge.

The real obstacle to rapid supply of articles is the lack of technical equipment to make these machine-readable spontaneously and transmit them subsequently in most libraries with otherwise satisfactory electronic support. It may be objected that telefax transmission has sped up conveyance considerably. This is unquestioned, but the quality of received facsimiles frequently betray the name. File transfer is the magic term in many a librarian's ears. The relevant protocols exist and workstations to employ them are being installed in more and more libraries.

Given the proper technical basis an ILL-system still may not work the way librarians and users would want to see it. It all needs a framework to channel information and requests as well as a graded description of conditions under which it may be used.

Veterinary interlibrary lending

In the field of Veterinary Sciences ideally a group of about eighty libraries would be sharing resources. A union list of serials of all these libraries in machine-readable

S. Bakker (ed.), Health Information Management: What Strategies?, 141-143.

format is highly desirable. About half of the optional number are participating in this project at present. A good number of European libraries are likely to join in 1996, which will make the number of participants approach 50. With so many libraries' holdings in a single specialised field there will undoubtedly be a large portion of titles possessed by nearly each of them, whereas others may only be found in a few or even just one. The two extremes will pose no problems, the situation, in which there are for example four libraries scattered around the globe hold a title, would cause confusion about where to direct an order and be served the most effective.

REGIONAL SERVICES

To get the most effective service it seems necessary to have preferences about the delivery of each title in the union list, so it will become clear for a library at location A that an order for an article from specific journal B should be sent to library C, if the ILL can be done in Europe for example, and that library D wanting an article from journal E would contact library F in North America and so on. The following table will illustrate this:

Title of Journal	Possessing library	Requesting library	ILL path
Journal of XXX	Univ. of Missouri	Vet School Hann.	
Journal of XXX	Univ. of Pretoria		
Journal of XXX	Univ. of Utrecht		
Journal of XXX	Vet. Univ. Vienna		X

Here it is assumed that the Library of the Veterinary University of Vienna was chosen or volunteered to serve requests inside Europe for articles from this particular journal. It is of no relevance in this model that the University Library of Utrecht is closer to Hannover. The ILL path is a convention. Utrecht could be the library to order from in another case, where it was chosen to serve request for another specific journal. In North America it would have been the Library of the University of Missouri, and in Africa the Library of the University of Pretoria. Such assignments also require the libraries with the respective holdings to guarantee delivery under the conditions agreed upon by the proposed Vet-ILL-Network.

URGENCY

A further differentiation should be made for the levels of urgency and - implied in this - mode of conveyance. It is sometimes necessary for a patron to have an article within the next 48 hours or faster. Practical considerations make it impossible to guarantee under all circumstances a delivery in less than 48 hours although in reality most orders would be satisfied in less than half the time, provided that telefax transmission or file transfer are used. It is self-evident that a request sent by surfacemail from overseas could not fall into this category. A medium time of delivery, which does not require the librarian in charge to rush for the document immediately upon receipt of the request, but makes use of electronic transmission, may also be wanted. More likely for not highly urgent requests is, what can be called the regular case, in which an article is delivered in reasonable time, 7 to 14 days. Here the distinction would have to be made for surface- or airmail, depending on the distance the document would have to travel.

The combination of aspects of region and urgency / mode of conveyance results in a number of different conditions, which require different actions and different costs. The categories given above are mere suggestions. They would have to be discussed on a broader level, but in principle a Vet-ILL-Network would arrive at some similar set of categories.

COSTS

As ILL will increase with the Vet-ILL-Network of the described structure, it will not be possible to have requests filled free of charge, as is done in most cases over the VETLIB-L nowadays by courtesy of librarians, because these requests are for the exceptional cases and it is assumed that serving and requesting will even out in the end. For a routine of such ILL, however, it would be optional for the participating libraries to agree on uniform terms regarding charges for delivery. If this cannot be accomplished, at least the charges should be made known on the union list. They would have to reflect the different categories outlined above as well as to cover expenses. These may be the following:

	regular, surface mail	regular, airmail	medium urgency	maximum urgency
continental				
intercontinental				

The blanks may be filled with the appropriate charges, which would have to be agreed upon.

Conclusion

The proposed Vet-ILL-Network, which would only be a logical development out of the union list of serials, would give interlibrary lending or rather document supply in the veterinary sciences a greater amount of certainty and reliability. It would be a great but also necessary step from union cataloguing.

ARIEL: INTERLIBRARY DOCUMENT DELIVERY ON THE INTERNET

Marc Walckiers, Université catholique de Louvain, Belgium

The origin of Ariel

The context of interlibrary document delivery is well known:
- the purchasing power of libraries is steadily falling, local resources are shrinking, more and more remote resources are used;
- new information and telecommunication technologies offer wonderful possibilities for information transfer, but librarians have to take care of their appropriate implementation for a better service to end users; at the time that bibliographic data are easily found on the web throughout the world, it is odd to see libraries sending each other millions of photocopies by ordinary mail.

In this context the Research Libraries Group (RLG, consortium of the main American academic libraries) developed a software working on off-the-shelf hardware for interlibrary document delivery on the Internet. The software was named ARIEL, as the servant of Prospero in Shakespeare's The Tempest, because, according to the words of this famous author: *"Ariel delivers as fast and faithfully as his master requires"*.

ARIEL was written for scanning, handling and printing documents and was released at the end of 1991; in 1994 replaced by a much better performing and more user friendly version: Ariel for Windows.

Functions

The document pages of original publications (bound or unbound) are scanned one by one, the document image is digitalized, compressed and temporarily stored in the PC until it is sent through Internet to the PC of the requesting library. After scanning, the process is completely computerized, including:
- automatic connection between both ARIEL workstations,
- up to 28 attempts per day for connection,
- transmission error detection and resend procedure,
- automatic printing by the ARIEL receiving workstation.

Equipment needed for ARIEL:

The appropriate workstation is a 486 PC with:
- 50 to 100 MB free on hard disk,
- an Internet connection,
- a scanner (usually HP),
- a laser printer working with 300 x 300 dots per inch.

S. Bakker (ed.), Health Information Management: What Strategies?, 144-148.

The scanning of articles is slightly slower than the photocopying: according to the recent LAMDA experience with 12.000 scanned articles, scanning one page takes 8 seconds on a HP scanner or 4 seconds on a more expensive Fujitsu scanner.

As ARIEL produces a bit-mapped image of the documents, it perfectly handles all kinds of graphic documents with all types of characters, drawings, photographs, etc. Thanks to the "dither" function, ARIEL handles and restitutes half-tones better than photocopy machines and ensures a better quality of reproduction; there is of course no comparison with the very poor reproduction by fax.

The receiving ARIEL workstation can also resent the document to another ARIEL workstation, e.g. in departmental libraries near the end user, which fastens the delivery to end users. The ARIEL workstations can simultaneously scan, send, receive and print documents. Low used ARIEL workstation could be used for other applications (word processing, e-mail...), but this is not recommended for very active ARIEL workstations.

The ARIEL software does not include any ordering procedure. Although most ARIEL libraries continue using existing ILL-systems, such as union-lists with teleordering system, orders sent by mail, e-mail, fax, phone, web site, as well as by ARIEL (sanned image of request form) are accepted by many libraries.

ARIEL software produces for each document a "header page" with identification of the document, the end user, the supplier, the number of pages, date and time of printing as well as any note added by the requester or the supplier. In addition, identification of document, end user and requesting library typed by the requesting library on teleordering systems such as RLIN, Docline or Pica can be transferred to the ARIEL workstation in order to avoid retyping of such data.

Costs and advantages of ARIEL

The ARIEL software is sold by RLG and its distributors for $ 789, with discount in case of multicopies orders. The full cost for hardware and software is $ 5000 or more, but ARIEL software can work on existing hardware and the equipment can always be used for other functions.

According to an in depth study carried out by experts in several American universities and published on the RLG web site in 1996, the running costs (staff, postage/telecom., etc.) for document delivery are lowest in the case of ARIEL than in the case of fax or mail.

ARIEL compared with photocopies:
- fast delivery, most often within 24 h.,
- better reproductions, especially half tones,
- time saving for library staff:
  . scanning is slightly slower than photocopying, but
  . ARIEL avoids the handling and despatching of the photocopies with enveloppes, addresses, postage...
  . ARIEL automatically keeps files of documents requested, sent and received.

ARIEL compared with fax:
- sending as fast as fax,
- a much better reproduction on plain paper,
- very much time saving for library staff:
  . photocopies are needed for fax transmission, not so by ARIEL,
  . ARIEL connection and sending process are automatic,
- no (extra) telecommunication costs.

Future of ARIEL

The main development announced by RLG (scheduled for February 1997) is a version of ARIEL enabling all ARIEL PC to send any documents by e-mail to any end users' workstation, so that they would receive their documents on their desktop.

A further step would be a more general software not only able to perform all ARIEL functions, but also to handle all documents available on the Web and to transmit them by electronic mail on end users workstations. This new software (announced by the National Library of Medicine and named "DocView") should be available next Spring.

Scanning of printed articles is obviously anachronistic: this cumbersome scanning could be bypassed if and when it is possible to transfer articles in their original machine readable form, e.g. electronic journals currently available in SGML format or ISI electronic library. In that case the whole ARIEL process could be automated.

Use of ARIEL

As ARIEL is a cooperative system, one cannot use it alone: you need a partner able and willing to use its own ARIEL workstation jointly with you. This was all right in the USA, because ARIEL was an initiative of the Research Libraries Group, but this is less easy in other countries.

ARIEL DIRECTORY

The ARIEL Directory, available on RLG's web site, lists about 700 ARIEL users in the world including 70% in USA and Canada. Other users are spread in 24 other countries:
- 33 ARIEL users in 11 European countries (12 in Finland),
- a number of ARIEL users in Australia, southern America, and Asia (mainly Pacific states and Israel).

However, the ARIEL Directory is often misleading because:
- these registered ARIEL users own the ARIEL software, but part of them do not accept any order or do not use ARIEL,
- an important number of genuine ARIEL users did not register in this ARIEL Directory, and we can guess that there are more than 2000 ARIEL workstations worldwide: e.g. the ARIEL Directory mentions 5 ARIEL users in Israel, but there are at least 30 Israelian university libraries using ARIEL.

USE OF ARIEL IN USA

The Health Sciences Libraries Consortium in Pennsylvania and Delaware are using ARIEL for all their interlibrary document delivery, further to a two month project in 1992; in addition, thanks to a joint use of ARIEL for quick supply of missing articles, two libraries of Pennsylvania University cancelled journal subscriptions and saved in one year twice the cost of their ARIEL workstation,

The University of Michigan set up seven ARIEL workstations for the same purpose in 1992.

Between member libraries of the Boston Libraries Consortium (including Harvard and MIT) 80% of the ILL traffic consists of ARIEL reproductions, as a result of a 25 week project launched in 1993 by 10 Boston libraries.

Since 1992, CISTI, the Canadian equivalent of the Document Supply Centre of the British Library, is sending by ARIEL 80% of the documents requested by the 15 branches of the Canadian Research Council; CISTI does accept orders for ARIEL reproductions from any ARIEL users in the world and reproductions are usually delivered within 24h.

EBSCODOC, the document delivery service of EBSCO, is doing the same and very efficiently: five articles requested last Friday at 5pm from Brussels were received on the same day!

The U.S. National Library of Medicine is also offering ARIEL reproductions and redirection of orders of foreign medical libraries for ARIEL reproductions could be considered through its Docline network.

USE OF ARIEL IN ISRAEL

After a successful pilot project of joint use of ARIEL by a science library and a biomedical library in Israel, the Ministry of Education funded 25 ARIEL workstations spread in the 25 main libraries of the 7 universities in Israel; this number has grown over 30 and all the document delivery between these libraries is now done with the ARIEL software.

USE OF ARIEL IN EUROPE

The first ARIEL project in Europe was funded by NORDINFO and carried out by 17 university libraries in the 5 Nordic countries in 1993. Special teletransmissions on the Danish network prevented Danish libraries to join the project.

The quick transmission and other advantages of ARIEL raised a strong interest; but the slow scanning was seen as a real problem, especially by the main suppliers. Nevertheless, the Finnish participants kept their ARIEL workstations in use so that there are now about 20 ARIEL workstations in use in Finland, at least one in each university; the main supplier is the National Health Sciences Library in Helsinki.

Another project was launched in 1993 by PICA in 14 Dutch libraries. To date, this project is still experimental and limited to these 14 libraries, mainly central university libraries, which are sending a few ARIEL reproductions per day. They have no technical problems, but there is still a lack of will to shift from photocopying to scanning.

The most recent ARIEL project in Europe is the LAMDA project, launched in 1995 by the Manchester university libraries, the University College London, the King's College and a few other libraries in London with funding from national academic authorities. During the first 31 weeks, 12000 articles have been sent by their 27 ARIEL workstations, including 9000 articles within 24 h.

ARIEL AT THE UNIVERSITY OF LOUVAIN IN BRUSSELS

The joint use of ARIEL by the medical libraries of the University of Louvain and the University of Rotterdam started in June 1995: ARIEL reproductions were regularly received within 24 h. until October 1995 when more and more frequent connection problems happening on the Internet forced us to stop. In the Spring of 1996, other partners were easily found: the National Health Sciences Library in Helsinki, the member libraries of the LAMDA project in London, CINDOC in Madrid, CISTI in Ottawa, EBSCODOC in San Francisco. The supply of ARIEL reproductions is working perfectly within 24 h. with these partners, and several hundreds of

documents have now been exchanged from June 1995 to September 1996.
In the near future there will be:
- a second ARIEL workstation working on the main site of the University of Louvain,
- and the use of ARIEL among Belgian libraries will be promoted by the announcement of an ARIEL option on the Belgian union list of current journals.

Conclusion

For reasons of the rapid supply of documents and many other advantages for end users and library staff, there are better chances for implementing the ARIEL system in libraries than previously for fax,
- but, therefor we need:
  . a will to train and manage the library staff as required by our "hi-tech" society,
  . a stronger demand of librarians for electronic document delivery by document supply centres.

With an Internet tool as ARIEL, one should consider international cooperation rather than national cooperation, and the main reason of this paper is to ask you if European health libraries would consider to launch such a project at European level or at world level, e.g. by:
  . a union list of current journals in European medical libraries using ARIEL,
  . a connection with the Docline network of the U.S. National Library of Medicine,
  . a cooperation with health libraries in the third world.

ARIEL has been in use in my library for 15 months. Based on this experience I have presented to you this appealing tool. I have to thank all American and European colleagues who gave me valuable information on ARIEL.

References

Ariel Directory: **http://www.rlg.org/aridir.html**

Beaubien A et al. Cost-effectiveness of Ariel for Interlibrary Loan copy requests, Summary of a report to RLG, 1996 **http://www.rlg.org/arifax.html**

Bennett V, Palmer E. Electronic document delivery using the Internet. Bull Med Libr Assoc 1994;82:163-167

Berger M. Ariel Document Delivery and the Small Academic Library. Coll Undergrad Libr 1996;3(2):49-56

Braid A. Electronic Document Delivery: Vision and Reality. Libri 1994;44:224-236

Brandreth M. & MacKeigan C. Electronic Document Delivery - Towards the Virtual Library. Interlend Doc Supply 1994;22:15-17

Friend F. Electronic Document Delivery through Library Co-operation. Interlend Doc Supply 1994;22:18-21

Friend F. LAMDA: Questions and some answers. Interlend Doc Supply 1996;24:27-29

Henry N, Dell E. Technology as a tool for cooperation. Bull Med Libr Assoc 1994;82:436-438

Jackson M. Document Delivery over the Internet. Online 1993;14-21

Lamda Newsletter 1996;(1)

Mickos E. The use of Internet in document delivery - a NORDINFO project. IATUL Proceedings 1994;3:266-275

Telraz M. Sending journal articles via Ariel. Inf Libr 1995;21:40-43

COPYRIGHT AND THE PHARMACEUTICAL INDUSTRY

Elspeth J. Scott, Glaxo Wellcome plc., Greenford, Middlesex, UK

Introduction

The pharmaceutical industry may be unique in its dependence on scientific, technical and medical (STM) literature. Published information is needed at all stages of drug development and post market surveillance.

We are heavy users of copyright material but also key contributors to the literature and to the revenues of STM publishers; it is vital that the pharmaceutical industry be involved in the debate on the future of electronic copying.

The industry has been at the forefront of use of technology to manage information. Today, as so much corporate knowledge resides in electronic form, the publishers' reluctance to grant anyone permission for management of electronic rights and the price tags attached when they do, pose serious threats to the management of external information.

This paper examines the current situation regarding electronic copying from the user viewpoint, some political and economic tensions in the publishing world, ongoing initiatives aimed at resolving the current impasse and some special pharmaceutical needs.

Needs of the pharmaceutical industry

Our usage of copyright material is twofold; the research scientists' needs are similar to those in an academic environment - to read current literature, confer and discuss papers, and to alert colleagues to key advances.

The needs at the other end of the R&D process are quite different. Regulatory authorities want the full text of papers referenced in submissions. Many companies are assembling submissions electronically requiring digitisation and handling of copyright material in-house. Much of the material is not available commercially in electronic format and if it were, format and compatibility problems may arise.

Another area of special use of copyright material is in product support. We have to supply information on the use of our products to the medical profession which requires companies to maintain indexed stores of product-related papers. Both types of re-use are essential for the pursuit of our legitimate business but neither is deemed to deprive publishers of hardcopy revenues. No extra sales of journals would result from these activities which focus on single articles. There may be potential for

S. Bakker (ed.), Health Information Management: What Strategies?, 149-151.

increased revenues from digital copying in the future, but any such charges should bear a relationship to the business benefit to be derived and not simply be based on the need for publishers to make big profits.

The current levels of royalties on individual papers are a huge disincentive to both the distribution of information to legitimate seekers and the uptake of new technology.

Current situation on electronic copying

Painting a coherent picture of electronic copyright is difficult; there are many different aspects, different players and legal issues. A few issues are, however, particularly important to the pharmaceutical industry.

Copyright law varies between countries and mostly does not cover electronic copying. The general view seems to be as in the USA, that existing laws can be adapted to cover the electronic situation. Any new law would have to be globally applicable rather than nationally based reflecting the multinational nature of both information and the pharmaceutical industry. The reality is that it takes a long time to develop and implement international laws and time is not on our side. The Internet is already a reality. We have pressing business needs for information to support our products and increasingly this is being done electronically.

Contracts may supersede copyright law to resolve current problems. This is certainly worth exploring but, in reality, there are too many publishers with whom we would have to interact. An estimate is that there are around 25,000 biomedical publishers and reports on our drugs could appear in any number of possible journals. The logical answer would be a clearing house for acquiring permission to handle copyright material in electronic form. Such 'Clearing Houses' already exist in the form of Reproduction Rights Organisations (RROs) but there are real tensions in their relationships with publishers. The RROs are not a homogeneous group, varying between countries in their activities and the national laws under which they operate. The US Copyright Clearance Center appears deadlocked; publishers, unhappy with the revenue from the CCC to date, seem unwilling to mandate them to negotiate electronic copying deals with pharmaceutical industry users until guaranteed future revenues; meanwhile pharmaceutical companies are unwilling to supply publishers with statistics on usage and enter open-ended deals without knowing the financial implications.

Ongoing initiatives

For too long, publishers have been lobbying the legislators and dictating the way forward. At last, it seems that the user community is becoming more organised and vocal, and publishers are now coming to understand that their customers must be involved in the debate and may even be part of the solution.

The Conference on Fair Use (CONFU) brought together a range of US users opposed to the recommendations of the Lehman report on the National Information Infrastructure.

The European Copyright User Platform (ECUP) is funded by the European Community (DGX111/E-4) and its objectives include: *"To continue discussing library privileges in electronic services and model clauses for licences for the use of electronic information rights owners and collecting societies"* and *"To reinforce the position of libraries in discussions about copyright issues with appropriate bodies"*.

Its steering group comprises representatives from different types of libraries including academic, public and industrial.

A specific goal of ECUP valuable to the pharmaceutical industry, is to secure libraries' right to digitise and store their own holdings not already available as electronic products.

The Association of the British Pharmaceutical Industry (ABPI) has established a task force to discuss electronic copying with the Copyright Licensing Agency (UK's RRO). We have drafted a 'wish list' designed as a basis for discussion with rights owners or their agents. Its key points are:

(i) A forum for discussion with rights owners

(ii) An understanding of the pharma industry's special needs

(iii) The right to scan and use copyright material in electronic form in-house

(iv) No payment for scanning of in-house holdings but payment for use thereafter

(v) Agreement on a fair price for (iii) above (the cost must not outweigh the benefit)

(vi) Any agreement must have a multinational effect

(vii) Flexible contracts

(viii) Rapid progress towards implementation of the above

Many publishers believe that they will be able to manage their rights directly through Electronic Copyright Management Systems (ECMS) but there are many technical, financial and security issues to be resolved before ECMS become a reality.

A further problem with contracts and licences is that they are difficult to draw up, agree and maintain and can consume an enormous amount of legal and administrative resources on both sides.

The way forward

The current uncertainties and lack of opportunity for meaningful debate are impeding information flow and uptake of technology which allows a greater efficiency in information handling; this ultimately impacts all healthcare product users and merits a concerted effort by our industry to tackle electronic copyright problems.

All information managers should participate in the debate, creating a common 'wish list' for our sector on which we can negotiate the future.

The way forward may be to participate in pilots or take out trial licences but at the very least to engage the publishing community in urgent dialogue.

STORAGE & DISSEMINATION OF ELECTRONIC JOURNALS

Chris C.P. Kluiters, Elsevier Science BV, Amsterdam, Netherlands

Elsevier Electronic Subscriptions (EES) in Europe

Every library customer requires different solutions to access information. Some want the capability to access information with almost immediate response; some will live with the rather slow(er) response times associated with the Internet. Some will want the capability to integrate the information with local, in-house databases and some don't. Some have development staff available to design information system solutions and some will rely on others. In other words you will need flexibility.

EES offers you a true building block to achieve a digital library concept of a local-remote solution for journal information with simultaneous access from every desktop. In 1995 Elsevier started introducing EES into Europe. The experiences of the TULIP project, resulted in a firm belief that with the introduction of EES a next step would be made towards helping build the digital libraries of ES customers.

One of the criticisms that came out of TULIP was the relatively small number of titles (43) in relation to a library's complete collection of title holdings and the fact that only libraries from the USA were chosen. This is the reason that for EES all the 1100-1200 journal titles are included and are offered to a worldwide audience. And for each and all of the journal issues and articles (estimated at 150.000 -180.000 per year) of these journal titles, the electronic production process results in so-called DATASETS containing four components. The whole process of electronic production and delivery of EES datasets are described and published in the IFLA Journal,[2] but can be summarized as follows:

1. *Page Image files*: Every scanned page results in *one* page image file. These page images are standard black & white single page TIFF 5.0 files with a scan resolution of 300 dots per inch (dpi). The maximum size is European A4 (210 x 297 mm). The compression method is the international CCITT Fax Group IV encoding scheme;

2. *Text files*: These are the result of Optical Character Reading procedures. These text files are referred to as "raw", since no keyboarding, editing and spell-checking is performed. The files contain only ASCII characters in the range from 32 to 126. Lines are variable and are in "stream mode". The text files contain the full text of the complete article with the exception of complex structures (displayed equations, matrices, tables, chemical formulae etc.) There is *one* "raw" ASCII text file per page issue;

S. Bakker (ed.), Health Information Management: What Strategies?, 152-155.

3. *SGML-coded bibliographic file*. This file contains for every article the bibliographic data and the abstract in SGML (=Standardized General Mark-up Language) format tagged and edited. Some 30-40 field tags can possibly appear in the article "heads" such as: article; author; dates; keywords etc;

4. *DATASET.TOC. file*. This is the main entry file in which all cross indexing reference data is provided. The directory structure follows a hierarchy that directly reflects the subdivision into journals, issues and pages. Journals are identified by their International Standard Serial Number (ISSN). This DATASET.TOC file is necessary to reconstruct journal issues and editorial items contained in it.

A fifth additional available component is a PDF-"wrapper", making it possible to use ADOBE's ACROBAT reader.

In the beginning of 1997 more standards ("true" PDF, SGML) will be added to complete the spectrum of open architecture based formats. In other words EES will not be limited in terms of formats, and be continuously upgraded. Datasets are profiled for each and every individual library and distributed via CD-ROM on a regular basis to every customer for local storage on their (image)server(s).

Remote versus local storage

The possibility of storing the Elsevier electronic information on a local system has lead to discussions with new customers on the topic of remote storage vs local storage. The discussion focuses on the necessity to build local digital collections. In many discussions the topic is remote storage and access as an *opposite* strategy to local storage and access. With the emerging new electronic information service from Elsevier Science: *ScienceDirect* tm[3] available in 1997, the discussion could focus more on how EES and this new service are complementary to another. *ScienceDirect* will provide additional options for EES customers, either giving them access to titles not held on their local networks or the ability to access everything remotely.

INTEGRATION AND PERFORMANCE

EES started off in a true open system standards fashion. The above described datasets are made available to customers without any search or front-end software. The market responded, not surprisingly, in two ways.

On the one side you have the *innovators*, libraries with a clear vision on the IT future of their organisation. They supported this approach warm-heartedly. Their arguments for developing their own information systems using EES, have to do with the flexibility and usability of the datasets. In a recent article in The Scientist,[4] the Chief Librarian of the Naval Research Library in Washington D.C., Laurie E. Stackpole comments: *"EES very much parallel what publishers have done in the past with print subscriptions. Once you subscribe to the EES then you have permanent rights to retain the material you receive. So if you were to cancel a journal, you would be allowed to continue providing your users with previously received information. That's not always true when you start to get into the electronic area with some publishers and vendors"*.

The delivered files are used for both an awareness and/or table-of-content service as well as for a full text service. By integrating the information into their already available services, one could argue that at least the end-user training and support can be maintained on the same level. There is a smaller need to train end-users a new system. Also the performance level of the information system such as the efficiency of the search engine, printing facilities, and fast (LAN-) access are arguments for this storage and integration strategy. It is also possible to add other publishers material. And finally it gives them the possibility to actively pursue collection developmènt for primary journals based on actual usage via logdata-analysis. Despite the option to choose from a variety of library systems, it will not come as a surprise that many libraries now choose a WWW front-end solution.

A second group of customers is interested in a *local* solution of EES, but do no want to get involved in developing a system. In the beginning of EES we could only offer them some advice on experiences gained within the TULIP project and of the first EES implementations. Collaboration was sought with The Tilburg Innovation Center for Electronic Resources (Ticer) to offer guidance and consultancy. And although this open standards approach with maximum flexibility is still very alive, we have now also added two other, "off-the-shelf" possibilities for local integration: OCLC's SiteSearch and ScienceServer from ORION Scientific Systems. SiteSearch is being used at the University of Toronto and ScienceServer at the Tohoku University in Japan.

These two possibilities have become available on the market in Europe recently and are targeted at customers that do not want to go a route where decisions on the search software and front-end software have to be made but still want to have the performance advantages of locally stored journals.

Remote storage however will be useful for several reasons. It doesn't seem logical even with the above integration & performance reasoning, to store digitally all the back issues of science journals of a particular library in the years to come. The archiving of this material could be solved by storing this remotely and only retrieved when needed. Current and other more frequently used collections could be held locally.

A number of studies have shown that the utilisation rate of journal material is, in general, very low.[5] But it is in many cases not very clear which journal titles of a library's collection are the truly high-usage ones. We have seen, and are seeing at the EES sites exactly how often journal titles are used and for what reason (browsing Table-of-Contents, Abstracts or Full text, and Printing, Downloading). Thus EES sites have enhanced collection development tools available.

The combination of titles available via a local "store" with lower-usage titles from a remote "store" may prove to be the optimal one for the next time-period. Migrating from there to a situation where end-users know exactly where and how to get their information fast and efficient could then be a next logical step in the development of the digital library.

END-USER ACCESS TO JOURNAL INFORMATION

At this moment we see tow types of implementation with regards to the access of the journal information.

First of all there is the "hierarchy browser". The journal titles available electronically are listed alphabetically on one of the service menu pages of the library. An end-user clicks on the Journal title and finds a list of recent and/or available issues. From there you click through to an issue where you find the table-of-contents of that particular issue. Then follows the abstract and from there you click to receive the full text. Although this way of journal disclosure is very basic, it at least provides a very specific group of end-users for their basic need: to browse their most favourite and wanted journal titles whenever an issue arrives in the library. The fact that the EES license provides for simultaneous, remote and campus-wide access enhances the appreciation of such a service. (No circulation of xeroxed t-o-c pages, or journal issues that may leave the library premises). A second reason why digital libraries go for this basic functionality is a more pragmatic one. In this time of pressure from faculty and board of governors/directors to develop digital libraries and offer better performance to library users, the development of this browser is relatively easy. In other words it is fast proof that the library is active in the forefront of information/library technology. Basically all the EES sites have installed a hierarchy browser.

A *second* model for integrating EES into the library services, is the linking of the full text with "Table-of-Content databases". But instead of using the journal hierarchy, a search-engine is used to retrieve information, e.g. via boolean searching. (The abstracts of the EES datasets can be integrated into such a database, to improve the efficiency of the search results). When the search is completed one can click through to the full text when an EES journal article is found.

A logical other linking similar to this, is the integration with other local available bibliographic databases such as INSPEC.

So far there is limited experience with SDI and other profiling services. But a number of sites are working on this, which will make it possible to alert end-users of newly arrived articles of their interest.

Conclusion

The implementation of EES requires a close collaboration of everyone involved. The integration and development of new information services as well as the necessary training and education of both library staff and end-users will lead to new roles for the librarians and information specialists of digital libraries. With the first EES libraries we will exchange ideas and discuss future roles at a seminar specially devoted to all the aspects of implementing the electronic journals of EES. The fact that many of these libraries have operational experiences will make this meeting of particular importance.

References

[1] TULIP Final Report, Elsevier Science 1996, ISBN 0-444-82540-1

[2] Kluiters C. Towards electronic journal articles: the publisher's technical point of view. IFLA J 1996;22:206-208

[3] Elsevier Science Press Release August 1, 1996

[4] Scientific publishers increasing electronic information offerings. The Scientist 1996;(August 19):19-20

[5] Tuck B. Document ordering and delivery systems in Europe: projects of the European Commission, services, conditions and prices. In: Electronisches Publizieren und Bibliotheken, 1996; pp 63.

FORMATION SUR L'USAGE D'UN CENTRE DE DOCUMENTATION POUR LES OMNIPRATICIENS

Maria da Luz Antunes, Centro de Saúde de Sete Rios, Lisboa, Portugal

Abstract

The General Practice Institute of Portugal South Area, is a governmental institution, which provides the General Practitioner with specific training (and there are about 3.000 GP's in this area). The Information and Documentation Center (IDC) lends assistance and attends to the needs of the GP's and researchers in general. The Institute promotes courses concerning documental research in Information Centers and Libraries about methodology in scientific work and papers such as: a thesis, un article, a report or a bibliography. Taking into account the database, its documental contents and the information net which has been developed by the APDIS, the IDC accomplishes an invaluable work of technic research, scientific assistance and bibliographical revision.

Introduction

L'Institut de Médecine Générale de la Région Sud est une institution gouvernementale responsable de la formation spécifique des médecins généralistes (les omnipraticiens) du midi portugais. Par ailleurs, il développe une composante assez importante de recherche médicale et d'épidemiologie. Le Centre de Documentation et d'Information (CDI) doit travailler dans la même ligne institutionnelle et avec les mêmes priorités. Plus que l'utilisateur, c'est le médecin qui a besoin de nous. C'est un utilisateur exigeant, toujours en recherche d'actualisation des connaissances.

FORMATION BIBLIOGRAPHIQUE

Cependant, le CDI a développé une autre stratégie d'utilisation en consonance avec la structure institutionnelle. Dans son plan de formation, l'Institut de Médecine Générale a consacré quelques heures pour le responsable de la documentation. Celui-ci fait des présentations, initiallement théoriques mais actuellement pratiques aussi, sur la méthodologie du travail scientifique, sur la présentation finale d'un travail scientifique (à plusieurs niveaux comme, par exemple, un rapport, un protocole, un article ou même une thèse), ainsi que sur la présentation et l'organisation d'une bibliographie.

S. Bakker (ed.), Health Information Management: What Strategies?, 157-160.

On présente deux ou trois hypothèses de normes bibliographiques plus utilisées en sciences médicales, comme Vancouver et Harvard. Ensuite, le CDI exécute le travail final: la révision méthodologique et bibliographique.

UN COURS DE RECHERCHE DOCUMENTAIRE

Les objectifs: l'application d'une méthodologie de travail et la réalisation d'une recherche bibliographique.

La méthodologie pédagogique appliquée:

1. La méthodologie en recherche:

- Comment choisir le sujet de la recherche?: Vérifier l'inclination personnelle, la possibilité de réussite, l'utilisation et l'opportunité, la délimitation du sujet et le caractère personnel du choix.
- Comment réussir la recherche?: Vérifier les conditions, les modalités et les méthodes théorique et pratique.
- Quelles sont les étapes à suivre?: L'observation, donner l'importance réelle à la lecture (quoi et comment lire), la réflexion, l'importance et la qualité de la réflexion.
- Acte d'écrire: Vérifier la vulgarisation, l'approfondissement et la clarification de l'écriture.

2. La recherche bibliographique:

- Le sujet de la recherche: comme objectif de travail, on demande une liste de documents de référence sur un thème spécifique.
- La recherche sur bases de données: procéder à la recherche sur les bases de données existantes au CDI (PORBASE, MEDLINE et DRUGDEX).
- Connexion avec le fonds documentaire: établir la correspondance des résultats de la recherche avec le fonds documentaire existant au CDI ou dans d'autres bibliothèques.
- Les résultats: présentation d'une bibliographie abrégée.

Evaluation du plan de formation:

1. La méthodologie en recherche: Présentation de huit sujets de recherche. Tenant compte des connaissances acquises, on procédera à l'élimination progressive des thèmes, jusqu'au sujet de recherche sélectionné par le formateur.

2. La recherche bibliographique: Du moins 75% des médecins généralistes doivent atteindre l'objectif de l'élaboration d'une bibliographie pareille à celle du formateur. Ainsi, on a réuni seize omnipraticiens dans une salle avec un ordinateur pour deux - on a encouragé la communication entre eux, la discussion des doutes, les possibilités de résolution du problème. Chaque ordinateur possédait trois bases de données: MEDLINE, DRUGDEX (base de données pharmacologiques) et PORBASE (Base National de Données Bibliographiques).

La méthodologie en recherche a été sélectionnée théoriquement, comme d'habitude, suivie des objectifs et du plan de travail. On a fait la présentation des huit thèmes de travail, en montrant l'inutilité de deux thèmes et le manque

1. Les coûts des soins de santé primaires.
2. L'indécision en médecine générale.
3. Le syndrome de mort subite du nourrisson.
4. Contrôle naturel des naissances.
5. Développement de la médecine générale en Mozambique.
6. L'hypercholesterolemie comme un facteur de risque pour l'accident vasculaire cérebral.
7. Les effets de l'informatique dans la relation médecin-malade.
8. Comparaison de deux modèles d'organisation de prestation de soins de santé nocturnes aux usagers du médecin de famille.

Tableau 1

d'originalité de trois autres (Tableau 1).

Pendant la session, on a prêté l'assistance nécessaire et urgente à chacun. Pour tous, la nouveauté consistait dans la recherche personnelle et totale, des bases de données jusqu'à l'élaboration d'un travail final, en passant par la lecture en diagonale des documents sélectionnés.

Le CDI se trouvait complètement à la disposition de ce groupe d'omnipraticiens pour la consultation immédiate des documents. On a leur enseigné son utilisation individuelle et particulière en expliquant: (1) la construction de la Table de Classification; (2) la construction des cotes; (3) la décodification des cotes; (4) l'arrangement des périodiques.

Pour les documents inexistants au CDI, les omnipraticiens ont établi la liaison avec d'autres bibliothèques et d'autres centres de documentation à l'aide du répértoire que le réseau APDIS a élaboré. La bibliographie finale a été, enfin, présentée et on a discuté avec chacun son choix et l'utilité de cette session. Il faut bien dire que les objectifs ont été accomplis avec une pourcentage de 82%; les normes bibliographiques avaient, cependant, beaucoup d'erreurs.

On peut donc constater l'inexistance d'une formation spécifique en documentation ou en recherche bibliographique parmi les médecins. Cette lacune doit être réflechie et changée.

LES MODULES DE RECHERCHE DOCUMENTAIRE DANS LE PLAN D'ÉTUDES MÉDICALES

Pour les américains il est très naturel que les médecins apprennent à utiliser les bibliothèques médicales pendant leur formation académique. C'est naturel mais ce n'est pas la réalité. Même si les bibliothèques développent un rôle important d'intérmediaire entre le chercheur et les sources d'information. Même si, de plus en plus, on constate le *boum* des bases de données en cherchant des réponses rapides et précises pour la prise de décision. Même si l'information est partagée sous une politique de coopération bien établie et bien assurée par les services documentaires. Les universités américaines identifient les services d'information médicale comme une composante essentielle dans le système des soins de santé.

Sous peine de faire l'apologie des États-Unis, on doit rehausser positivement les initiatives de l'Université de Columbia, dont la bibliothèque organise la formation sur les techniques de recherche en ressources electroniques; des Bibliothèques des Universités de Cornell, de Johns Hopkins, de Rochester et de Washington qui développent la formation en management de l'information et en recherche sur bases de données.[1]

La Bibliothèque d'Utah a pris les devants: avec le Département d'Informatique Médicale elle étudie la possibilité d'intégrer ces modules dans le curriculum scolaire.[1]

Aussi bien que la bibliothèque des sciences médicales de la Faculté de Médecine de l'Université de Pittsburgh qui, dès 1992, développe un programme d'information en premier année du cours relation médecin-malade, en utilisant du matériel audiovisuel, des sources d'information informatiques et, sur place, de la présence d'experts.[2] Elle privilégie la recherche individuelle. Les résultats sont excellents et les étudiants sont impressionnés par les sources d'information et aussi par le rôle des bibliothècaires.

Un autre cas est celui de la bibliothèque de la Faculté de Médecine de l'Université de New Mexico.[3] Depuis 1993, elle développe un programme d'éducation bibliothécaire pour les étudiants, lequel est intégré dans le curriculum. Les étudiants apprennent à consulter le MeSH, l'Index Medicus, les catalogues 'on-line' et à sélectionner les sources d'information les plus importantes. Cette formule assure une bonne utilisation des ressources documentales. Les documentalistes ont adapté leurs services aux besoins éducationnels des étudiants.

De même, la Bibliothèque de la Faculté de McGoogan (Nebraska) est responsable du module d'Introduction à la médecine.[4] Leurs documentalistes familiarisent les étudiants avec les sources d'information: les textes de référence, les bases de données et les systèmes multimedia. Les résultats présentent des étudiants avec un niveau de connaissances très élevé.

En France, les Facultés de Médecine de Lyon et de Nancy ont proposé des modules de recherche documentaire et le Ministère d'Education Nationale, de l'Enseignement Supérieur et de la Recherche étudie la proposition d'intégration d'un module de recherche documentaire dans le plan d'études médicales.[5]

Conclusion

Finalement, on doit reconnaître le rôle d'éducateur du documentaliste. Les bibliothèques et les centres de documentation sont responsables de la prise de connaissance des utilisateurs. On constate que cette relation entre chercheurs et documentalistes n'est pas difficile. Les codes documentaires sont parfois complexes pour les médecins, mais la relation fonctionne, parce que le professionnel de l'information aide et instruit constamment le demandeur avec humilité et diplomatie. Les deux connaissent l'autorité et le pouvoir de l'information sur le savoir scientifique.

Bibliographie

[1] Florance V, Braude RM, Frisse ME, Fuller S. Educating Physicians to Use the Digital Library. Acad Med 1995;70:597-602

[2] Schilling K, Ginn DS, Mickelson P, Roth LH. Integration of information-seeking skills and activities into a problem-based curriculum. Bull Med Libr Assoc 1995;83:176-83

[3] Eldredge JD. A problem-based learning curriculum in transition: the emerging role of the library. Bull Med Libr Assoc 1993;81:310-5

[4] Satterthwaite RK, Helms ME, Nouravarsani R, Van Antwerp M, Woelfi NN. Library faculty role in problem-based learning: facilitating small groups. Bull Med Libr Assoc 1995;83:465-8

[5] Accart JP. Santé publique et aide à la décision: le rôle des bibliothèques et services de documentation. Documentaliste 1996;33:161-6

IMPACT OF LIBRARY AND INFORMATION SERVICES ON PHYSIOTHERAPISTS' DECISION MAKING

Maggie Ashcroft, Instant Library Ltd, Loughborough, UK

Context for the study and survey population

This paper is based on the findings of a study undertaken in 1995, commissioned by the British Library, as one of a series of United Kingdom "Impact" studies. The programme was supervised by Professor Joanne Marshall, who had used the methodology for a study of clinicians in Rochester, New York.[1]

The study focused on physiotherapists in National Health Service (NHS) hospital trusts in the Northern and Yorkshire region of England. Physiotherapists are the largest group of Professionals Allied to Medicine (PAMs), but make up only 5% of NHS employed health care professionals and are therefore a specialist minority amongst much larger and more demanding groups of health care library users. Physiotherapists have an increasingly important role as decision makers in patient care.

Findings

Table 1. Value of information received

Relevant	74%
Accurate and current	88%
Refreshed memory	75%
Substantiated prior knowledge	66%
Provided new knowledge	87%
Information was of clinical value	81%
Better informed clinical decisions	74%
Contributed to better quality care	74%
Saved physiotherapist's time	75%

Previous research on physiotherapists has studied patterns of information use, and this study confirms what is already known. Physiotherapists' experience of hospital library services has not previously been studied in the same way. The findings indicate that a significant majority of professional practitioners value information, as well as perceive significant impact of information on patient care. The conclusions drawn from other evidence provided by the study are not so favourable. Some physiotherapists apparently experience barriers to access to library and information services, which are not necessarily the fault of library service managers. Improvement of specialist access and provision policies could be through a variety of developments - some of which are discussed.

S. Bakker (ed.), Health Information Management: What Strategies?, 161-163.

Physiotherapists as users of health care libraries

The study found that only 4% used the library, regularly once a week; 31% used it once a month; 51% used the library less than once a month, and 14% had not used the library at all during the last year. Other sources of information are normally preferred to hospital libraries: journals, colleagues, personal and departmental collections are all convenient and easily accessible. When asked to evaluate the importance of information received for a specific enquiry, physiotherapists ranked the importance of hospital libraries lower than university libraries and discussion with colleagues. They rated the Chartered Society of Physiotherapy even lower.

Table 2. Aspects of patient care changed

Advice given to patient	59%
Choice of treatment	53%
Amount of treatment received	35%
Criteria for treatment	39%

Table 3. Avoidance of adverse effects

Greater amount of in-patient treatment	16%
Additional out-patient hours	24%
Ineffective/inappropriate treatment	55%
Inappropriate referral	29%

Physiotherapists had a lower appreciation of the value of information than the clinicians in the Rochester study,[1] but this result is likely to be related to significant differences between clinicians and physiotherapists in the level and type of patient care decisions they make (Table 1). Many physiotherapists (74%) believed that information received had led to a change in their care of patients (Table 2) and avoidance of adverse effects (Table 3).

Interpretation of survey findings

Although there was strong evidence of the impact and value of information supplied by health care libraries, the more circumstantial evidence was disappointing, both to library managers and to the physiotherapy profession. The response rate was low, indicating that there is a need for different methods for collecting evidence on impact.

The study raised doubt about the transferability of the method of data collection, and the use of "critical incident" research methodology - with users who are less committed to library use than the clinicians previously studied, and who experience serious barriers to accessing hospital library services. Comparison of results is also difficult, due to different types and levels of decision making.

In the context of service delivery, the survey findings indicate the need for change and development.

Role of library and information services for physiotherapists

Policies and practice need to be developed, particularly to improve:
- access to evidence, to improve evidence-based practice
- access for practitioners who are distant and isolated from library facilities
- relationships between health care professionals and information specialists as colleagues
- effectiveness of specialist departmental resource collections, alongside centralised multidisciplinary collection policies
- the use of electronic networking for access to national and international bibliographic resources and professional discussion groups

- the role of the national professional body, the Chartered Society of Physiotherapy, in setting standards for information use and access.
- training and development of information retrieval skills for specialist users of multidisciplinary libraries.

Future developments

The Chartered Society of Physiotherapy is already taking a lead in providing a series of workshops around the country, to develop critical appraisal skills amongst senior professionals. The role of libraries in providing access to the necessary tools is heavily emphasised in the programme.

The CSP are very concerned by the findings of this study, and are prepared to take up the challenge and influence those who purchase physiotherapy education and training, to ensure satisfactory levels of library support are available.

Inadequate funding for health care library services is a fundamental cause of poor levels of provision and access. Funding streams for education and research are particularly relevant. The National Health Service is in the process of developing more robust funding mechanisms for library provision, and the specialist professions need to monitor policies to ensure the needs of their members are met.

Reference

[1] Marshall JG. The impact of the special library on clinical decision making: the Rochester study. Bull Med Libr Assoc 1992;80:169-178

LOCAL MEDICAL INFORMATION DATABASE: AN INDISPENSABLE COMPLEMENT TO GLOBAL INTERNATIONAL SEARCH

Jorge Crespo, Hospitais da Universidade de Coimbra, Portugal

Summary

Searching literature and information is, nowadays, indispensable for decision making in medical practice. Databases like Medline, Cancerlit or Micromedex are fundamental for searching what's new at the top of medical knowledge. No one dispenses them when looking for an actualized point of situation regarding any medical subject. They are fast and up-to-date, letting medical doctors be well informed on what scientific community is doing or looking for. However, each country has its own reality that cannot be forgotten. There are genetical, epidemiological and all other sorts of local differences that make medical practice and patient responsiveness somewhat different, too. Ignoring this is to forget a basic principle of medical practice. That's why in countries where the number of internationally indexed journals are sparse, it is important to provide a local medical information database including all local publications from the health area. They allow health professionals from different centers to know better each other and their works, the same way they do with international ones, but with additional local advantage regarding cooperative tasks, medical meetings and regional knowledge.

S. Bakker (ed.), Health Information Management: What Strategies?, 164.

INFORMATION SUPPORT FOR CLINICAL DECISION MAKING IN PRIMARY HEALTHCARE

Frances E. Wood, University of Sheffield, U.K.

The use of information in clinical decision making by general practitioners

This paper presents findings of an investigation of information use by general medical practitioners (GPs) in their clinical decision making.[1,2] Twenty seven interviews were conducted with GPs. Participants were asked about the last time they had sought information to assist in the decision-making process related specifically to their treatment of a patient. GPs commented that they needed information most frequently about drugs which they found by using drug compendia. Other information sought included details of hospital referral systems or from hospital patient records: medical opinions; the results of laboratory tests or x-rays; treatment protocols and other agencies' procedures. Sources in the practice which were used were drug compendia, reference books, journals, disease protocols, the practice library and colleagues. In most of the incidents information was obtained from outside the practice by asking hospital, social services or professional association staff and community pharmacists. Use of sources outside the practice always involved contacting people by telephone. Table 1 outlines the critical incidents.

The GPs' assessment of the value of the information

In all except one case the information was considered by the GPs to be of good quality. In almost all cases the GPs thought that it had enabled them to give higher quality care. Over two thirds of the GPs definitely or probably handled the situation differently because of the information. In over half the incidents the GPs said the information helped them decide not to arrange additional tests, referral to a consultant or admission to hospital. Two GPs said that, as a result of the information, the patient had recovered when s/he might not have done and 11 GPs said that the patients' health status had improved when it might not have done without the information.

The GPs use of external libraries

None of the GPs used libraries in dealing with the critical incidents described. Less than half of the GPs had used an external medical library within the previous six months. Although none of the library use was related to an immediate patient problem

S. Bakker (ed.), Health Information Management: What Strategies?, 165-167.

some was in connection with the treatment of specific illnesses. Some of the GPs had not used a medical library for 15 or more years but most of those who could remember had used one within the last four or five years. Physical access to the nearest medical library, especially parking, was regarded as a major problem by several GPs.

Information support for clinical decision making by GPs

In planning improved information support for GPs' clinical decision making it seems sensible to see what can be done to improve the effectiveness of GPs' current information seeking behaviour rather than trying to change it.

The most frequently used sources of information are paper or online drug compendia. Some similar compendia are being developed to provide online access to the medical information GPs need. Critical reviews and other evaluations of medical practice will become available in machine readable forms which the GP can access on his or her desk. The extent to which the content of these publications is relevant to medical practice in primary care remains an issue.

GPs often need information from hospitals. This information is obtained over the telephone, sometimes only after several calls. In future the results of tests may be transmitted by EDI (Electronic Data Interchange) although sometimes GPs may still want to discuss aspects of the results with hospital staff. E-mail is a more reliable way than the telephone to contact known members of hospital staff. Hospitals could improve access with better directories of their staff and services.

A preferred source of advice and information directly related to the medical aspects of the care of individual patients is hospital staff. At present the advice or information is based on knowledge and experience but is not necessarily 'evidence-based'. In future hospital staff could be a major channel through which 'evidence-based' information could be given to GPs.

Other ways in which GPs currently gather information are by attending meetings and reading journals especially, in the UK, the British Medical Journal. The use of these sources in the care of individual patients depends either on the GP remembering what was said at a meeting or in a paper, looking up the notes or the journal issue, or searching in the practice library or on a database. These ways will continue to help GPs to keep up to date and thus contribute to patient care. However, new journals and databases focusing on relevant evidence based practice possibly delivered in electronic form may be more effective.

There is a range of services which medical libraries could supply to GPs in support of their existing information seeking behaviour such as, advice on the choice of information sources to purchase, guidance on developing a practice library or collection, customised searches on particular topics and training in information seeking. It should also be possible to provide electronic access.

The preceding paragraphs outline ways in which GPs information seeking can be supported and enhanced. The General Medical Council of the UK in its recommendations for undergraduate medical education is promoting a shift towards more problem-based teaching and learning which should lead to a greater emphasis on the critical appraisal of the literature. This should mean that the next generation of GPs will be better able to utilise information in the service of their patients.

Acknowledgement. This project was funded by the British Library Research and Development Department.

References

[1] Wood FE, Wright P, Wilson T. The impact of information use on decision making by general medical practitioners. London: British Library Research and Development Department Report, 1995; pp.97
[2] Wood FE, Palmer J, Bacigalupo R, Simpson S, Wright P. General practitioners and information: evidence based practice explored. Curr Perspect Healthcare Comput 1996;543-48

Table 1 The critical incidents in detail (27 critical incidents)

Location	Access	Source	Information sought or action needed
1. Hospital	Telephone	Consultant biochemist	Advice
2. Hospital	Telephone	Consultant biochemist	Advice
3. Hospital	Telephone	Consultant biochemist	Advice on tests. Calls separated by some weeks. Appointment with a specialist
4. Hospital	Telephone	Drug Information Pharmacist	Written information - to support opinion
5. Hospital	Telephone	Registrar and consultant	Advice patient to wait for urgent appointment at clinic
6. Hospital	Telephone	X-ray Department staff	Results
7. Hospital	Telephone	Pathology Lab. staff	Results of test
8. Hospital	Telephone	Psychiatric Unit staff	Urgent appointment
9. Hospital	Telephone	Clinic appointments staff	Appointment and name of consultant
10. Hospital	Telephone	Registrar	Recently discharged patient had problem. No helpful information obtained
11. Hospital	Telephone	Registrar, appointments clerk, doctor	Urgent referral
12. Hospital	Telephone	Admissions, consultant's secretary, patient records	Identification of medication prescribed by the hospital
13. Hospital	Telephone	Colleague in practice, protocol, registrar	On analgesia, drug treatments, tests to do and HRT
14. Hospital	Telephone		What services offered by a clinic and an appointment
15. Hospital	Telephone		Advice on treatment
16. Hospital	Telephone	Call routed to five different people	Urgent appointment
17. Hospitals	Telephone	Several calls to doctors & receptionists in 3 hospitals	About a particular unit, its services, who was in charge
18. Hospice	Tel./meeting	Consultant	Second opinion, domiciliary visit, meeting patient+family
19. Pharmacy	Telephone	Pharmacist	Advice on the availability of a special drug
20. Soc.Serv.	Telephone	Staff	Arrange meals for housebound patient
21. Practice	Reading/lecture	Practice protocol, meeting (earlier) journals, BMA	Developing a management plan for a patient
22. Practice	Asked	Colleague	Decision to biopsy
23. Practice	Looked up	Monthly Index of Medical Specialities	Constituents of a contraceptive pill
24. Practice	Looked up	British National Formulary	Drug dosage information
25. Practice	Looked up	Drug compendium	Dosage for a child
26. Practice	Looked up	ABPI Data Compendium	Side effects of a drug
27. Practice library	Looked up	Book	Confirmed diagnosis

UN BULLETIN BIBLIOGRAPHIQUE EN SANTE PUBLIQUE A DESTINATION DES PAYS FRANCOPHONES

Chantal Lheureux, Patricia Goddart-Degove, Virginie Halley des Fontaines and Bernard Pissarro, Faculté de Médecine Saint-Antoine, Paris, France

Summary

"Santédoc" is a public health bibliography for professionnals and institutions in 15 countries (North Africa, Middle East, South-East Asia). Readers can order for free articles and books so as to implement their own documentation. The Public Health Documentation Center, of the Social Science Department in Saint Antoine Medical School (Paris) realizes scientific work: document selection and analyses. As a matter of selection policy, we have privileged scientific review, issues diversity and dialogue with the readers. Needs expressed by some of them induce to revalue the selection of subjects for each bulletin in order to satisfy our correspondents' request together with searching universal documents to meet the majority of desires, even the silent ones.

Présentation de "Santédoc"

"Santédoc" est un bulletin bibliographique analytique et sélectif, composé d'analyses d'ouvrages et d'articles écrits en langue française sur l'ensemble des thèmes consacrés à la santé publique et plus spécialement l'épidémiologie, la médecine sociale et la promotion de la santé. Santédoc est à destination de professionnels et d'institutions de 15 pays (Afrique du Nord, Moyen-Orient et Asie du Sud-Est). Chaque numéro présente 35 articles et 16 ouvrages, soit 51 notices comprenant des indications bibliographiques, un résumé et des mots-clés. Le premier numéro est paru en 1993.

Une des grandes originalités de ce bulletin réside dans le fait que les lecteurs peuvent commander gratuitement 2 ouvrages et 18 articles par numéro. Il s'agit non seulement de diffuser l'information sous une forme condensée, mais aussi de fournir les documents primaires aux lecteurs afin qu'ils puissent constituer un fonds documentaire à titre personnel ou dans le cadre de leur institution.

La sélection des documents et le travail documentaire sont réalisés par le Centre de documentation en Santé publique du Service de médecine préventive et sociale de la Faculté Saint-Antoine à Paris. La mise en page du bulletin et la diffusion des documents sont assurés par le centre de documentation BDPA. Le financement provient du Ministère des Affaires Etrangères français, qui est à l'origine du projet.

Résumé des activités en 1995: 300 correspondants sont inscrits, mais on peut estimer le nombre réel des lecteurs à plus de 5 000, grâce aux prêts inter-services (Enquête d'impact auprès des correspondants, 11/94). Pour chacun des deux numéros

S. Bakker (ed.), Health Information Management: What Strategies?, 168-169.

parus en 1995, plus de 1 100 articles et près de 100 ouvrages ont été commandés.

La politique de sélection des documents et les besoins des lecteurs

Santédoc est un projet conçu par une administration centrale, ce qui sous-entend une détermination des besoins, à la place des lecteurs. De plus, ces lecteurs ont des professions, des situations et des environnements professionnels très divers, dans des pays de différents continents. Quels peuvent être les thèmes d'intérêt d'un médecin épidémiologiste d'un institut de recherche universitaire du Maghreb et quels sont ceux d'un directeur d'hôpital rural au Vietnam? En bref, comment répondre aux besoins des lecteurs? La réponse a consisté à faire de la sélection une étape essentielle du processus documentaire et à instaurer un dialogue permanent avec les lecteurs.

Comité de sélection. Nous avons mis en place un comité de sélection pluridisciplinaire comprenant des médecins ayant de nombreuses expériences de missions humanitaires et d'enseignements dans les pays du sud, et une documentaliste. Nous avons défini des critères de qualité des documents: qualité scientifique, intérêt de la recherche, intérêt thématique, et nous avons cherché à diversifier les approches (document technique, innovation, validation des pratiques professionnelles) sur des thèmes jugés importants et intéressants. Les désirs exprimés par les lecteurs nous ont parfois désorientés ou ont remis en cause certaines de nos positions. Ainsi, nous pensions au début que les lecteurs seraient surtout intéressés par des expériences ou des données concernant leur pays, à la limite les pays limitrophes. Mais grâce à un dialogue continu avec nos correspondants, via leur courrier, les enquêtes d'opinion ou les envois spontanés de documents, nous nous sommes rendus compte que ceux qui s'exprimaient, désiraient dans la plupart des cas des documents d'envergure internationale, des guides pratiques et des manuels d'enseignements.

Les critères de sélection. Nous avons, alors, réévalué les critères de sélection pour mieux répondre aux attentes des lecteurs, tout en conservant une attitude pédagogique vis-à-vis des thèmes importants. La marge doit être assez grande que chaque lecteur trouve son compte en lisant Santédoc. Le comité de sélection se réserve le droit d'introduire des thèmes qu'il juge importants, même si aucune demande à propos de ce thème n'a été formulée. Nous essayons de trouver un équilibre entre les besoins exprimés par les lecteurs sans léser la majorité silencieuse. Nous cherchons des documents à la problématique et aux solutions suffisamment universelles pour plaire au plus grand nombre. Par exemple, un article sur une expérience de prévention du choléra au Pérou dans un quartier défavorisé fut un des articles les plus demandés. Le Pérou ne fait pas partie des zones géographiques destinataires de Santédoc, mais le programme de prévention exposé était transposable dans d'autres pays et continents.

Conclusion

Nous avons réussi à établir des échanges entre les lecteurs et le comité de sélection et à considérer les lecteurs comme des correspondants. En bref, nous avons amorcé une réseau de santé publique international. Mais le bulletin Santédoc tel qu'il vient d'être présenté, est interrompu depuis cette année pour des raisons financières. Il va continuer sous une forme différente: il sera diffusé biannuellement par la revue française "Santé publique". Cela signifie un nouveau lectorat, donc une nouvelle politique de sélection à peaufiner, à réévaluer selon les voeux et attentes des lecteurs.

A EUROPEAN INFORMATION NETWORK FOR ETHICS IN MEDICINE, HEALTH PROFESSIONS AND HEALTH CARE

Ute Elsner, Ute Meinecke and Stella Reiter-Theil, Akademie für Ethik in der Medizin, Göttingen, Germany

Actual status

In 1994 we started a system analysis - an analysis of actual needs and of existing information sources in the field of bioethics - as basis for the establishment of a European Information Network. We asked 158 scientists from 26 European countries via questionnaires what they do in case they need information on bioethical questions.

Figure 1. Present information patterns of people interested in biomedico-ethical problems

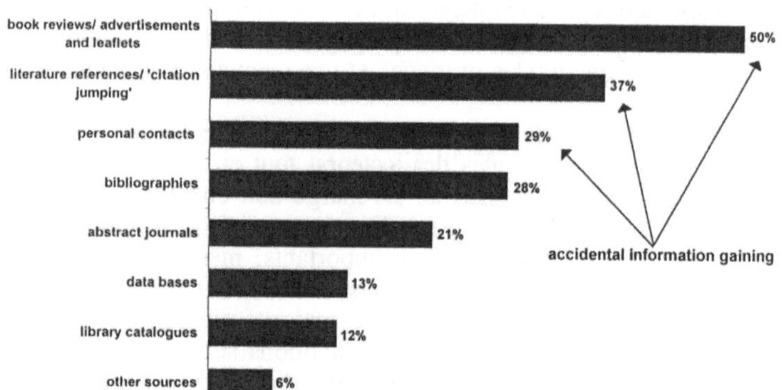

As figure 1 shows we found that the "ordinary scientist" uses an unsystematic way of information searching. The systematic using of e.g. bibliographies, abstract journals, databases and library catalogues is rather sporadical among scientists and academics.

As problems during information searching 50% of the scientists mentioned "not enough time" and 40% "not enough personnel". The lack of a central drop-in center and of an adequate database was regretted by 31% and 47% of the scientists. They even felt dissatisfied with the accidental results they got by their usual searching methods. At the time the analysis was realized, this considerable demand for the systematic reference of European literature could not be satisfied, since it exceeded the informational content of the currently operating databases (MEDLINE, BIOETHICSLINE, EMBASE, PHILOSOPHERS INDEX and RELIGION INDEX). The only professional on-line databases existing for the field of bioethics are BIOETHICSLINE of the Kennedy Institute of

S. Bakker (ed.), Health Information Management: What Strategies?, 170-172.

Ethics, Washington D.C. and ETHMED of the Information and Documentation Center for Ethics in Medicine at the Academy for Ethics in Medicine, Goettingen, Germany. BIOETHICSLINE mainly contains American literature references, whereas ETHMED mainly contains German literature. This very insufficient professional information infrastructure in Europe is reflected in the interest of the scientists in the future information network.

Fig. 2. Interest in foreign publications and expected use of an information network

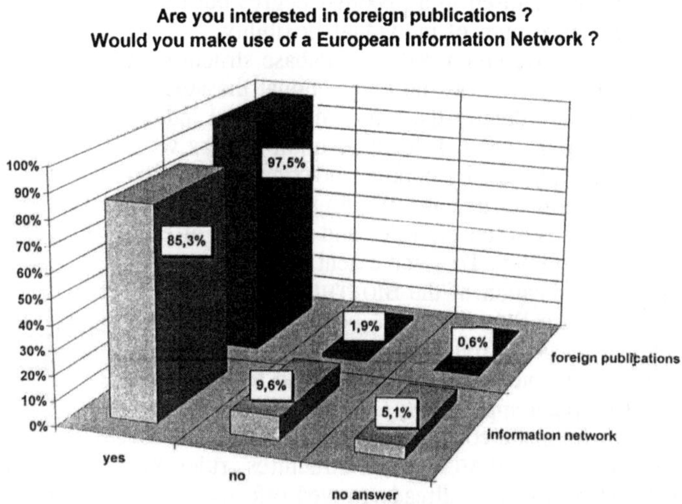

Figure 2 describes the interest of the scientists in foreign publications and in the information network. The questions "Are you interested in publications published in other countries?" and "Would you make use of a co-operative, European Information Network that would allow easy access to medical ethics literature of other countries?", were answered positively: 85% were interested in foreign publications and would welcome a European Database Network as reliable and competent resource of information.

INFORMATION PRODUCTION

Within the last years the increase in discussions on medico-ethical topics has resulted in an exponential increase of publications. We analysed MEDLINE containing world-wide medical literature references, but mainly English literature. Only a small part of the literature analyzed by MEDLINE since 1970 comes from European countries. The majority represent the non-European literature. This increase in publications makes it difficult for people interested to get specific information about specific topics. Another aspect is the interdisciplinarity of the field "Ethics in Medicine". Disciplines such as "medicine", "biology", "law", "theology", "philosophy" and "social sciences" are concerned. Often someone is a specialist in his or her own field. Nonetheless one does not know much about the other fields influencing the own field.

The project

In order to set the basis for a professional and competent exchange of information among the people in need of information, the European Commission decided to support the establishment of a standardised, labour-dividing European Information and Database Network in their BIOMED-2-Programme. France, Germany, the Netherlands, and Sweden joined to realize such a European Database (see insert). This project primarily aims at the establishment of a common European Database containing references for journal articles, books, unpublished documents, conference reports, dissertations and legal documents of interdisciplinary fields concerned with biomedical ethics. The national databases will be joined into a unified database network that will provide various information services.

The unification of the four already existing national databases will be realised to a maximal degree but on the condition of a maximum of individual flexibility.

As a first step we compared the database structures and cataloguing rules as well as the four national thesauri and indexing rules. To identify the status of the usual indexing methods of the four national documentation centers we realised an indexing test by parallel indexing and writing abstracts of several documents. We found that there was a good conformity between the rules and standards of each national partner center. To some extent, this advantage is owing to the application of the BIOETHICS-Thesaurus of the American database BIOETHICSLINE being taken as basis for their national thesauri from the Dutch, German and French Documentation Center. For this reason and for the purpose of a trans-European applicability, the European Database Network will be made compatible with the online databases BIOETHICSLINE and ETHMED. Their structures, rules and keywords (Thesauri) have already proved effective.

User acces to information from European countries

Persons in need for information from European countries have the possibility to ask their national Documentation Center or, in case there is none, the Project Coordinator IDEM for: (1) literature searches on individual topics; (2) bibliographies of specific topics; (3) copy services of the original literature; (4) lending services (at present offered only by the Swedish documentation center).

Apart from the conventional communication facilities the user can ask the National Documentation Centers via E-Mail and Internet for information and will get the information, if needed, immediately. The databases BIOETHICSLINE, ETHMED and SPRI-LINE are already searchable via World Wide Web. A direct online access via telecommunication facilities (e.g. Internet) to the European Database is planned for the future, and the diffusion of the whole European Database by national hosts will be taken into consideration. Also, the production of a CD-ROM will be discussed.

At this stage of the project the services are offered according to the national charging conditions of each documentation center. For other BIOMED-II-projects literature searches in the national databases of each center are offered free of charge.

Contact addresses:

GERMANY:
Project Coordinator:
Information and Documentation Center for Ethics in Medicine (IDEM)
Academy for Ethics in Medicine (AEM) at the Institute for Ethics and History of Medicine
University of Göttingen
Humboldtallee 36
37073 Göttingen
Tel. +49-551-393966
Fax +49-551-393996
E-Mail:
UTE@ethik.med.uni-goettingen.de
Ute Elsner (Dipl.-Doc.)
Ute Meinecke (Dipl.-Doc)

SWEDEN:
SPRI Swedish Institute for Health Services Development
Hornsgatan 20
Box 70487
107 26 Stockholm
Tel. -46-8 702 47 81
Fax -46-8-702-47-99
E-Mail: arne.jakobsson@spri.se
Arne Jakobsson

THE NETHERLANDS:
Katholieke Universiteit Nijmegen (KUN)
Faculty of Medical Sciences
Department of Ethics, Philosphy and History of Medicine
Geert Grooteplein 21
P.O. Box 9101
6500 HB Nijmegen
Tel. +31-80 61 53 20
Fax +31-80 54 02 54
Prof.Dr. Henk ten Have

FRANCE:
Centre de documentation en éthique des sciences de la vie et de la santé (CDEI)
Service commun no. 12 de l'INSERM
Faculté de Médicine Necker
156, rue de Vaugirard
75730 Paris Cedex 15
Tel. +33-1-40-61-54-59
Fax +33-1-40-61-55-88
Dr. Paulette Dostatni
Dr. Jean-Claude Buxtorf

BIBLIMED: A NEW SPANISH DATABASE IN CLINICAL MEDICINE

María Angeles Zulueta, Luz Moreno, María Bordons and Manuela Vázquez, Consejo Superior de Investigaciones Científicas, Madrid, Spain

Introduction

In spite of the large amount of medical journals generated in Spain, only a few of them are covered by the largest international databases. In 1995, approx 500 medical journals were published in Spain, but only 5 were included in Science Citation Index, 35 in Medline, and 60 in Excerpta Medica.

Health Sciences is a broad area that comprises many specialties, spread in a wide basic-clinical range. Although nobody questions the international scope of basic science, this is not the case for some clinical areas, which address mainly domestic issues, and are specially useful for national practitioners.

With the aim of making Spanish literature widely accessible, it was planned to build the BIBLIMED database, including clinical aspects of medical practice as covered by the most prominent Spanish medical journals.

Project objectives

BIBLIMED was designed to include documents published in 50 high quality Spanish journals, covering 28 different medical specialties, from 1992 onwards. A selected subset of journals should be retrieved in a full text form, while only a bibliographic format including abstract and keywords would be displayed for the remaining journals.

The project is oriented towards the health care professionals at the primary health care level. It aims to satisfy their needs for reliable and immediately available information in their own language and to provide support for the decision-making process inherent in their daily clinical practice.

The database is conceived as a service to be provided by the Spanish Medical Association (Organización Médica Colegial, OMC), main financing body of the project, for all its members. A close collaboration has been established between the Centre for Scientific Information and Documentation (CINDOC), that belongs to the Spanish Research Council, and a well-known Spanish medical publisher. CINDOC is responsible for the initial assessment and selection of journals, as well as for the subject indexation of documents, while all technical questions are the publisher's responsibility. The project started in january 1995, and should be finished by june 1997.

S. Bakker (ed.), Health Information Management: What Strategies?, 173-176.

Project development

DATABASE COVERAGE

We tried to include in BIBLIMED the best journals of the most clinical specialties. Professional needs of physicians, mainly defended by the OMC, and quality of journals, judged by the publisher and the CINDOC, were assessed trying to achieve a balanced selection. A special questionnaire was designed to assess formal and scientific aspects of the journals. Only articles, case reports and reviews were included in the database.

DOCUMENT MANAGEMENT

Database structure. The following bibliographic elements were included in the database: document title, authors, address, journal title, volume, issue and page, publication year, author abstract and keywords.

Subject indexing of documents. This was based on the thesaurus developed by the Latin American and Caribbean Health Sciences Information Center (BIREME), that produces -through a cooperative network structure- the database LILACS (Literatura Latinoamericana e Caribe em Ciencias de la Saude). The main principles of the controlled vocabulary follow closely those established by the U.S. National Library of Medicine (NLM) for Medline, though adapted to Spanish medical terminology.[1,2]

TECHNICAL ASPECTS

Software and hardware requirements. The database was built on ORACLE, using the Unix operative system, since this was the software used by the OMC in their other electronic products, all of them accessible through INTERNET.

Searching capabilities. The following facilities are foreseen:
. displaying of MeSH (alphabetical and permuted list, tree structure)
. index of journals
. searching: all fields are searchable; boolean logic, field selection, explosion of tree-structure and storing of search profile are possible capabilities of the system.
. output: variable formats, downloading capability.

HUMAN AND ECONOMIC RESOURCES

Subject indexing was carried out by 3 medical information scientists: 1 full time and 2 part time scientists were involved in the project and working at CINDOC. One computer specialist was in charge of programming and technical developments, while working for the OMC. The experts made use of the infrastructure of their institutions.

The task of the information scientists

SELECTION OF JOURNAL TITLES

The most relevant journals were selected attending to national and international standards.[3-5] A special questionnaire was designed including different type of criteria:

Formal criteria. Information available about the journal and publisher: full and abbreviated journal title, ISSN, no.issues/year, price, table of contents.

Scientific quality. Description of the scientific committee; Foreign members in the scientific committee; Articles submitted to referees; Type of publisher: commercial or scientific; Impact according to SCI; References analyses.

Dissemination criteria. Direct: number of subscriptions, presence in national and foreign library catalogues, etc.; Indirect: presence in international databases, documents co-authored with foreign researchers, etc.; Abstract and keywords in Spanish and English.

Specialty. The journals were divided into specialties, and only the best ranked journals in each specialty were selected, trying to keep an equilibrium among the different medical specialties.

SUBJECT INDEXING OF DOCUMENTS

The subject indexing of documents was based on the controlled vocabulary Descriptors in Health Sciences (DeCS),[1] and using the Manual of Indexing as a guide.[2] The vocabulary of the DeCs is trilingual: Spanish, Portuguese, and English. It includes more than 14,000 terms referring to the health sciences, grouped in categories.

Two different type of descriptors were used: primary descriptors, indicating the main topic of a document, and secondary descriptors, that describe aspects of secondary interest. Descriptors were drawn from the DeCs list, and their meaning can be narrowed using subheadings, like in the Medline database.

The DeCS list was developed attending to the Spanish used in Latin-American countries, sometimes different from that used in Spain (see Table I).

Current state of the project

BIBLIMED is presently accesible on-line, through INTERNET, to all members of the OMC subscribed to the OMC Plan Telemático. However, the project is still under development, and the current coverage of the database is not comprehensive -it includes 8,000 documents, 65% of them with indexing terms- and some of the searching and retrieval facilities foreseen are not available yet.

Different problems were found in the development of the project:

Technical problems, related to the introduction of the subject indexing terms and making possible the retrieval using the Thesaurus.

Cooperative issues: (1) To establish collaboration contacts with BIREME. They have kindly provided their Thesaurus in printed and CD-ROM version. (2) To reach an agreement with Spanish medical publishers to make their journals available in a full text format. The medical publishers readily agreed to include their journals in BIBLIMED in the short bibliographic format, but were reluctant to accept the full text format.

Terminological questions: (1) Different Spanish vocabularies for Spain and for the South American countries. These language differences could have a negative impact on the retrieval process. (2) The terms corresponding to the newest diseases or drugs or the latest scientific findings are usually missing in the Thesaurus due to the delay in the updating process.

Future challenges

On the short term it is planned to have BIBLIMED fully available, with all searching and retrieval facilities working by june 1997. An evaluation of the project should then be carried out.

On the long term up-dating of the database has to be planned. Implementation of a new project involving not only the OMC, but also other professional associations, i.e. those of the pharmacy and odontology fields. Another development will be to include BIBLIMED in the LILACS database. Subject indexing of documents was done according to the BIREME standards, being aware of the future interest of comprising all medical literature from Iberoamerican countries on the same database.

References

[1] Descriptores en Ciencias de la Salud. Sao Paulo: Centro Latinoamericano y del Caribe de Información en Ciencias de la Salud, Organización Panamericana de la Salud, 1992

[2] Manual de indización. Sao Paulo: Centro Latinoamericano y del Caribe de Información en Ciencias de la Salud, Organización Panamericana de la Salud, 1988

[3] National Research Council of Canada. Indicators of quality for research journals. Report. Canada, 1981.

[4] ISO. Documentation and information: ISO Standards Handbook 1. 3 rd ed. Geneve: ISO, 1988

[5] AENOR. Documentación. Normas fundamentales: recopilación de normas UNE. Madrid: AENOR, 1994

Table I. Non-correspondence between medical terms as used in Spain and Latin-American countries

USA	Latin-American countries	Spain
Neoplasm	Neoplasma	Neoplasia
Lithotripsy	Litotripsia	Litotricia
Hybridization	Hibridizacion	Hibridación
Urinary reservoirs	Reservatorios urinarios	Reservorios urinarios
Quadriplegia	Cuadriplegia	Tetraplegia
Blocking agents	Bloqueadores	Bloqueantes
Absenteeism	Ausentismo	Absentismo
Tissue donors	Donadores de tejidos	Donantes de organos
Monitoring	Monitoreo	Monitorización
Ulcerative colitis	Colitis ulcerativa	Colitis ulcerosa

DOCUMENTALISTE DANS UN SERVICE D'INFORMATION A SPECIALISATION MEDICALE ET PHARMACEUTIQUE

Armelle Martin and Sylvie Guillo, Pharmacie Centrale des Hôpitaux de Paris, France

Summary

The role of the Service d'Information Médico - Pharmaceutique (SIMP) of the Pharmacie Centrale des Hôpitaux de Paris (Assistance Publique) is to give an adequate answer to the documentary needs of health professionals belonging to the institution (mainly physicians and pharmacists) and more widely to hospital practitioners. That is why the SIMP give them access to an information of good quality: essential condition for all evidence - based decision making.

In this context, we deliberated on the originality of the function of the information scientist in an information center adressed to a public composed of different but nonetheless complementary professionals. We detailed the different documentary tasks in this unit, taking into account the impact of the new technologies and the specificities of the service related to his status and history. In this way, we tried to show how the function of the information scientist in such a structure involves a great diversity of professional activities. Then, we attempted to evaluate a profile of skills required by an information scientist to provide quality work and be recognized in that type of professional unit.

Service d'Information Médico-Pharmaceutique (SIMP)

L'Assistance Publique-Hôpitaux de Paris (AP-HP) est le plus grand centre hospitalier d'Europe. Il regroupe 50 établissements (29511 lits) et 5 services généraux dont la Pharmacie Centrale des Hôpitaux (PCH). La Pharmacie Centrale des Hôpitaux a pour mission principale de fournir aux établissements de l'AP-HP l'ensemble des biens consommables dont les médicaments, les dispositifs médicaux, les réactifs. Ses activités sont organisées autour de 4 pôles: achat, distribution, production et un pôle scientifique dont fait partie le Service d'Information Médico-Pharmaceutique (SIMP).

Le Service d'Information assure diverses missions:

- mission documentaire, à travers la Documentation Médico-Pharmaceutique PCH-ADDM;
- mission d'information / consultation avec notamment un secteur répondant à des questions ponctuelles sur le bon usage du médicament.
- mission d'assistance à la Commission du Médicament de l'AP-HP et de relation avec les Comités Locaux du Médicament: instruction scientifique des dossiers,

S. Bakker (ed.), Health Information Management: What Strategies?, 177-180.

proposition d'amélioration du service médical rendu hospitalier, bulletin du médicament.
- enfin, mission de pharmacoépidémiologie et de pharmacoéconomie: cellule de pharmacovigilance et réévaluation des produits PCH, études de consommation des médicaments à l'AP-HP.

Le SIMP participe activement à un décloisonnement dans l'accès à l'information et à l'assurance qualité du circuit du médicament à l'hôpital par la diffusion d'information et par la mise à disposition d'une documentation spécialisée aux médecins prescripteurs, aux pharmaciens et au personnel de soins.

Les exigences augmentent sans cesse pour les professionnels de santé (augmentation du nombre de patients, accumulation des connaissances, contrôle des dépenses de santé...) et la pratique clinique doit tenir compte des changements rapides qui peuvent intervenir dans les méthodes diagnostiques et thérapeutiques, c'est pourquoi la recherche d'information doit être intégrée dans la pratique médicale. Ces différentes contraintes expliquent que l'accès à l'information soit devenu d'une importance stratégique pour le corps médical.[1] Le secteur de santé est de plus très gros producteur d'information (articles, résumés d'articles, références bibliographiques, dictionnaires, traités...) et la qualité, l'importance de ces publications intervient à plus d'un titre dans la progression de carrière et dans la reconnaissance professionnelle des praticiens hospitaliers. Il s'avère donc crucial pour garantir l'efficacité des services et la qualité des soins à l'hôpital de recueillir, organiser la documentation mais aussi de pouvoir diffuser l'information "utile" le plus rapidement possible aux publics concernés afin qu'elle soit source d'aide à la décision.

Les documentalistes

Le documentaliste est un agent de transfert des connaissances et il doit faire parvenir l'information avec une affinité suffisante pour qu'elle puisse être intégrée au mieux c'est à dire permettre de décider, réaliser, innover... de manière éclairée. Il sera d'autant plus efficace s'il connaît bien ses destinataires et leur travail, s'il sait s'adapter à des solutions évolutives et surtout s'il participe à la vie de l'entreprise.

Bien que le centre soit spécialisé dans le secteur médecine-pharmacie et qu'il s'agisse d'une structure relativement importante (25 personnes: pharmaciens, médecins, documentalistes, bibliothécaires, secrétaires, magasinier), il n'y a pas eu éclatement de la chaîne des fonctions documentaires. Les fonctions de repérage, collecte de l'information et des documents, traitement et exploitation, recherche et diffusion ne sont pas cloisonnées. Chaque documentaliste reste polyvalente avec des tâches variées réparties au mieux des aptitudes de chacune.

COMPÉTENCES DES DOCUMENTALISTES

En ce qui concerne les connaissances, une triple compétence s'avère nécessaire pour toute intégration d'un documentaliste au sein du service:
- formation Bac + 4 minimum, avec spécialisation au domaine d'activité (médecine, pharmacie, biologie...)
- maîtrise des outils et des technique documentaires
- maîtrise de l'anglais. Environ 80% du fonds documentaire est en langue anglaise et l'interrogation des banques de données biomédicales suppose une bonne connaissance de cette langue.

Le centre possède une importante bibliothèque qui propose une collection de 700 périodiques biomédicaux avec un pôle d'excellence en pharmacie-pharmacologie. L'orientation des dernières années a été de maintenir les collections ultérieures à 1975 directement accessibles aux lecteurs.

Un service d'accueil avec conseil et orientation des lecteurs permet de répondre aux besoins du public interne (services PCH) ou externe (professionnels de santé hospitaliers essentiellement) et d'identifier ses priorités grâce à un dialogue établi avec les intéressés. Des questionnaires sont ainsi régulièrement diffusés: (1) pour choisir les meilleures voies de diffusion de l'information et (2) pour solliciter les lecteurs quant à leurs suggestions d'acquisition.

Une réunion d'information hebdomadaire a lieu au sein du centre. L'ensemble des cadres du service y est convié. Les nouveaux projets et les divers problèmes sont évoqués, les nouveaux achats sont discutés (ouvrages, périodiques, équipements informatiques...) et les nouveautés scientifiques sont présentées. Les documentalistes participent activement à ces réunions qui permettent de faire circuler plus efficacement l'information dans l'ensemble du service. Par une meilleure connaissance des projets en cours, des attentes en information de chacun, le documentaliste est alors plus à même de mettre en place une veille informative et de mieux transmettre une information adéquate aux bonnes personnes, au bon moment avec fourniture de documents (articles, normes, ouvrages, périodiques...) ou d'informations informelles.

LES PRODUITS D'INFORMATION

La production de banques de données internes participe également à ce concept de "veille" par le dépouillement d'une presse spécialisée. Le centre produit ainsi deux banques de données:

- MedocAP: médecine clinique. Mises au point, articles de synthèse de 41 revues dont 28 françaises; congrès et numéros spéciaux parus dans l'ensemble des revues du service.
- Bibliographif, accessible sur Minitel (3617 APHIF): thérapeutique médicamenteuse, matériel médico-chirurgical, hygiène, pharmacie hospitalière, parmi 63 revues indexées dont 30 en langue française.

Un gros travail d'homogénéisation des mots-clefs avec utilisation de lexique contrôlé ou de thesaurus est en cours et un système d'assurance qualité est mis en place avec des réunions régulières et une mise en oeuvre de procédures d'indexation. Ces deux banques de données sont interrogeables gratuitement au sein du service et apportent ainsi une forte valeur ajoutée à l'information disponible sur place.

Depuis 1994, l'ensemble des acquisitions d'ouvrages est informatisé. Des recherches multicritères sont ainsi possibles et les ouvrages diffusés dans les services PCH sont facilement localisés. Une liste des nouvelles acquisitions est diffusée tous les deux mois aux utilisateurs internes et externes.

En matière de législation pharmaceutique, le Journal Officiel est dépouillé quotidiennement et une diffusion sélective de l'information est faite pour les différents services de la PCH. Un questionnaire avait été diffusé en 1993 afin de mieux définir les besoins et les thèmes des profils. Une enquête de satisfaction concernant ce produit est en cours d'élaboration afin de mieux en déterminer la pertinence et de le réajuster éventuellement.

L'intégration des nouvelles technologies s'est faite progressivement au niveau du centre, tout d'abord par l'informatisation de la gestion documentaire (logiciels Datatrek, Texto). L'apparition des réseaux informatiques a permis ensuite de travailler en réseau local (Novell), d'avoir accès en ligne aux banques de données biomédicales internationales, de mettre en réseau les CD ROM (Medline, IPA, Micromedex), et enfin d'avoir accès à Internet (modem en réseau) que l'on utilise actuellement comme une source complémentaire d'information et de documentation. Ces nouveaux outils ont fait évoluer les méthodes de travail en donnant un accès facilité aux ressources documentaires à l'ensemble du personnel de documentation mais également aux praticiens hospitaliers du service (médecins, pharmaciens) dans le cadre de leur pratique professionnelle.

LES APTITUDES

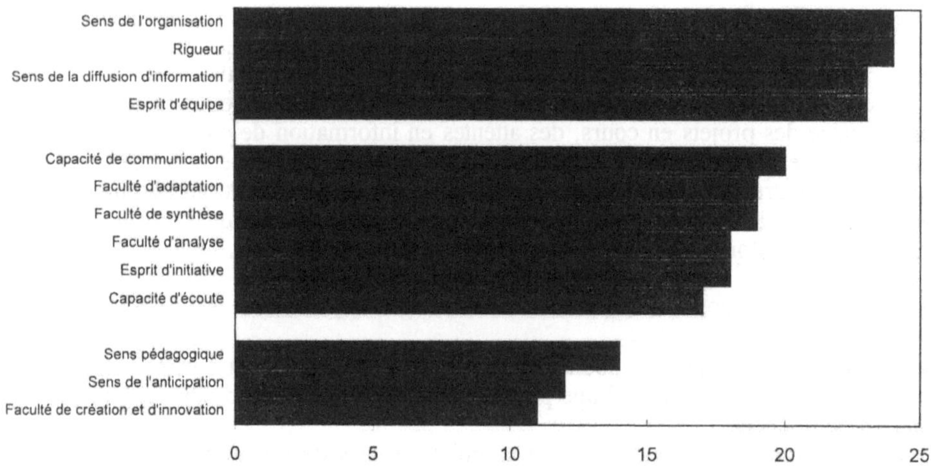

Figure 1. Aptitudes

Grâce aux référentiels ADBS[2,3] nous avons alors tenté de définir les aptitudes requises pour effectuer un travail de qualité en tant que documentaliste dans ce service. La figure 1 présente les aptitudes retenues classées par ordre d'importance.

En reliant ces aptitudes aux connaissances décrites précédemment, il a été possible de dégager un cadre de référence qui pourrait par exemple être utile lors d'une embauche ou pour mieux évaluer les besoins en formation.[4]

L'analyse approfondie de nos activités nous a également apporté une vision plus globale de notre fonction, permettant ainsi une réflexion plus prospective sur son évolution ainsi que sur celle du centre.

Références

[1] Ministère du travail et des affaires sociales, Direction des Hôpitaux. L'information et la documentation à l'hôpital. Paris: Hôpital Expo (Journée d'étude 28 Mars 1996), 1996

[2] Association des professionnels de l'information et de la documentation, Commission des statuts. Référentiel des fonctions des personnels de documentation et d'information de l'administration. ADBS, 19 janvier 1996

[3] Association des professionnels de l'information et de la documentation. Guide pour la caractérisation des profils de compétence des professionnels de l'information et de la documentation. Première partie: Caractérisation des savoirs et savoir-faire. Paris: ADBS, 1995

[4] Sutter E. Les profils de compétence des professionnels de l'information et de la documentation. Documentaliste 1994;31:168-73

NEED AND USE OF TOXICOLOGICAL INFORMATION IN OCCUPATIONAL HEALTH SERVICE

Merja Jauhiainen, Finnish Institute of Occupational Health, Helsinki, Finland

Do databases used in medicine and occupational health cover the needs for toxicological information? What is the role of Medline, in this respect?
There is a growing demand of toxicological information in occupational health services because of (1) increased production of chemical substances, (2) growing awareness of adverse effects of chemicals and (3) changes in legislation. In Finland about one million people are exposed to chemicals and more than 60 000 chemical products are used in industry.

An analysis of the search requests during the past five years, 1991-1995, in the Information Service Centre of The Finnish Institute of Occupational Health has been conducted; 141 searches in toxicology were analysed, which is 12% of all searches in occupational health and safety. Of search requests 83% deal with adverse health effects of chemicals including specific effects on specific organ systems in and 17%. relate to an employee being exposed to chemicals resulting to a specified symptom or disease. The databases used in a CD-ROM network: MEDLINE EXPRESS, TOXLINE and OSH-ROM (SilverPlatter), with the bibliographic databases NIOSHTIC, HSELINE and CISDOC, TOMES PLUS, MICROMEDEX, including RTECS, HSDB, REPRORISK and MEDITEXT, CCINFO (Canadian Centre for Occupational Health and Safety, f.ex. database CHEMINFO). The databases used on-line: EMBASE, BIOSIS. The searches were divided into seven groups based on adverse health effects: adverse effects in general, allergy, respiratory tract diseases, nervous system diseases, carcinogenicity, skin diseases, poisoning. The relevance of obtained references were not assessed.

The most frequent topic of searches deals with adverse effect in general following allergy. The number of databases used for each search showed that searches conducted for adverse effects in general and for carcinogenic effects were few (in average 2.6) compared to other topics (in average 3.8). MEDLINE, TOXLINE and NIOSHTIC were the most usable databases (in more than 60%). They are thus the essential databases as evaluated by the information scientist. Factual databases are applicable in the case of specific topics of adverse effects. The database NIOSH is useful in search for professional related information. Factual databanks HSDB, RTECS, CHEMINFO, REPRORISK and MEDITEXT provide information for risk assessment, first aids and reproduction wich are not so frequently asked for by occupational physicians. In most of the cases the bibliographic databases MEDLINE, TOXLINE and NIOSHTIC provide enough information. The highest degree of applicability is achieved when the search request is well specified and the source is correctly chosen.

S. Bakker (ed.), Health Information Management: What Strategies?, 181.

INFORMATION FOR PEDIATRICIANS: A NEED TO BE SATISFIED?

*Manuela Colombi, Vanna Pistotti** and Giovanna Zuin***, *Schering-Plough S.p.A., **Information consultant, ***Pediatric Department IV University of Milan, Italy

Dissemination of information

A pharmaceutical company has the moral obligation to produce scientific knowledge and distribute it to the scientific community, especially to doctors, family physicians and clinicians, in a way that best suites their needs. The Company had already started some targeted training initiatives for some categories of physicians, such as cardiologists, dermatologists and gastroenterologists. As to pediatricians, the problem was difficult, as the pediatrician is not interested in just one specialty, but for patients within a given range of age, he has to be informed at the same time about gastroenterology, cardiology, infections, endocrinology, dermatology, etc.. Therefore, it was necessary to provide for a reactive service rather than a proactive one, in order to answer the questions physicians have to face from time to time. Moreover, in Italy there are more than 10000 pediatricians and in order to reach all of them it was necessary to study proper solutions.

Aware of the needs of its many associates, The Italian Society of Pediatrics (SIP) asked Schering-Plough to evaluate a proposal for the distribution of information in the shortest time. In co-operation with a company of services skilled in the definition of informatic solutions, Schering-Plough has developed a suitable technical solution. It is based on the installation of a free phone line 'Linea Verde'(green line), where the physician can make his questions, and the starting of the 'Postel' service for a quick forewarding of answers. The service 'Postel' is delivered from the Italian Post Office for the electronic/paper forwarding of correspondence. Furthermore, to a selected group of opinion leaders, a special phone equipment was offered acting as terminal for the direct connection to the operative centre. This was called the 'PILOT' project (Pediatric Italian Link on Telenetwork). As to the scientific contents, the choice was made together with the Company library to adopt the well-known databases Medline, Embase Pediatrics and Current Contents which are already available in an electronic format.

Operators were documentalists graduated in scientific disciplines who answered to the calls in 4 hours' shifts for 5 days in a week for 50 weeks in a year. They were subject to the supervision of a pediatrician and of a senior documentalist.

Through its own scientific sales representatives, Schering-Plough distributed about 9500 identification cards to pediatricians thus offering them the possibility of requiring information about the most different topics. After two years of activity, persevering calling physicians were still about 1750, thus showing a high interest in

S. Bakker (ed.), Health Information Management: What Strategies?, 182-185.

this kind of initiative. Thus, a survey was suggested with the aim of assessing the frequency and reason of calls, the kind of requests and the opinions of interviewed persons about the quality of the received information. The opportunity was taken to assess the presence and the owning of libraries in structures where physicians were active.

Materials and methods

The sample interviewed during the 1995 spring was selected among the users of 1994, equally subdivided into the three Italian geographic areas - North, Centre, South - and exactly shared between family physicians and clinicians. Two-hundred-forty physicians were thus contacted, equal to 13,7% of the users of the Linea Verde Pediatrica (LVP, Pediatric Green Line). Then, 30 users of the PILOT service were contacted, corresponding to 33,3% of the installations.

Two different questionnaires have been preprared for the two groups:
The *LVP questionnaire* aimed at determining the frequency of requests, their topic and reason (update, urgency, congress, drawing-up of scientific articles). An opinion about the material obtained was then asked as well as information about its use. General questions were made to assess the existence and owning of a library at the working site and to know whether and how frequently the physician used updating instruments different from LVP. To the last two questions, the physician had to give his opinion about the usefulness of the service and its future use, if any.

The *PILOT questionnaire* first assessed the physical location of the apparatus as well as the number of potential and actual users. Users had then to assess the services offered, among following ones:

1. bibliographic research concerning topics they themselves required;
2. list of the future national and international congresses, taken from specialized journals and specific databases;
3. SDI from the contents of the top-ten pediatric journals;
4. possibility to exchange messages among the centres involved in the initiative;
5. consultation of the yearbook of the members of the Italian Society of Pediatrics;
6. consultation of the addresses, if and when available, of the specialistic centres.

It was then asked who was the user of the phone equipment and how the user used the answers obtained. In this case, too, the last questions concerned the opinion about the material received and the existence of a library at the working site of the physician together with an opinion about its owning. Further questions concerned the use of other services for scientific documentation.

For the statistical analysis, the data obtained with the questionnaire were collected in three-dimensional tables of contingency and analysed through a two-way-linear model (assignment per geographic area) for categorical data.[1] The parameters of the linear model were assessed by the minimum squares method while the statistical comparisons between parameters were carried out with the Wald method which is distributed as an asymptotic chi-square.[2] The data were processed through CATMOD procedure of the SAS statistical package.[3]

Results

The primary aim of the statistical analysis in the present study is to assess the existence of a significant difference (if any) between the physicians' answers in relation with both their assignment (clinician or family physician) and their geographic location (Northern, Central or Southern Italy).

RESULTS OF THE QUESTIONNAIRE LINEA VERDE PEDIATRICA

Provided that all doctors interviewed had called at least one time, one notice that 53,3% called from 2 to 4 times, with a maximum of 61,3% in the South but without significant differences. The requests were to obtain bibliographic searches (80,8% in the center and 80,4% among hospital physicians). It is interesting to note how the family pediatrician needs information about specialistic centres.

Analysing the reasons for the request two phenomena can be observed: without detriment to the need for updating (94,6%) felt from the family as well as from the hospital physician, it appears how the family physician requires material in case of medical emergencies, while the clinician working within the hospital structure needs the information to support the preparation of scientific articles.

It has been observed how the family pediatricians, and mainly those working in Southern Italy, are satisfied with the quality of the given answers. Though it is not statistically significant, these data show some criticism on behalf of the family physician working in Northern Italy, about the specificity of the answer obtained. This fact does not annul the remarkable and marked satisfaction for the results achieved.

The recieved material was used differently: it can be observed how it is generally enough for the family pediatrician to read an abstract, while the clinician mainly of central Italy looks for the complete article.

Analysing the anwers about the existence of a library at the working site, it can be noted how in the South only 57,5% of those interviewed have a library at the working site, in comparison with 82,5% in Northern and 67,5% in central Italy. The owning of said library is considered by 50% insufficient in the South versus 35% of good in the North. This difference is statistically significant.

In Northern Italy, the presence of journals in English is remarkable, while it decreases in Southern Italy where 43,5% of the texts is still in Italian.

Clinicians make use of libraries and databases to find information, while for family pediatricians the alternative to libraries consists in personal subscription to journals. In central Italy both categories make use of public libraries; in Northern Italy clinicians make good use of the services offered by pharmaceutical companies. This is partly due to the fact that companies are mainly located in Northern Italy and to the fear for the long time needed for information to reach the most extreme areas of the country. The frequency of use of this kind of services is high, tending to be higher in the South than in the North and Center. Nevertheless, in Northern and Central Italy the percentage is higher of those making use of the service from 7 to 15 times a year. In this case, the difference observed turned out to be statistically significant. All the persons interviewed confirmed the usefulness of the given service.

RESULTS OF THE PILOT SERVICE

From the interview to the users of the PILOT services, the statistical evaluation was impossible owing to the small sample and professional homogeneity; all those users are clinicians. For purposes of information, we report only some data we deemed more significant. A marked interest is confirmed in bibliografic searches, to which 72% of those interviewed attributed the maximum score. An even greater interest is shown in SDI (contents from the top-ten journals on pediatrics). In this case, too, it turns out - thus confirming the data obtained from the interviews to clinicians, users of the LVP service - that the material obtained is used for updating purposes and to solve medical emergencies and to draw up articles. The opinion on the quality of the answers is good and excellent in 96% of the cases.

Taking into account the fact that the PILOT service is offered to quite important hospitals throughout the territory, it turns out that 20% of them do not have a library or that their owning is considered rather fair but rarely excellent (4%).

Conclusions

If it is not enough to observe by which sort of assiduity do physicians contact both the LVP and the PILOT service even after three years of service, interviews confirm the interest of Italian pediatricians in these two services offered from Schering-Plough. Usefulness arises from the fact that in some Italian areas, information can be found with difficulty, both from their primary and secondary sources. The great interest in the SDI service, wherefrom it derives the remarkable request for articles, further confirm the datum.

Between the two categories of physicians considered - family and hospital physicians - the first turns out to need more information even owing to the fact that these physicians do not work in organized centres.

In Southern Italy, though in their structures they do not have appropriate libraries (only 33% of those interviewed answer yes to the question concerning the existence of such service) as many as 62% of the interviewed physicians make use of them. The owning of said libraries is mainly in Italian and the fact that the library is consulted more often than databases, where the data are exclusively in English, confirms once again the situation already reported elsewhere of a poor knowledge of English to be ascribed to a great extent to the Italian school.

Thus, though the infrastructure of Italian services has made remarkable steps forward in the offer and distribution of scientific information, areas still exist where the private intervention makes up for an institutional lack. Nevertheless the physicians turned out to be able to assess the quality of the service offered, as shown from the assiduity of phone calls throughout the years, thus urging the company to continue investing in favour of culture.

References

[1] Grizzle JE, Starmer CF, Koch GG. Analysis of categorical Data by linear model. Biometrics 1969;25: 489-504

[2] Wald A. Tests of statistical hypotheses concerning general parameters when the number of observation is large. T Am Math Soc 1943;54:426-482

[3] S.A.S. Institute Inc.: SAS/STAT Guide for peronal computers, Versio 6.Ed. by SAS Institute Inc., Cary NC, p.191-282

[4] Macagno F. Il ruolo dell'ospedale nella formazione del medico specializzando in pediatria. Riv Ital Pediatr 1995;21:419-424

[5] Bausano G. ?L'ho letto sul dinosauro'. Come si aggiorna il medico italiano. Recenti Progressi in Medicina 1995;86:375-377

[6] Gorman PN, Ash J, Wykoff L. Can primary care physicians' questions be answered using the medical journal literature. Bull Med Libr Assoc 1994;82:140-146

[7] Massey Bowden V, Kromer ME, Tobia RC. Assessment of physicians' information needs in five Texas counties. Bull Med Libr Assoc 1994;82:189-196

Thanks are due to Multimedia System for the operative management of the service and for the interviews carried out, as well as to Dr. Erminio Bonizzoni for the qualified statistical analysis.

MARKETING LIBRARY SERVICES TO PRACTISING VETERINARIANS

Raisa Iivonen and Sinikka Suckcharoen, University of Helsinki, Finland

The exhibition of the annual meeting

The Veterinary Library in Finland has participated twice in the exhibition of the Annual Meeting of the Finnish Veterinary Association at the Helsinki Fair Center. Practicing veterinarians gather once a year for three days in the name of continuing education. At the same time and place there is an exhibition, where all the industry related to the veterinary practice is presented i.e. drugs, pet foods, cars etc. There are also stands for the Museum of Veterinary History and the Student Association, and all the animal welfare associations. The two big Finnish bookshops, and some smaller publishers are there, too.

FIRST PRESENTATION IN 1994: CD-ROMS

Our library brought up the new ways of presenting veterinary information to the practising veterinarians for the first time in 1994. We started by introducing VETCD and BEASTCD. All the necessary equipment was brought there, and we made some demonstrations of how to seek information from databases, and how to use the CD-ROM edition. We thought it is the most important thing to bring up, and the vets must be really interested in it. But maybe it was something too unattended - first, a library in a fair (!) and second, something to do with computers.

As a "side product" we also brought all the publications of the College of Veterinary Medicine to be browsed, and we prepared some order forms to be filled in. That was a success, the vets preferred to touch real books and buy them (they were cheap comparing to the prices of our two big bookstores ...) more than look at the computer screen. The consequence was

FINNISH VETERINARY ASSOCIATION
ANNUAL MEETING
Helsinki Fair Center, september/october

Stand of the Veterinary Library 1995:

* PC with modem
  - demonstration of the OPAC catalogue of Veterinary Library (VTLS)
  - borrowers cards
* PC with CD-ROM reader
  - demonstration of VetCD/BeastCD
  - prints
* leaflets
* price-lists
* possibility to buy Publications of the College of Veterinary Medicine (ceased 1995)

S. Bakker (ed.), Health Information Management: What Strategies?, 186-187.

that the library had to sell all the publications from 1995 on. (The other side effect is that the library gets some income of it!)

SECOND PRESENTATION IN 1995: ONLINE CATALOGUE

In the year, 1995, we introduced HELKA, our on-line catalogue, in order to tell our customers that their library has finally changed to the computerized era. For example, our well working service to send books by post directly to practicians, needs that all clients are recorded in the VTLS circulation system. So we made borrowers' cards in situ!

On our stand of 3 m^2 there was also again PC for VETCD and BEASTCD, and the selling stand for the publications, especially the 50-years history book of the college.

Last year the practicians were not so afraid of computers anymore - maybe there were more younger vets, and maybe the need for computerizing small practices is growing. And there are several answers to that need!

Those three days at the Helsinki Fair Center are very interesting, sometimes fun, sometimes quite hard for us. We meet several customers that have been only names on the requests or voices on the phone. Also our "own" teachers and doctors from the Animal Hospital see "their" library in another view. And perhaps one of the most important reasons to be there also in the future is that all the vets in Finland will not anymore be graduated from our faculty. As a member of European Union, Finland accepts examinations from the European veterinary colleges and faculties. All the vets in the field do not know what are their information services in Finland, all the vets do not read properly the journal of their association where we have been writing every now and then about our services.

ARTO TO BE PRESENTED IN 1996

This year, 1996, the Annual Meeting is earlier, i.e. in the end of September. We will bring three PC's to the Helsinki Fair Center, now introducing ARTO, the Article Index of Finnish Journals. Veterinary Library is indexing all the articles about veterinary medicine and animal welfare appearing in Finnish journals. We also index all the articles and monographs written by Finnish veterinarians, whether they were published in national or international journals.

Exchange of ideas and experiences

We would like to hear/read comments from our colleagues whether anybody else have been doing anything of this kind and what kind of experiences they have? What kind of techniques are brought out of the library (we had a modem and direct connection to the Computer Center of the University of Helsinki). What kind of demonstration material do they have, posters, leaflets etc.

MEETING THE CHALLENGE OF THE YEAR 2000 - INFORMATION SUPPORT FOR DECISION MAKERS IN THE DEPARTMENT OF HEALTH

Ian Snowley, Department of Health, London, England

Introduction

Department of Health (DH) Library and Information Services (LIS) exists to meet the operational and strategic information needs of 4,500 Department of Health staff, located throughout England. There are 43 staff in 4 libraries in London and Leeds which are stocked with approximately 200,000 books and pamphlets and 2,000 current periodicals on key areas of Departmental interest in health service management, public health and the personal social services. LIS use a wide range of online and CD-ROM services meet user needs. Departmental staff are linked by a mature Office Information System (OIS), which provides access to a standard suite of Windows software and e-mail.

Levers for change

The Department of Health, in common with all other UK Government departments has been going through a period of contraction for some time now. However, this pressure on staff numbers and budgets has coincided with a period of increased awareness of the value of information in support of decision making (evidence based decision making), and increased demand from end-users for access to information services.

In view of the benefits to be gained from addressing this demand, despite pressure on resources, a decision was taken to maximise the impact of LIS resources by applying a distributed approach to information management. Providing staff direct access to a range of information sources on the desktop. These services are managed centrally by Information Management branch which is therefore able to maintain an overview of all information services provided.

As a result of this all staff now have desktop access to a bespoke Staff Location Database, a Noticeboard, a Press Index, an index to Hansard, travel information and an electronic guide to who does what in the Department. Icons for these items appear together in an 'Information' group on the windows desktop, which will also be used to provide an natural home for future services, such as networked access to CD-ROMs and other databases.

At the same time there has been a recognition that it is not possible for the Department's LIS to hold all the information resources which DH needs and that an

S. Bakker (ed.), Health Information Management: What Strategies?, 188-190.

'access rather than holdings' strategy is now required. One practical example of this is that the Library database (called LION) now includes records of stock borrowed from other libraries in order to facilitate easier re-borrowing in the future.

The aim of this approach is to release Library staff time to work more closely with staff to help them to navigate their way through the mass of information, by providing tailored support for their information seeking activities and to ensure that effective searching and retrieval mechanisms are used.

One spin-off from this policy change is that despite the pressure on resources, some additional money has been found because the value of this work has been clearly recognised.

It is clear that these new approaches require new skills and a new philosophy for training staff. We are starting work on identifying the skills which staff will need to develop to ensure that they can handle the additional demands for information analysis and evaluation which will be required in this new environment.

Cooperation

In order to maximise the staff and other resources available to the Department we have also begun to look around for strategic partners to develop new or existing products. The first of these alliances has been with the National Institute of Social Work (NISW). For a number of years the LIS published and sold on subscription a monthly abstracts bulletin Social Services Abstracts (SSA). In 1995 we decided that it was wasteful to try to compete with NISW's CareData Abstracts and instead reached agreement that we would stop publishing SSA and that they would supply Caredata at a discount to the Department.

The next stage of this process will be for NISW to supply their catalogue records for input to DH-data, thereby reducing the staff effort required on cataloguing and data input. We plan to extend this process to our other abstracts bulletin - Health Service Abstracts (HSA), but will probably link up with a partner from the commercial sector as we don't feel that there is another organisation already active in this area with an existing product.

New sources of DH Information

There was also a recognition that with limited resources the only way the Department could assist the UK Health Information Community in an effective way was by making existing information sources available either through new media such as the Internet or by commercial/cooperative partnerships.

Internet Home Page

The Department has had a presence on the Internet for some time now and has gradually increased the amount of information available, the Library contributes to this and now provides a list of recent DH publications. In addition to these the site provides access to DH press releases via the COI.

There is a great deal of interest in publishing on the Internet within the Department and a policy for this is currently being drafted, as a result there should be an increase in the information made available in the coming year.

HEALTH CD

This is a very important project which the Department has been working on for about a year now in partnership with TSO and Silver Platter. The product will be in the similar to OSH-ROM and will provide the full text of DH publications from 1994 (with some earlier works) onwards.

The disc will be sold on quarterly subscription and the launch is planned for the end of the year. We hope that this will prove to be an important Health resource, both in UK and Europe, and would like to extend its coverage as new issues are released.

HMIC CD

I hope that some of you will have heard of the Healthcare Management Information Consortium (HMIC) which consists of the Libraries of DH, Kings Fund and University of Leeds Nuffield Institute for Health. HMIC was set up in 1992 with the aim to "promote the co-ordination and development of healthcare management Library and information resources"

The three libraries have been working together for a number of years and have recently been working to produce a CD-ROM of their databases (DH-data; HELMIS; KF Library database). This project is coming to fruition and it is likely that Silver Platter will be producing this disc during 1997. This disc will consist of three separate bibliographic databases, although it will be possible to search across all three databases.

The consortium is also working on a joint Thesaurus which is intended to cover the core areas of the three libraries and should consist of between 9,000 and 10,000 post-co-ordinated terms. We hope that this can be included on future issues of the disc, the NHSweb and be used by the healthcare information community as well.

Conclusions

This rather brief snapshot of developments in the Department has, I hope, given you a flavour of the changed world which we will rapidly have to adapt to.

I believe that we can make our own future, but to do so we will need to:

* respond to our changing world
* change our philosophy
* develop new skills

This approach will, I believe, lead us into new roles and a brighter future.

CONTENTS TABLES OF BIOMEDICAL JOURNALS VIA E-MAIL

Marianne Gretz, Peter Stadler, Doris Baumann, Ernst Mernke and Martin Thomas, Boehringer Mannheim GmbH, Germany

Introduction

The central library of Boehringer Mannheim (BM), a research-based pharmaceutical company in Germany with sites at Mannheim, Tutzing and Penzberg (Upper Bavaria), provides its services for some 6.500 employees engaged in therapeutics, diagnostics and biochemicals at the Mannheim site. Besides the library three information departments (Medical Information, Chemical-pharmaceutical Information and Diagnostics-related Information) ensure comprehensive supply of information in Mannheim, while the central library's task is to supply the original literature.

Two decades ago, the central library routed journals to its clients. With the advent of copiers, there was a switch towards copied tables of contents. However, due to recent cuts in staff this service could no longer be offered. The electronic supply of tables of contents was considered as an alternative.

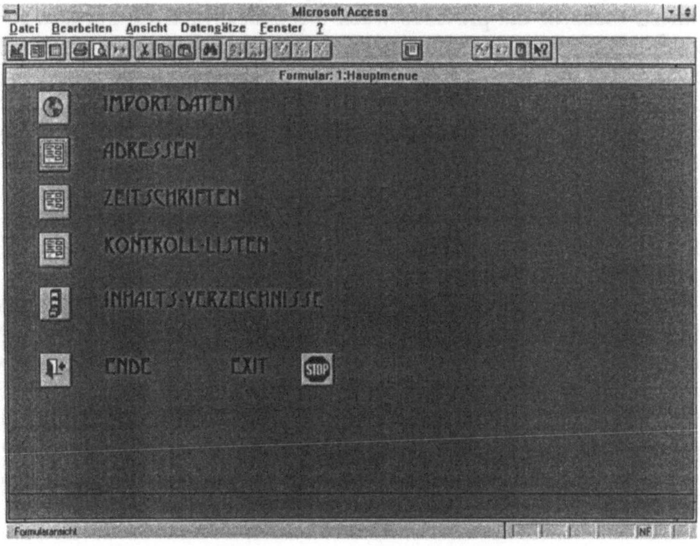

Figure 1. Main menu of the MS-Access component of BM-SwetScan

The "raw" product SwetScan and preliminary work by the library

As BM has been cooperating with Swets for more than 10 years, their product

S. Bakker (ed.), Health Information Management: What Strategies?, 191-193.

"SwetScan" was tested.[1] SwetScan contains the tables of contents, scanned and automatically processed, of more than 14.000 scientific journals of all fields.

BM selected some 300 titles of journals the library is subscribing to. BM-SwetScan is the combination of: SwetScan raw data, MS-ACCESS database and cc:Mail.

SwetScan raw data on disk are delivered once a week. A feature which both processes the raw data and assigns them to the respective addressees has been programmed by the information technology department. Whenever the new data are imported those of the previous week are overwritten on purpose so that only the most recent data are available for dispatch. Some preparatory work by the library was necessary for the MS-ACCESS application to function properly. A file containing the addressees' names identical to the one in cc:Mail had to be produced (fig. 2), and files containing the journal titles including the International Standard Serial Number (ISSN) and BM-internal codes (fig. 3). Then a link had to be established between the addressees and the journal titles selected, and the preferred mailing system (cc:Mail, BM internal surface mail, facsimile) had to be entered. For the MS-ACCESS application five menu options were created in order to approach all functions.

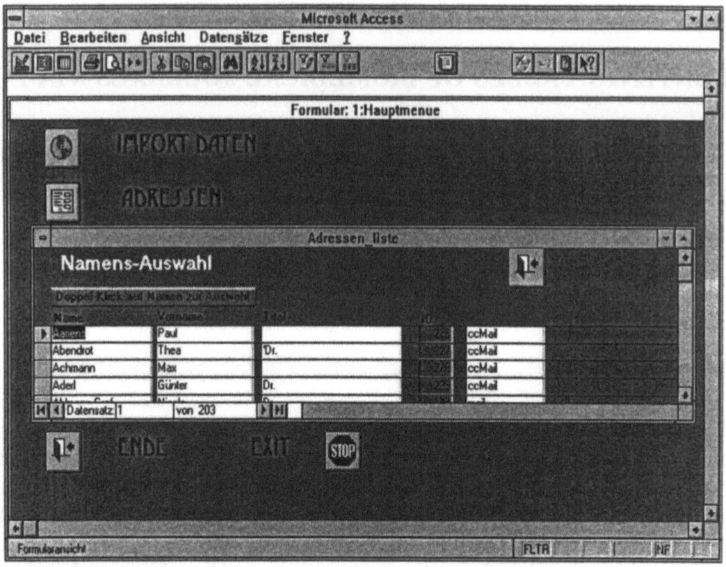

Figure 2. File of addresses in the MS-Access component of BM-SwetScan

While the programming and the preparatory work in the library were under way all clients on the list for "traditional" photocopied tables of contents were made aware of the forthcoming change by a letter explaining the project and suggesting the switch. The response was excellent; quite a number of new clients who had not received copied tables of contents in the past showed great interest in this new service. The subscription fees for the electronic tables of contents of one journal are at present DM 14 per year, irrespective of the number of contents pages per journal or per year. This is a practicable solution simplifying the payment procedure with Swets & Zeitlinger considerably.

Results

At present the BM-SwetScan package comprises roughly 340 journals for roughly 200 different clients. Importing the raw data into the MS-ACCESS application, processing the data and dispatching them to the individual clients takes about half an hour per week. The electronic mail is much faster than the internal mail, so one of the most important criteria - speed - has been fulfilled. Clients are given an information package tailored to their individual needs and preferences. Moreover, once the service is installed they do not have to ask actively for information, but rather "automatically" find in their computers a message from the library containing the tables of contents chosen. Each delivery from the library contains an integrated header referring to the originator, the central library, of this information service. The user has to make his or her own copies; however, with exceptions in urgent cases.

An electronic order function has not yet been installed, because shortage in staff in the library does not allow such a copying service. Moreover it was our aim to prevent the library being flooded by copy requests for articles revealing themselves as useless later on. The same reasons may prompt the library at the University of Heidelberg to introduce fees for electronic document delivery service once the test phase is over.[2]

The electronic mail system is being extended worldwide to all sites of BM. This could open up new opportunities for the library to act as centre of competence.

Although the new service has been well received, there are some critical points. Only the header tells the reader what journal the table of contents belongs to. There is nothing left to help the reader to recognize the familiar layout of e.g. "The Lancet". Differentiations in typesetting like different sizes or types of characters helping to structure and to evaluate the contents of a journal no longer exist.[3]

Conclusion

BM-SwetScan is a valuable service tailored to individual needs; it is flexible and economical. Contacts between library and clients are intensified by regular electronic deliveries. The regular service reminds users constantly of the library and its services. The library stands out as a forward-looking centre of competence for fast and efficient provision of information and literature.

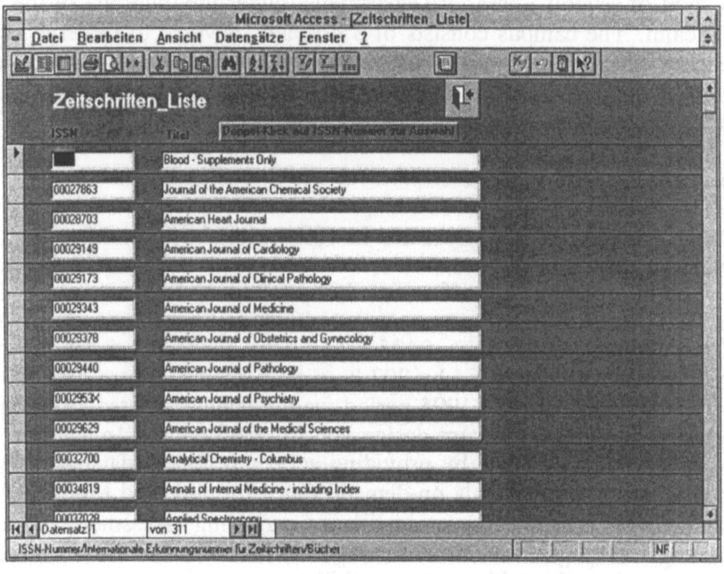

Figure 3. List of journals in the MS-Access component of BM-SwetScan

References

[1] Lampe K. SwetScan: ein neuer InhaltsverzeichnisService für Bibliotheken Liber Q 1994;4:88-95

[2] Eckes A, Pietzsch E. Electronic Document Delivery an der Universitätsbibliothek Heidelberg: elektronische Bestellung und Lieferung von Zeitschriftenaufsätzen. Bibliotheksdienst 1995;29:1797-1802

[3] Kallner H, Modan M, Modan B, Wolman M. Contents page format in scientific journals - effect on efficiency and ease of scanning. Meth Inf Med 1977;16:106-110

INTERNET ACCESS AND UTILIZATION IN BIOMEDICAL RESEARCH AT THE VALL D'HEBRON HOSPITALS

Marta Jordà-Olives, Hospitals Vall d'Hebron, Barcelona, Spain

Vall d'Hebron Hospitals

The Research and Teaching Department of the Vall d'Hebron Hospitals was formed according to a government bill issued on December 12, 1990, recommending the creation of several Research Departments under the umbrella of the Catalan Institute of Health. The campus consists of 3 hospitals devoted to General Medicine, Materno-Pediatry, and Traumatology, and 4 buildings for central services: Blood Bank, Microbiology, Anatomical-Pathology, Central Administration and Research Department. The number of beds is 1,453; the number of staff is 6,800 (1,319 medical).

Information Unit

The Information Unit was created in 1994 to establish an infrastructure to cover the medical researchers' information needs and to serve these 571 potential users.

The information unit offers email, ftp, telnet and net navigation tools. Also we deal with web page assessment, user training and help desk. By December 1995 48 PCs, implying a minimum of 125, users were connected to the network and 44 training seminars, attended by 202 hospital personnel, were offered.

The activities for the 1995 period were computer-related like connection of PCs, software installation, system design and troubleshouting. In addition we dealt with information-related work by providing access to remote databases (eg. Genbank), printing electronic journals on-demand (eg. Mortality and Morbidity Weekly Report), managing the internal discussion list and providing assessment and support for building web pages. Our user training activities were centered on the elaboration of user manuals and teaching internet skills.

Conclusions

The electronic mail is the best known internet tool and helps to improve professional opportunities. However internet navigation is seen to be less worthwhile than the media says and it is not possible to confirm the quality and reliability of the information obtained through this media. Although there is no credibility regarding practical applications, there is a social interest in navigation.

As people are demanding better internal information infrastructures, Intranet is anticipated to be useful in broad areas of every day internal work.

S. Bakker (ed.), Health Information Management: What Strategies?, 194.

SETUP AND USE OF THE WEB-SITE OF THE LIBRARY KNAW

Joop Dijkman and Janine Lentz, Library KNAW, Amsterdam, the Netherlands

Introduction

The Library KNAW, one of Europe's largest specialized libraries for the biomedical disciplines, is used by a wide range of people inside and outside the Netherlands. The World Wide Web (WWW) is a very powerful medium for offering information access to such a widely dispersed group of users.

The Web-site of the Library KNAW not only contains brochure-like information about the Library, but has links to other biomedical sites on the Internet, and also contains 'content', including different (bibliographic) databases, some developed by the Library KNAW exclusively for presentation on the Web. The results can be seen at: **http://www.library.knaw.nl**

Presenting databases on the Web

Several options exits to present databases on the Web. To make use of specifically developed client-software is not user-friendly as the customer has to retrieve and install the client on his/her computer; another disadvantage would be that the Library KNAW had to develop this software. The option to offer databases with a telnet interface would bypass the advantages of Internet connections.

The most convenient option for our customers was to make use of a general web browser, leading to the following approach:

User side (client)	*Library side (server)*
- General Web browser (Netscape etc.)	- HTTP Deamon
	- CGI scripts
	- Search engine (PLS)
	- Databases (OPAC etc.)
	- (normal) HTML pages

(The 'Z39.50 gateway' solution was far from stable at the time this approach was developed, so this option was excluded.)

This Web client-server system is quite different from most stand-alone software and OPAC's used in libraries. It is possible to browse through databases and to search in specific fields, but always with the restriction that you get only 'one page'

S. Bakker (ed.), Health Information Management: What Strategies?, 195-198.

at a time. After this 'one page' you can easily jump to another Web-site.

However, with CGI scripts it is possible to create a rather sophisticated user-interface. These scripts are very flexible and a skilled programmer can easily make adjustments. A major drawback is that any change in server software or search engine and for each new database format adjustments to the CGI scripts have to be made.

Notwithstanding the 'one page' restriction a user interface was built for several databases, with some powerfull CGI scripts. Search screen, search and browse options are tailored to each database and indexes are made by the search engine.

Presentation of the Web-site

The actual presentation on the screen depends on the Internet connection, the hardware, software and the browser adjustments of the user. It is presumed that most customers make use of a Windows operating system, with a minimum of a 486-microprocessor, 28K8 modem and 256 colours.

The Web-site was tested with several versions of Netscape, Mosaic and the Internet Explorer.

WHAT IS PRESENTED AND HOW

During the first few months after the launch of the Web-site the main focus was on 'what to present'. As the Web-site became more complex the presentation of the main index was changed and a graphical designer was recruited to bring visual unity into the myriad of Web pages: each 'page' got the same background image (with a specific color for each main group, see below) and each 'page' got an image on top (the header) with the following options:

- go to the main index
- search for a specific page
- a mail address
- a general help funtion

Although the design of the Web pages is very important, even more important is the logical structure. The Web-site of the Library KNAW is divided into 4 main groups:

General information. This group contains information about the library, prices, employees, organization etc. (like in a brochure).

Services of the Library KNAW, e.g.:
- The **OPAC**: bibliographic data (26.000 serials, of which 10.000 current, and a large number of books, reports and dissertations) converted and presented on the Web.
- The **table of contents** from approx. 750 international biomedical journals from 1994 onward is put into a database, in which an article can be searched either directly, or via journal title and the table of contents of a specific issue.
- A database with the **table of contents** of approx. 70 Dutch medical journals. Although database structure and presentation is the same as for the international journals, a new method was developed to scan the contents and to load the data.
- The **'Dutch Dissertations'** database gives a colourful presentation of otherwise grey literature, i.e. Dutch biomedical dissertations from 1994 onward. Not only the bibliographic data are shown, but also a picture of the front cover, a summary and the reference list of the articles on which the dissertation is based.
- A **directory of biotechnological research** with research descriptions and institutional addresses in Europe (BIOREP).

- A **document order form** to which results from a bibliographic search can be automatically copied and only name and address have to be filled in.

Links to other (medical) sources on the Internet. A searchable database is build with data collected from these sources.

Presentation in cooperation with Dutch biomedical organizations of a number of relevant Web-sites

While building a Web-site many problems, some technical, some organizational, will be encountered, but most difficult is the dillema between presenting too much information on one page and making too many hypertext links. The structure of the Web-site should be clear and each page should have some links to other relevant pages and a link to the main index. The presentation of the main index and the number of hypertext-links on this index are of crucial importance.

User survey

Statistics show that every week approx. 10.000 Web-pages are consulted by approx. 1.500 different IP-addresses. Feed-back was received from quite a number of these users, but a more structured user survey was necessary as a public opinion poll. This survey consisted of three parts:

A *questionnaire* regarding the hardware and software used, and user characteristics.
An *observation* of users carrying out 10 (known item) searches and navigation tasks.
A *structured interview* to get an impression of what the user thinks of the Web-site.

Twenty-six persons took part in this user survey: 13 librarians and 13 medical specialists. Most surveys lasted approx. 2 hours and took place at the workplace and -station of the users.

Results from this user survey and tips for building a Web-site

In general, users were impressed by the features of this well maintained Web-site (not many dead links) with a lot of services and an elegant graphical design. About one third was very enthousiastic, 50% was positive, but had some critical remarks and one sixth was rather negative.

NAVIGATING THE WEB-SITE

Navigating such a large Web-site was for most people rather difficult. It took some time before they understood the structure of the Web-site. The most heard complaint was about the main index. Originally the main index showed only 4 groups, each with a link to a detailed list. After the implementation of the new design and the reorganization of the index, the whole main index was presented on one page. Instead of giving an overview, this presentation turned out to be very confusing to the users; therefore the old situation will be restored (but with the new layout).

GRAPHICAL DESIGN & IMAGES

Know the characteristics of your Web-site users, take this into account when making the graphical design and, above all, tell your designer! There is a great difference between Web surfers who like fancy images and researchers who prefer no-nonsense and easy-to-use screens. Uniform and elegant designed Web pages are appreciated if not bringing down response time (when loading) or taking too much screen space (for scrolling). The main index will be revised as the survey showed that loading took too much time. Experienced users are impatient and will go to another site, even when the lack of speed is due to their own hardware, software, or internet provider.

Loading images is time consuming. Do present text alternatives for 'functional images', and whenever clickable text is used within an image, make sure it is self-evident to everyone. (e.g. presentation like a command button).

HELP FUNCTION

By seeing a 'Help-button' users expect context-oriented help. As this is very difficult and time-consuming to make, in-build help functions will be limited.

SEARCHING IN DATABASES

Although (free) access to so much information is convenient, for most users the many different search screens before reaching the information is rather confusing. All search screens are based on the same concept, with only slight differences adapted to the database. To have a results-page model presented at the beginning of a database search was not appreciated; the user preference of only one (or a few) integrated search screen will be granted and implemented soon. The search screens are easy enough to work with, well presented and offer sufficient options to limit a search.

About 20% of the search questions/navigation tasks was unsuccessful. Most difficulties occurred when searching for authors; a specific author-index would be greatly appreciated.

The user survey showed - not unexpected - differences in searching by librarians and biomedical researchers/physicians. Librarians use Boolean operators (especially AND) and word truncation more often and are unique in using index terms. Both groups were in favour of splitting the search screens into two versions: a simple one for beginners and another for advanced searchers.

As long as the results comply with user's expectations, the search algorithm (a combination of Relevance ranking and Boolean logic) does not seem to matter.

Users find it very convenient that the result of a bibliographic search can be uploaded automatically to the Document Order Form.

Conclusion

In the Netherlands the Library KNAW Web-site is often referred to as a good example showing Internet possibilities. The results of the user survey will be taken into account by making improvements notwithstanding technical limitations. Nevertheless the main objective still is and will be the creation of a user-friendly Web-site.

SILENT REVOLUTION IN THE LIBRARY: ELECTRONIC MEDIA REPLACE PRINTED PRODUCTS

Martin Thomas, Marianne Gretz and Peter Stadler, Boehringer Mannheim GmbH, Mannheim, Germany

Objective

The pharmacopoeias at Boehringer Mannheim Germany (BM) serve as an example to demonstrate the switch from printed products to electronic media. Preparatory work, economy and the actual procedure at the central library are analysed.

Pharmacopoeias are typically delivered as loose-leaf editions with supplies or basic editions with supplements. Multiple subscriptions have to be initiated and cared for, and supplements must be incorporated into the already available collections. Filing away new supplements is often delegated to employees without knowledge of librarianship. Difficulties in updating and searching are therefore almost inevitable.

Would work become easier and more efficient both for the library and the respective departments if printed versions were switched to electronic ones? Would savings in working hours be compensated for by higher costs? How would customers accept the new service?

Methods

To compare the vast amount of (often differently structured) information regarding printed and electronic versions, a form sheet was developed (Fig. 1).

A five-year period was chosen to clarify the economy of a potential switch. For the costs of the first year, the number of subscribers is multiplied by the price of the basic paper edition. Then the number of subscribers is multiplied by the costs of the supplements for one year and by four to cover four years. Adding these two figures results in the overall costs of the printed version for a period of five years. Increases in price are not considered in this calculation. The prices of the network versions for the first year and for the updates for four subsequent years were calculated likewise with prices pertaining to the number of potential concurrent users.

Results

Loose-leaf editions can be handled much more easily in electronic form compared to paper editions. The number of subscribers and thus the number of deliveries can be reduced. Invoices and claims will decrease. For ensuring smooth running of the

S. Bakker (ed.), Health Information Management: What Strategies?, 199-202.

applications, specialist data-processing knowledge has to be available, especially during vacations or in case of illness.

Electronic databases are current, provided that producers supply updates regularly and in time. Compared with paper editions one single entity of data can be searched in electronic versions while with paper editions a search might include several supplements. Filing away supplements or loose leaves is no longer necessary. This saves the end-users a lot of time and ensures completeness. Often entire loose-leaf editions had to be bought again, because of filing mistakes. Electronic versions also help saving shelf space, as most paper editions consist of several files.

BM subscribes to more than a thousand loose-leaf editions for 170 different departments. Each year approximately 2,500 loose-leaf supplies are received. Supposed that filing away one such supply takes only 15 minutes on average, this will add up to 78 workdays of 8 hours each. With an estimated savings potential of only 50% of this time, as not all loose-leaf editions will be replaced by electronic versions, 39 workdays can be saved: i.e. roughly 2 months of working hours. On the other hand, time will still be needed in the library for registering deliveries, paying invoices or sending claims. However, working hours (wage costs) and original costs (see 5-year comparison) will be saved to quite an unexpected extent. The qualitative improvement in searching electronic media goes along with actual savings.

More than 50% of the subscribers to paper editions of pharmacopoeias returned the completed form sheets. For 5 out of 7 items the subscribing departments were willing to pay for the respective network versions. For two pharmacopoeias the decision has been deferred.

Surprisingly, departments not yet having subscribed to paper editions, wished access to the electronic version and agreed to pay their share. The initiative to switch media has aroused new interest and met a demand not evident beforehand. In addition, the form sheet revealed who else needed the same literature and dealt with similar work.

Discussion

Provided that technical requirements are fulfilled (availability of network and suitable PCs), our analysis revealed that even a partial replacement of printed pharmacopoeias by electronic media clearly improves the library's service to end-users and saves considerable costs for the company. However, costs for acquisition and maintenance of PCs and network have not been included in the calculations.

The confronting display of costs for a five-year period shows the unambiguous savings potential of electronic media. All users profit, since updating and searching information is made much easier by electronic versions of pharmacopoeias. Installation and maintenance of the data processing equipment (network server) require considerable technical know-how.

End-users must have certain knowledge in handling PCs and software. At present almost every CD-ROM unfortunately requires a different approach. For those using CD-ROMs only rarely, this can be a real drawback. Accessing electronic data depends considerably on the way search functions are represented on the screen. Very often end-users are not aware of the underlying search mechanisms. A well elaborated help function available online seems indispensable, in particular, as by accessing databases via networks user manuals are seldom available.[1]

The acceptance by the end-users is a critical point. Potential savings connected with the introduction of the electronic versions have convinced most of those responsible for budgets. However, these persons are not the ones actually using the system. Filing away loose leaves used to be a task delegated to rather unqualified people; with electronic media, know-how in handling PCs and in particular handling electronically processed literature is necessary. Training people in this respect takes more time than showing them how to file away leaves. Librarians are expected to support their clients in this new area. Several studies showed that inexperienced or untrained users found only a fraction of the information on CDs compared with experienced and well-trained searchers.[2,3] The investment in time and money will be compensated for by better searching and actually finding information. The employees need certain qualifications and the willingness to work with electronic media. Then innovations induced by the library are likely to be accepted and well-received by end-users, much more so, once the increased efficiency and the decreased workload become obvious.

Conclusion

The use of electronic databases instead of printed loose-leaf editions means a considerable improvement in the supply of information within the company. Using the electronic versions instead of the paper editions leads to clear cost savings. By supplying and taking care of the databases the library keeps the overall charge in its most genuine field and creates a distinctive image as a modern and efficient provider of service. The central availability of the data allows access from almost any workplace within the Boehringer Mannheim site. Even end-users needing such information only rarely thus have (almost) unrestricted access. Standardisation of search and display screens is desirable, thus increasing the user friendliness of the systems. Nevertheless, the switch from print products to electronic media is an asset for end-users indeed. They appreciate the services rendered for them by the library.

References

[1] Goedert W. Multimedia-Enzyklopaedien auf CD-ROM: Eine vergleichende Analyse von Allgemeinenzyklopaedien, Informationsmittel für Bibliotheken, Beiheft 1. Berlin: Deutsches Bibliotheksinstitut, 1994

[2] Cannell S. User reactions to CD-ROM in a medical library. In: SCIL 89. Proceedings of the Third Annual Conference on Small Computers in Libraries, London, 1989:115-118

[3] Lancaster FW, Elzy C, Zeter MJ, Metzler L, Loew YM. Searching databases on CD-ROM: Comparison of the results of end-user searching with results from two modes of searching by skilled intermediaries. RQ 1994;33:370-386

Figure 1: Form sheet for comparison of printed vs. electronic versions

Central library (TF-MLB) 10th February, 1996
Peter Stadler, phone 2376

To all subscribers of printed pharmacopoeias or reference books

Switch from printed to electronic versions

Bibliographic data

Title	**United States Pharmacopeia / National Formulary**	
Printed version:	**Basic edition with supplements**	
Publisher:	**US Pharmacopeial Convention Inc.**	

Prices

Basic edition Print	225 US$	
Supplements Print	241 US$	
CD-ROM net	4000 US$ (for 5 concurrent users)	
Update net	4000 US$	

Subscribers within Boehringer Mannheim (Paper edition)

Department, Name	TF-CA Dr. S.	
	TF-GS Library	
	TF-MLB Central library	
	TF-MP Dr. B.	
	TF-RA Mrs. S.	
	TF-RAU Mr. R.	
	TH-CK Mr. D.	
	TH-PDT Mr. B.	
	TQ Prof. K.	
	TQ-A Dr. W.	
	TQ-BK Dr. V.	
	TQ-BS Dr. S.	
	TQ-E library (Mrs. L.) 9 copies	
Total:	**21 subscriptions**	

Economy (ratio print vs. electronic version

Paper edition / expenses for 5 years		**CD-ROM / expenses for 5 years**		
21x US$225=US$ 4.725 (1st year)		1 x US$4.000 (1st year)		
21x $241=5061x4 yrs=US$20.244 (4yrs)		4x$4000=US$16.000 (4 yrs)		
Sum	**US$ 24.969**	**Sum**	**US$ 20.000**	

OMNI: QUALITY BIOMEDICAL NETWORKED INFORMATION RESOURCES

*Sue Welsh and Betsy Anagnostelis**, *National Institute for Medical Research, **Royal Free Hospital School of Medicine, London, UK

Introduction

It is surely a sign that the Internet is maturing that so much effort is being devoted to improving access to its content. In May this year that most style-conscious of Internet journals, Wired, devoted its cover piece to the subject of indexing the 'Net, and significantly dismissed library science as 'almost no help'[1]. It is a problem which simultaneously challenges the imaginations of the Internet's brightest minds and its novices; while Stanford graduates[2] and Digital researchers[3] try to answer everyone's query with a single retrieval system, every new medical school webmaster lists a few hand-picked sites as a starting point for their own users.

In between these two extremes are services providing small databases of materials selected on the basis of quality, subject and sometimes country of origin. These subject based information gateways do not aim to give undifferentiated access to every site on the Web (as automated search engines do) but rather provide enhanced search and browse facilities to a few hundred/thousand items.

The OMNI Project began work over a year ago on a service targeted at the UK higher education and research community. Our aim is to provide selective access to biomedical Internet resources world-wide, plus a comprehensive database of UK resources. One of the first things we did was to come to the last EAHIL conference in Prague to announce the project, in the hope of making contact with other initiatives in Europe. The purpose of this paper is to explore the relationship and the possibility of collaboration between the various European gateways.

Review of Current Activity

There are of course many listings of biomedical resources across Europe. The examples that follow are not a comprehensive list but are intended to be illustrative. The gateways that exist presently can be divided into:

Resources listed by country. There is perhaps a perception that large US based services such as Yahoo fail in their coverage of non-US resources, these services seek to redress the balance. The Hopitaux de Rouen[4] offers such a resource for French sites, and there is another example at Frankfurt University[5] in Germany.

Quality resources from around the globe. Many more, however, cover resources from around the globe such as the Anatomish Institute at the University of Oslo[6], and

S. Bakker (ed.), Health Information Management: What Strategies?, 203-205.

MIC-KIBIC at the Karolinska Institute in Sweden[7] (who are recommended by the Whole Internet Catalogue[8]).

Euro search engines. Occasionally subject-based services offer search facilities (for example OMNI[9]) but most rely on well organised browsable lists to guide their users to appropriate resources.

In addition to these subject specific gateways, there are a few search engines which offer non-subject specific access to European resources, for example, Euroferret[10] claims to index only European resources, while HotBot[11] offers the option to restrict to European domain names (.uk, .de, etc).

There are no Europe-wide, collaborative projects that we know of at this time. However, the European Union is funding research in the area of resource discovery and retrieval. The DESIRE[12] (Development of a European Service for Information on Research and Education) Project, part of the EU's Telematics Application Programme will be looking at solutions to some of the problems faced by researchers finding information on the Web, including indexing/cataloguing and quality control for subject based information gateways.

Diversity of Approach

The examples listed above indicate that there is much work being done, especially at the institutional or departmental level. We may identify some key features:

Scale. There is a great diversity of scale ranging from tens to many hundreds of resources.

Arrangement. There are almost as many ways of classifying resources as there are attempts to classify them! Local services arrange their services in such a way as to address the needs of their own particular community, while national services may use a recognised library classification scheme or medical thesaurus.

Metadata. Information about the resource listed is absent from most services. Some services supply a link only while some offer a brief description

Mode of access. The distinctive nature of many of the listings we have looked at reflects not only the perspective of the communities they are intended for, but also the amount of time available to the author, and the complexity and maturity of the Internet scene in that country.

In contrast to the apparent variety described above, the nature of the activity which constructs these databases and resource lists is very similar. It can be summarised as:

(i) *Discovery.* We are all Internet users and in the course of our work, whether by serendipity or design, we find new resources.

(ii) *Evaluation.* An assessment of the resource ensues, which may be formal or informal. Few services make available their evaluation criteria, which implies an informal approach is practiced in most cases.

(iii) *Inclusion or discard.* As a result of (ii) the resource is included or excluded.

Co-operation

The aim of co-operation between services must be to combine our individual efforts and thereby create something that is greater than the sum of the individual services. This might be a Europe-wide gateway, or an enhancement of the various national services (by an increase in depth or range.)

We should aim to offer easier access, to more resources, for more of our users, and to create a new and different service, not a replacement for the individual listings which are now in place. The local list of key sites will always be of value, despite the existence of a European-wide list, just as everyone maintains a personal hotlist even though their institution has a local listing. The most effective access to information on the Web by an individual is the result of an appreciation of the various levels of access, which of us uses one search tool for every query?

The challenge which is the result of this diversity is finding routes to collaboration even though we are all doing, quite rightly, "our own thing".

The barriers to creating a Europe-wide service are real and should not be dismissed casually.

Diversity. A diversity of approach dictated by different audience requirements and by lack of database and metadata standards.

Time and opportunity. Many of us are not full time Internet gurus! It will take time and effort to bring our disparate activities together. As for opportunity, EAHIL is one example of a forum that offers us scope to meet, while the Internet itself makes face to face communication unnecessary.

Language. The language barrier is a real challenge. It may be acceptable to all of us that this conference is being conducted in French and English, but if we were similarly restrictive on the Internet, how many of our prospective audience would we exclude or alienate?

Conclusion

The Internet is a key new resource for health librarians. Many individual efforts to improve access on a local or national basis are underway, but these initiatives do not often achieve global visibility. By pooling our resources we may at the very least benefit from sharing experience and may be able to collaborate to improve access to resources across Europe, thus answering our critics in Wired and elsewhere, and proving that librarianship has a role in the newest information environment.

References

[1] Wired. 1996;(May):108
[2] See Yahoo. <URL:**http://www.yahoo.com/**>
[3] See Alta Vista. <URL:**http://www.altavista.digital.com/**>
[4] <URL:**http://www.chu-rouen.fr/dsii/html/servsant.html**>
[5] <URL:**http://www.klinik.uni-frankfurt.de/findex/index.htm**>
[6] <URL:**http://www.med.uio.no/imb/anatomi/biomed.htm**>
[7] <URL:**http://www.mic.ki.se/Diseases/index.html**>
[8] <URL:**http://www.gnn.com/gnn/wic/index.html**>
[9] <URL:**http://omni.ac.uk/**>
[10] <URL:**http://www.muscat.co.uk/**>
[11] <URL:**http://www.hotbot.com/**>
[12] <URL:**http://www.surfnet.nl/surfnet/projects/desire/desire.html**>

MEDICAL NETWORKED INFORMATION IN THE CZECH REPUBLIC

Otakar Pinkas, National Medical Library, Czech Republic

CESNET (Czech Educational and Scientific Network), the most effective and most widely used computer network in the Czech Republic, aims to assist the sphere of education and research but is open also to other commercial and non-commercial organizations. It became operational in 1992. Through CESNET nearly 30 Czech towns are interconnected. The number of CZ domain nodes exceeds 15,000. Information on CESNET is available on **http://www.cesnet.cz/**.
Health Informatics Programme, projected by the Ministry of Health, includes: Communication networks, National Health Information System (personal data, communication, standards); health statistics; information systems of health establishments; electronic patient record; health libraries. Financial means are allocated for purchase of hardware and software and for Internet participation. However, there is no special programme centrally funding a computerized network in the field of health care. The still continuing transformation of health services in the CR makes that most of finances is spent on local information systems in hospitals.
CESNET information sources. Czech medical information resources with WWW service may be divided as follows: government resources, faculties and health establishments resources, resources of other institutions. The major part of Web pages is accessible in English and most servers support code selection of Czech texts (see: **http://www.cesnet.cz/html/cesnet/cesnet-resources.html**).

Government resources offer a rich scope of information on their own activities but also health directories, methodical instructions, legislative regulations, drug lists, references to other sources in the CR and abroad. The Web server of the Ministry of Health (**www.mzcr.cz**) is the most prominent source of medical information.

In the CR 7 medical, 2 social health and 2 pharmaceutical faculties have altogether 9,000 students. The scope of information differs from site to site, usually including information on the history and organization of the faculty, its training and Internet resources etc. The site of the 2nd Medical Faculty in Prague **www.lf2.cuni.cz** is one of the best. A few servers can be found in teaching hospitals and research institutes. In 1996 the first primary medical journals have appeared on Czech WWW servers.

About 20 university libraries and 10 municipal or governmental libraries offer information on the web (see: **www.cbvk.cz/libracz.html**). The most important ones are: The National Library, Prague (**www.nkp.cz**), The Moravian Library, Prague (**www.mzk.cz**), The Faculty of Medicine, Brno (telnet://**knihovna.muni.cz** LOGIN: TINLIB, PASSWORD:-, CATALOG: 4) and the National Medical Library, Prague (**www.nlk.anet.cz**).

S. Bakker (ed.), Health Information Management: What Strategies?, 206.

WEBIS, IBIS, AGMB, MEDIBIB-L: INTERNET PROJECTS IN GERMANY

Oliver Obst, University of Münster, Germany

Internet projects in Germany

WEBIS

The main purpose of WEBIS, WEB (Bibliotheks) Information System, is to guide the user to the German library which owns most books and non-book material in the subject area in question. There is no single library in Germany as great and comprehensive as the British Library, the Library of Congress or the Bibliothèque Nationale; instead 35 libraries cooperate and acquire with financial support from the German Research Association, book and non-book material in 113 areas of human knowledge. Until now one had to go to the library for the specialized collection. A Bavarian chemist has to travel 500 km to the library of Hannover which is responsible for this very subject area, and a Saxonian clinician has to travel all the way through Germany to the Central Medical Library to Cologne. WEBIS eases access by providing a unique Internet entry point to these specialized collections and information services (**http://wwwsub.sub.uni-hamburg.de/webis**). There you will be able to search each library's OPAC, download a list of recent acquisitions, take a look at specialized CD-ROMs and request searches in them, make questions to the subject specialist by Email, order documents or mail suggestions for acquisition. In the future you will also find links to Internet sources in each subject area. For example, if you choose medicine & psychology from the main menu you will be guided to the subject area of medicine, which provides detailed definition of the subjects covered. There you will find a link to the German National Library of Medicine.

IBIS

Whereas WEBIS is devoted to electronic access to more or less traditional services, IBIS (Internet-Based Information System) offers electronic access to Internet sources (**http://www.ub.uni-bielefeld.de/ibis.html**). The goal of IBIS is quite the same as that of OMNI with two differences worth mentioning: First, IBIS will cover not only medicine but all subject areas, and second, IBIS will be funded in hardware and software but not as to the staff. Instead of being dependent on volunteers and dedicated staff, IBIS will be cooperatively maintained at each university library as a part of the routine work of the subject specialists. This project is supported by the

S. Bakker (ed.), Health Information Management: What Strategies?, 207-209.

German Ministry of Education, Science, Research and Technology as well as by the federal state North-Rhine Westphalia.

IBIS selects, evaluates, annotates, indexes, and catalogues Internet sources of local, regional, national, and world wide origin (in that order). The catalogued and indexed Internet sources could than be searched side by side with traditional media in one of the greatest German union book catalogues (**http://www.hbznrw.de/hbz/Komma.html**). The Internet sources are subject indexed with MeSH as well as classified according to the "Regensburger Classification".

Although acquisition and archiving are still unsolved problems, they will also be a major part of this service in the near future. Because of the gigantic task of providing a selected access to Internet sources the success will heavily depend on the widest cooperation possible, may it be German-wide, Europe-wide, or world-wide.

In contrast to these two previously mentioned projects, the following two projects were initiated by myself because I felt responsible to facilitate information exchange between German-speaking medical librarians.

MEDIBIB-L

When I started my job in 1993 there was no framework for information exchange between medical librarians beside the annual meeting. At first I thought of a printed newsletter to keep the members of the profession informed, but gave it up because of the accompayning problems. Later on when I was more familiar with the Internet it occurred to me that an electronic discussion list would perfectly meet this information need beside being free of charge and easy to manage. So in early 1994 I started MEDIBIB-L (Medizinbibliotheken-Liste). Although somewhat slow in the beginning, MEDIBIB-L has today about 160 members and is quite successful as a communication forum for German-speaking medical librarians. Interestingly, many medical librarians from outside Central Europe subscribe to MEDIBIB-L - probably out of interest for German medical librarianship. In many ways MEDIBIB-L serves today as a center of competence for questions regarding information needed in medical libraries (**http://medweb.uni-muenster.de/zbm/medibib.html**).

AGMB-HOMEPAGE

The announcement of the homepage of the Medical Libraries Association (USA) convinced the Association for German-speaking Medical Librarians (AGMB) of the multiple benefits of such an Internet presence. The homepage of the AGMB should be devoted to several purposes:

1. Information and communication forum for members of the association as well as for clients.
2. Promotion by presentation: through their presence on the web the AGMB participates on the overall positive Internet appeal.
3. Clearinghouse for themes of interest for both medical librarians and their clients.
4. Corporate identity.
5. Recruiting new members.

Instead of maintaining lists of Internet sources at each library homepage, every library can benefit from one single cooperatively built index. Through their presence on the web, the AGMB is able to distribute information to its members and clients very easily and promptly (**http://medweb.uni-muenster.de/agmb**).

Dangers and drawbacks associated with the Internet

One of the greatest dangers of the information highway is that access to useful, value added information will only be fully accessible by an information elite. Important prerequisites for controlling the information environment, i.e. newest hard- and software, profound knowledge, time and money, are owned by a small percentage of the world population. One solution to this dangerous imbalance is that libraries offer free access to the Internet - like to every other information source - to anyone who is in need of it. If this happens the library has also the great responsibility - in my opinion - to take care of its accompayning problems like for example: information overload, the scattering of interests and thinking, the undermining of the social function of libraries, the social isolation of users, the addiction to the Internet, and its dark sides, which are just one mouse click far away.

The great advantage of the library are the Internet and information experts, who can guide the users and teach them information literacy, for example how to use Internet sources. This can be done by giving them tools for selection of useful and high quality information. Through the interaction with a librarian the users can become aware of their real needs and what they really are looking for. Librarians could add value to the Net and - last but not least - preserve the human touch.

INTERNET DIDACTIC NETWORK FOR THE MASTER ON HEALTH SERVICES MANAGEMENT AND ADMINISTRATION

*Maria Camerlingo and Rosita Bacchelli**, *CINECA, Bologna; **Regione Emilia Romagna Agenzia Sanitaria, Bologna, Italy

The Internet didactic network

The project consist of an Internet network based system able to supply didactic and management continuity to all activities related to the Master. One of the project aim is to expand the didactic effectiveness over every constraint of time and place, improving Master's purposes.

General project goals:

- better information exchange between people involved in the Master;
- network Master management;
- international spreading with the aim to broaden the teaching activities;
- easy access to the documentation produced by the Master activities.

In details, the project will provide to the subjects involved, the following services:

- e-mail tools
- hypertext internet style access to the management information;
- hypertextual access through Forms in HTML language, to the database containing the teaching documents, with various levels of search complexity;
- teledidactic tools to make easier relationships between teachers and students;
- control tools for the documents with limited accessibility, allowing users enabling or setting up users profiles.

S. Bakker (ed.), Health Information Management: What Strategies?, 210.

RECHERCHE ET FILTRAGE DE L'INFORMATION DANS LA BIBLIOTHEQUE VIRTUELLE

Jean-Pierre Lardy and Pascal Bador, Université Claude Bernard-Lyon I, France

Introduction

L'Internet connaît depuis les années 90 un développement impressionnant. La messagerie individuelle et de groupe (Listes et News) est devenue le premier outil de communication informelle des chercheurs. Les services de publication tels Gopher puis W3 permettent de diffuser de manière rapide, massive et à peu de frais l'information produite dans les universités, les laboratoires de recherche etc..

La diffusion électronique de l'information secondaire par les bases de données existe depuis plus de 30 ans. L'Internet a introduit de nombreuses innovations:
- la diffusion des documents en texte intégral est devenue courante alors que les bases de données commerciales sont encore essentiellement bibliographiques (Medline, Embase, Biosis, Pascal ...),
- le multimédia mêlant texte, image fixe ou animée et son fournit une information plus riche et plus agréable à consulter. Le domaine biomédical est un fort producteur de telles ressources.
- l'appropriation de ces outils par l'utilisateur final pour consulter l'information mais aussi pour la diffuser. Ce dernier point est capital car il remet en cause toute une structure où l'utilisateur était réduit au rôle de producteur.

Cependant les caractéristiques même de l'Internet qui ont permis ce développement présentent des inconvénients qui peuvent limiter fortement l'utilisation de cette information. Nous retrouvons ici les problèmes classiques de la recherche documentaire informatisée qui nécessite toujours des intermédiaires humains pour être efficace et ceci à différents niveaux: classement, indexation, interrogation.

Mais l'Internet est aussi de par son ouverture et du volume des données en jeu l'objet de développements importants d'outils automatiques de gestion et recherche d'information. Cependant retrouver l'information sur l'Internet est plus compliqué que dans les bases de données traditionnelles. Il est indispensable de connaître les différents outils disponibles, leur constitution et principes de fonctionnement.

Caractéristiques de l'information sur l'Internet

- C'est une *information dispersée*: contrairement à la dizaine de serveurs de bases de données commerciales dans le monde (Questel-Orbit, Dialog, Datastar, STN ...), c'est par dizaines de milliers que se comptent les serveurs sur l'Internet. Un simple

S. Bakker (ed.), Health Information Management: What Strategies?, 211-213.

micro-ordinateur suffit et de nombreux logiciels serveurs sous Windows ou Unix (Linux) sont gratuits. La tentation d'être sont propre éditeur et serveur est grande.

modes d'accès		sources	outils
l'utilisateur va chercher l'information sur un serveur	effort important	serveurs ftp: fichiers divers Gopher, W3: documents	humains: · guides · répertoires classés
		en texte intégral News: messages, textes	automatiques: · robots + moteurs de recherche
l'utilisateur reçoit l'information diffusée automatiquement	effort minimum	messagerie serveurs de Listes de discussion	outils de filtrage: · à la source · sur le poste de travail

Tableau 1.

- C'est une *information d'origines variées à la durée de vie* plus ou moins brève: il y a encore 5 années, l'information était issue essentiellement des universités et des laboratoires de recherche publique. Mais on trouve de plus en plus d'informations de nature technique et commerciale, issues des entreprises.
- C'est une *information très hétérogène* dans son contenu et dans sa présentation: l'information scientifique côtoie l'information publicitaire. Là où certains privilégient la rigueur, d'autres jouent sur la forme. Les formats de fichiers sont nombreux.Une information peu validée: un des reproches adressés à l'information trouvée sur l'Internet est son défaut de validation. Mais ce n'est pas toujours vraie car une thèse, un rapport de recherche sont des documents publics validés. De même pour les journaux électroniques dont les articles commencent à être signalés dans les grandes bases de données bibliographiques comme CAS ou Medline.
- C'est une information le plus souvent *gratuite mais protégée* par le droit d'auteur: gratuit ne veut pas dire sans auteur et sans reconnaissance.

En conclusion l'information sur l'Internet est très hétérogène, très dispersée et en grand volume. Ces caractéristiques rendent sa recherche difficile surtout dans la mesure où les outils de recherche sont essentiellement automatiques sans intervention humaine comme pour les bases de données.

Les outils de recherche d'information

De nombreux outils ont été créés pour identifier et localiser des ressources documentaires. Ils sont tous gratuits et répondent aux différents besoins et modes de recherche d'un public très large d'utilisateurs. Le tableau 1 donne les différents types d'outils selon le mode d'accès à l'information.

Les outils humains. Des listes de ressources par domaine ont été constituées depuis quelques années: basées à l'origine sur un travail essentiellement bénévole, elles sont de plus en plus l'oeuvre de sociétés commerciales. La diffusion électronique en permet une mise à jour régulière, souvent très rapide mais inégale d'un auteur à l'autre.Les guides de l'Université du Michigan en sont un bon exemple; en effet plus de 170 guides thématiques couvrent l'ensemble des connaissances. Ecrits par des professionnels et des étudiants, ils sont classés en une dizaine de domaines.

Les catalogues ou répertoires tiennent à jour des listes de ressources classées par grandes catégories. Les plus connus sont Yahoo, Galaxy et Magellan. Ce dernier se particularise par une analyse du contenu conduisant à une notation et à la rédaction d'un résumé.

En général deux modes de consultation sont disponibles:
- pour une recherche générale, on partira de la catégorie principale qui conduit à une liste de sous-catégories et enfin aux ressources.
- pour une recherche plus fine, on peut interroger un index.

Les outils automatiques: robots et moteurs de recherche. Connus sous le terme de "moteurs de recherche", ces outils sont des bases de données constituées automatiquement grâce à des logiciels appelés robots. Ces derniers scrutent à intervalles réguliers les serveurs (Web, Gopher, FTP ou autres selon le produit) déclarés sur Internet. Ils en indexent mot à mot le contenu. Selon le robot, les index portent soit sur le titre ou l'entête des documents, les URL (Uniform Resource Locator) et les zones hypertextes, soit sur le document complet. Le résultat de cette indexation est une gigantesque base de données qui associe à chaque uniterme l'adresse (URL) des documents le contenant. Les termes anglais les plus fréquents sont filtrés grâce à un dictionnaire de mots vides.

Ces outils très utiles sont maintenant assez nombreux. Issus de travaux universitaires, ils ont très vite été sponsorisés car ils deviennent des produits d'appel pour des entreprises. Cependant d'une manière générale la consultation en est gratuite. Les exemples sont nombreux: InfoSeek, Alta Vista, Lycos ....

Les outils de filtrage. Les volumes de plus en plus important d'information échangée et diffusée sur l'INTERNET rendent son utilisation problématique. Sans une nouvelle culture de la sélection de l'information à l'aide d'outils facilitant le filtrage, l'INTERNET risque de devenir un labyrinthe virtuel.

Un système de filtrage est un système qui lit et filtre les documents que l'on reçoit sur l'Internet. Il doit être capable d'identifier uniquement les textes qui traitent les sujets intéressant l'utilisateur qui a préalablement décrit ses centres d'intérêt.

Deux méthodes sont actuellement explorées:
- le filtre sur un serveur d'une université américaine: c'est le principe de la Diffusion Sélective de l'Information bien connu des utilisateurs de bases de données commerciales. L'usager s'inscrit au service, définit ses besoins d'information et décrit son profil. Le service envoie à intervalle régulier via le courrier électronique, les messages répondant au profil. Ces outils fonctionnent actuellement essentiellement sur les systèmes de News et ont pour nom SIFT, DejaNews ...
- le filtre tourne sur le poste de travail et traite les informations stockées sur le disque dur: Infoscan en est un exemple.

Conclusion

L'Internet souffre du fait que les outils de recherche d'information n'ont pas été pensés au moment de la définition des services de diffusion d'information comme le Web. La gestion décentralisée des réseaux et la croissance vertigineuse de ces dernières années impliquent l'utilisation d'outils automatiques. Mais la nature hétérogène des données rend ceux-ci peu précis. Il faudrait s'orienter vers une combinaison de la recherche et du filtrage pour affiner les résultats et réduire le bruit.

ONLINE DRUG INFORMATION SYSTEM

Christo Mutafov, Medical Information Centre, Sofia, Bulgaria

The drastic changes in social life had a great impact over the business orientation of the Medical Information Centre (MIC). As a result one of the main products of MIC is already worked up. This is the On-line Drug Information System (ODIS) aimed to keep presenting the Bulgarian medical society with current pharmacotherapeutic information on drugs registered for sale in Bulgaria. In the course of two years time a team of professionals planned, programmed, and fed information into the database ODIS. By the end of 1996 it will be taking part in the broad spectrum of information activities. The 1994-WHO anatomo-therapeutic classification is embodied as a semantic base for the system's structure. Its five levels include: the anatomic and therapeutic group, the therapeutic and chemical-therapeutic subgroup and the subgroup of the active substance.

The classification of therapeutic agents in ODIS is represented in divisions referring to the respective organ systems and some specific drug effects.

The information on every drug starts with its *International Nonproprietary Name (INN)* and is classified within 10 main subject headings:
1. Physical Properties, Pharmacokinetics, Mechanism Of Action; 2. Indications; 3. Contraindications; 4. Side Effects; 5. Dosage; 6. Drug Interactions; 7. Overdosage; 8. Precautions; 9. Proprietary Names and Presentation; 10. Law Information.
The information contained in ODIS will be offered to the physicians, chemists and pharmaceutical firms, students and postgraduates in the following forms:

•Periodical publishing of up-to-date references (the whole Database or separate sections). The first edition of the whole reference is expected in 1996-1997. It will present about 2500 items within a volume of 4000 pages. Untill now a number of headings (subheadings) have been published.

•Information retrieval for customers on their themes and questions. Results are provided on printed materials and diskettes. Further development of the retrieval strategies is also possible by using well-known pharmaceutical information sources.

The advantages of ODIS are: written in Bulgaria; cheaper for the Bulgarian users; it includes only drugs registered in Bulgaria; relatively small in size, which enables an easier information retrieval; it refers mainly to the practice, partially satisfying research tasks; it provides an easier operation that helps students' and specialists' education and self-education. ODIS contains more data than already published in Bulgarian pharmaceutical reference books. The most contemporary Bulgarian and foreign pharmacotherapeutical publications, monographs, references and other manufacturers' databases have been used for the preparation of ODIS.

S. Bakker (ed.), Health Information Management: What Strategies?, 214.

LES SERVEURS WEB DANS LE DOMAINE PHARMACEUTIQUE

Pascal Bador and Jean-Pierre Lardy, Université Claude Bernard-Lyon 1, France

Introduction

Ce travail a pour objectifs de présenter succintement une sélection de serveurs Web permettant un accès direct ou indirect à des informations pharmaceutiques plein texte, validées pour la plupart par un comité d'experts et qui peuvent être consultés pour répondre à des questions relatives à la pratique quotidienne des professionnels de santé.

Serveurs Web répertoriant et classant par thème les bases de données pharmaceutiques

Ce type de serveurs ne produit en général pas lui même les bases de données qu'il signale, il permet l'accès, grâce à des liens hypertextes, à plusieurs dizaines ou centaines de bases de données classées par thèmes.

PHARMINFONET

Pharminfonet est produit par la compagnie américaine "Pharmaceutical Information Associates, Ltd" qui est spécialisée dans la communication d'informations scientifiques aux professionnels de santé (**http://pharminfo.com/**).

Ce serveur, qui représente une importante source d'information en matière d'actualités pharmaceutique et thérapeutique, propose neuf thèmes dont les plus représentatifs sont les suivants: Disease Centers qui présente des informations scientifiques classées en fonction des différentes spécialités médicales; Drug information qui offre une base de données sur les médicaments (index à partir duquel on accède à une description très succincte d'un médicament donné mais aussi grâce à des liens hypertextes à des articles du Medical Sciences Bulletin); un Drug FAQ qui fait la synthèse des questions et réponses les plus intéressantes sur les médicaments; la revue électronique Medical Sciences Bulletin qui publie des articles sur les nouveaux médicaments et les nouveaux moyens thérapeutiques avec un accès par classes pharmacothérapeutiques; enfin un module plus commercial qui offre des liens vers des organismes, des entreprises, des fournisseurs et des consultants du secteur de la pharmacie.

S. Bakker (ed.), Health Information Management: What Strategies?, 215-218.

THE VIRTUAL PHARMACY CENTER

Ce site (**http://www-sci.lib.uci.edu/~martindale/Pharmacy.html#PP3**) fait partie plus généralement du Virtual Medical Center développé par Jim Martindale aux Etats-Unis. Le menu général est très dense et parait assez confus, il est difficile lors des premières consultations de se repérer dans cette quarantaine d'écrans extrêmement chargés qui demandent à chaque fois un temps de chargement assez long pouvant devenir dissuasif. Le Virtual Pharmacy Center est certainement le site le plus complet qui renvoie donc au plus grand nombre de ressources pharmaceutiques du monde anglo-saxon.

Il permet d'accéder à plusieurs glossaires et dictionnaires en huit langues avec des définitions dans les domaines de la pharmacologie, la biotechnologie et diverses disciplines médicales et chimiques. Il fait le lien avec de nombreuses bases de données médicales et pharmaceutiques et notamment avec de très bons guides d'utilisation et guides de cours consacrés à l'usage des médicaments.

Il renvoie également vers des banques d'images et d'animations 3D par exemple. Il renvoie à la liste la plus complète des revues biomédicales électroniques présentes sur le Web (accès aux sommaires et aux résumés d'articles le plus souvent, très rarement aux articles plein texte). Enfin il permet d'accéder à des adresses d'organismes, d'associations et d'institutions pharmaceutiques américaines.

Ce site a donc pour intérêt de répertorier un nombre incalculable de serveurs pharmaceutiques intéressants mais il ne produit pas lui-même des bases de données avec des informations en tant que telles. Son principal inconvénient reste quand même le fait que, lorsqu'on revient à l'écran principal, le temps de chargement reste beaucoup trop long à mon sens!

THE WORLD WIDE WEB VIRTUAL LIBRARY: PHARMACY

Ce site (**http://157.142.72.77/pharmacy/pharmint.html**) est comparable au précédent car il propose un classement par thème des sites intéressant le secteur pharmaceutique, mais il ne les décrit pas ou de façon très succincte ce qui présente l'avantage de ne pas ralentir le chargement. On peut ainsi accéder à un grand nombre de facultés de pharmacie classées par pays, à une liste d'organismes, d'institutions et d'associations pharmaceutiques, à une vingtaine de revues (sommaires ou résumés d'articles essentiellement). Ce site propose également des offres d'emplois, des liens vers une vingtaine de bases de données, et une trentaine de laboratoires pharmaceutiques industriels ainsi que des liens vers des sites commerciaux. Il renvoie de plus vers une vingtaine de listes de diffusion pharmaceutiques.

PHARMWEB

Ce serveur très convivial (**http://www.pharmweb.net/**) est produit par l'Université de Manchester. Il a le mérite d'avoir été le premier serveur structuré d'informations pharmaceutiques sur Internet puisqu'il a été créé en 1994. Il permet l'accès à de nombreuses bases de données mais sa spécificité est basée sur la mise en place et la gestion de listes de diffusion accessibles aux pharmaciens en fonction de leur type d'exercice (officine, industrie, hôpital, université) et de leur nationalité. Son objectif est de favoriser l'échange d'information et la confraternité entre les pharmaciens du monde entier. Ce serveur sera présenté en détail par M. Antony d'Emanuelle au cours de la session plénière.

SERVEUR DU CENTRE HOSPITALIER UNIVERSITAIRE DE ROUEN

Ce serveur (**http://www.chu-rouen.fr/**) est le site français le plus complet dans le domaine de la santé (il offre de plus une version en anglais). Il donne la possibilité de faire une recherche par mots clés et bien sûr une recherche thématique. Il propose spécifiquement la liste des serveurs en France et francophones dans le domaine de la santé avec un accès par spécialités médicales. Il permet également l'accès aux listes de diffusion biomédicale, il donne la liste des serveurs des hôpitaux et des universités, des organismes et des institutions importants. Il permet l'accès à des ressources documentaires et à des journaux électroniques.

Exemples de bases de données pharmaceutiques plein texte et permettant un accès direct à des informations sur les médicaments ou la thérapeutique

MANUEL MERCK DE DIAGNOSTIC ET THÉRAPEUTIQUE

Il s'agit de l'ouvrage de référence, texte intégral, en langue anglaise bien connu des praticiens et consultable en ligne gratuitement après une inscription préalable. (**http://www.merck.com/!!rRJsq2ojNrRJsq2ojN/pubs/mmanual/html/sectoc.htm**) Sa structure hiérarchisée en chapitres et sous-chapitres permet une consultation aisée dans le cadre de la pratique quotidienne du médecin et du pharmacien. Les liens hypertextes permettent de plus d'accéder à d'autres parties de chapitres également pertinentes ainsi qu'aux tableaux, figures et schémas de l'ouvrage.

BIAM

La BIAM ou Banque d'Information Automatisée sur le Médicament est une banque française d'information sur les 2600 principes actifs commercialisés en France (**http://cri.ensmp.fr/biam/acceuil.html**). Après une recherche sur un nom de substance ou un nom commercial, on obtient pour chaque médicament les renseignements suivants: moyen d'identification, mécanisme d'action, propriétés pharmacologiques, indications, effets indésirables, précautions d'emploi, contre-indications, posologie et modes d'administration, etc. Le module interactions entre différents médicaments permet une analyse d'ordonnance et signale les différents types d'interaction entre les médicaments pris deux à deux.

L'Index des laboratoires pharmaceutiques industriels permet d'obtenir la liste des médicaments commercialisés par chaque laboratoire. L'option substance non active permet d'obtenir la liste des médicaments contenant un excipient donné (jaune de tartrazine par exemple), il s'agit d'informations difficiles à obtenir par ailleurs. L'Index alphabétique des spécialités étrangères répertorie les équivalents de médicaments étrangers d'environ 80 pays.

La BIAM, que l'on peut consulter sur le Minitel français depuis de nombreuses années, présente des informations fournies par les laboratoires pharmaceutiques industiels. Cette version sur Internet utilise toute la puissance des liens hypertextes et permet d'obtenir très facilement et de façon très conviviale des informations ponctuelles et des listes de médicaments répondant à des caractéristiques précises. Elle présente un intérêt certain pour les praticiens francophones d'autant plus qu'elle est la seule de ce type en langue française accessible sur Internet.

BANQUE ADM (AIDE AU DIAGNOSTIC MÉDICAL)

Elle présente en langue française pour chaque médicament une liste très détaillée de ses effets indésirables avec indications des sources bibliographiques (**http://www.med.univ-rennes1.fr/adm.dir/menu.html**) (2400 effets indésirables sont ainsi répertoriés).

Conclusion

Cette communication avait pour objet de faire connaître une sélection des principaux serveurs Web pharmaceutiques. A l'issue de ce travail et après de nombreuses heures passées à naviguer sur le Web, un certain nombre de points importants nous sont apparus:

- Tous ces serveurs sont liés entre eux c'est-à-dire qu'ils offrent des liens hypertextes permettant l'accès à un serveur à partir de tous les autres, si bien qu'en fait le choix initial de l'un d'entre eux au détriment des autres n'a que peu d'importance. Ainsi, seul le temps d'accès sera différent et dépendra au départ du chemin plus ou moins direct emprunté par l'utilisateur.
- Ces serveurs d'origine anglo-saxonne et américaine pour la plupart répertorient à l'aide d'un classement par grandes rubriques thématiques plusieurs centaines de sites qui dans un second temps devront être consultés afin d'accéder à l'information ponctuelle recherchée.
- Ces serveurs sont tentés de vouloir signaler le plus grand nombre de sites possibles ce qui fait que certains d'entre eux proposent jusqu'à une trentaine de page-écran comme écran initial. Cela entraîne des temps de chargement qui peuvent être dissuasifs si l'on revient souvent à l'écran et au menu de départ. De plus, le choix et l'accès à la base de données susceptible de répondre à la question du moment sont souvent difficiles en raison de la multiplicité des bases de données disponibles sur Internet.
- Les serveurs américains représentent l'immense majorité des ressources disponibles sur Internet pour l'instant et il est urgent que les autres pays mettent en place rapidement les serveurs d'information électronique spécifiques à leurs propres publics nationaux.
- Enfin il faut bien avoir conscience que les serveurs Web sont en évolution constante, que certains changent d'adresse, d'autres sont accessibles mais n'offrent que des pages dites en construction et que certains ne sont pas mis à jour régulièrement et proposent des informations complètement obsolètes.

En fin de compte, c'est bien sûr à l'utilisateur de repérer les sites qui lui paraissent les plus performants et qui peuvent répondre de façon optimale aux demandes d'informations résultant de sa pratique quotidienne.

PHARMWEB - PHARMACEUTICAL INFORMATION ON THE INTERNET

Antony D'Emanuele, Department of Pharmacy, University of Manchester, UK

Introduction

The development of the world wide web (WWW) has transformed the interface to the Internet from that involving a UNIX command line into a user-friendly graphical interface. The WWW has developed rapidly into a hypermedia rich system with technologies evolving that not only enable simple text and graphics to be delivered to users, but real-time sound and vision. The WWW has made the Internet a fully interactive communications resource.

PRESENT LIMITATIONS OF THE INTERNET

A number of isues remain to be resolved if the Internet is to realise its potential. The growth in usage and interest is exceeding the capacity of the current network infrastructure. The bandwidth of the networks will have to be upgraded if it is to develop into the communication medium of the next millennium. This problem is being addressed with significant commercial investment. Improvement is bandwidth may one day allow users to communicate in real-time with high quality sound and vision. Indeed, in the future we could be using Internet addresses to contact people rather than telephone numbers! The present system using IP addresses is presenting problems as the Internet is running out of new addresses, however the Internet protocols are being developed to accomodate the expected growth.

The security of the Internet has been a source of criticism and concern regarding information being sent securely and the vulnerability of computers to attack from both viruses and hackers. Computer systems can be protected appropriately by the installation of software (firewalls) and careful system management. Data can be transmitted securely using encryption. Indeed, it is already possible to make purchases on the Internet with several companies selling their products electronically. Further improvements in security will occur when the proposed development to the Internet protocols result in automatic encryption of all 'transactions' at the packet level. The governments of a number of countries have prevented the implementation of high level encryption technology with concerns regarding the free exchange of information by criminals.

The Internet is proving problematic for drug/medical regulatory bodies, particularly concerning the product information that companies may wish to present. Regulations of countries differ regarding the information that may be made public

S. Bakker (ed.), Health Information Management: What Strategies?, 219-222.

available and the range of conditions that a particular medicine may be used for. Now users from different countries cannot be prevented from accessing this information.

FINDING INFORMATION ON THE INTERNET

A growing problem concerns the vast amount of information that is available. It is becoming progressively more difficult to find useful and reliable information. Several search engines have now been developed which aim to catalogue the entire Internet, however, searching these databases often produces either lengthy results, or results that bear no relation to the sought after information. In particular, these search engines often do not discriminate the source or quality of information. This situation is likely to worsen in the future. Health professionals are unlikely to want to 'surf the Internet' and waste time searching for information. Professionals using the Internet simply as an information resource will wish to go to a particular site where they know they can locate useful information rapidly. It is likely that specialist sites will develop and become important sources of information in different subject areas such as medical information and pharmaceutical information. It was with the anticipated growth and development of the Internet that PharmWeb (figure 1) has evolved.

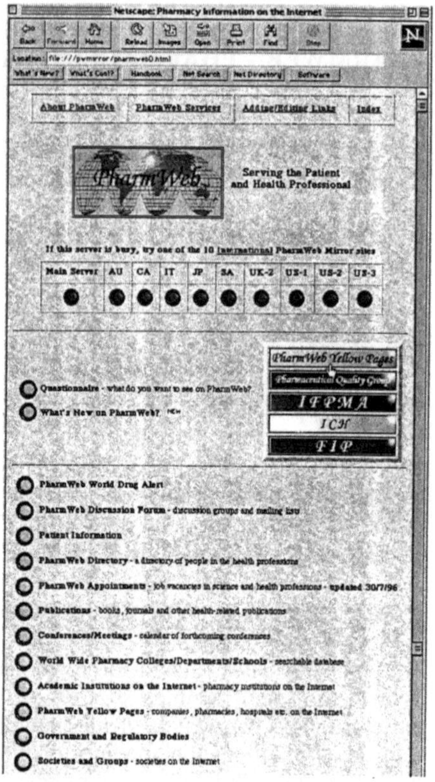

Fig. 1 Top of the PharmWeb Home Page

PharmWeb

PharmWeb has developed into one of the main sources of pharmaceutical information on the Internet (**http://www.pharmweb.net/**). It was the first structured site for pharmaceutical information (1994), and including the development of the first pharmaceutical society pages and the first directory of health professionals (PharmWeb Directory). The site has developed as an Internet provider for pharmaceutical and health-related information with several organisations maintaining their pages on the PharmWeb server. Presently the site has 10 mirror sites (figure 2) around the world ensuring fast access irrespective of a users location. The UK servers alone have been accessed by over 100 countries and are receiving some 18,000 page requests per week (figure 3). A comprehensive series of links to other pharmaceutical sites are maintained on PharmWeb. Examples are:

Newsgroups. A pharmacy newsgroup called **sci.med.pharmacy** has been operating for several years. Messages are posted by pharmacists and the general public. The group is unmoderated and gnerally not the best forum to discuss professional issues.

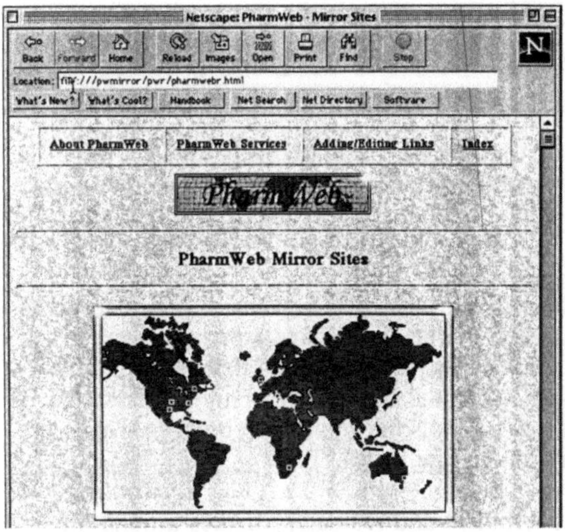

Figure 2. Location of PharmWeb Mirror Sites: Australia, New Zealand, Canada, Japan, South Africa, United States (3), UK (2).

Discussion groups/mailing lists. Several discussion groups have been established, the first was a general pharmacy discussion list set up at DeMontfort University and restricted to pharmacists and workers in related fields. Several more specialised discussion groups have been developed in topics such as pharmaceutical care, managed care, and pharmaceutical science and technology. Additionally, pharmaceutical societies are developing mailing lists to deliver information to their members. The International Pharmaceutical Federation (FIP) was the first society to develop such a list and regularly disseminate information to their members using e-mail.

Societies. Over 20 pharmaceutical societies and groups have established pages on the WWW. These sites can provide a wide range of information including details on membership, conferences and latest news. The first on the Internet (1994) was the United Kingdom Controled Release Society (UKCRS) shortly followed by the American Association of Pharmaceutical Scientists (AAPS) and the FIP.

Conferences. The Internet is being used to advertise conferences and meetings. Up to date meeting programs can be viewed together with information on registration and accommodation.

Drug information and medical databases. Several useful drug information databases are starting to appear with many more certain to follow. Services such as Medline are available and as bandwidth increases the Internet will be routinely used to access information databases.

Education resources. Several academic institutions are developing educational resources and the Internet promises to be a powerful medium for the delivery of continued and distance learning material. Students may interact with their tutors on-line, and in addition, it is possible to have a multiple choice examination paper marked in a matter of seconds.

Directory of health professionals. The first directory of health professionals on the Internet was developed on PharmWeb. People may register on the directory by simply filling a form on a Web page with their name, contact details, and e-mail address. A person can then be found by entering a keyword such as a surname or company name, and a person may be contacted by simply clicking on their e-mail address which than automatically generates an e-mail form. Over 1,000 people have registered on the PharmWeb Directory.

Patient information. The provision of patient information on the Internet is an area of growth. Information on the use of medicines and a range of specific products can be found on various web servers.

Schools database. FIP developed the first searchable database of its kind on the Internet with the FIP World Wide List of Pharmacy Schools. Schools are found by entering a keyword, and if the school has a web site a hypertext link to that particular school is also provided.

Directory of companies and pharmacies. Eli Lilly was the first major pharmaceutical company on the Internet in 1994. Nowadays, virtually all have a presence on the Internet. These web sites vary from a simple company profile to detailed product information. Companies are also starting to use the Internet as an aid to marketing. Many hospital and community pharmacies have also developed web pages. Links to these sites maybe found on the PharmWeb Yellow Pages.

Government and regulatory bodies. Government and regulatory bodies around the world are also developing web sites. Included in these is the Food and Drug Administration, the European Medicines Evaluation Agency, the Japanese National Institutes of Health, and Health Canada.

New sites. New pharmaceutical sites are appearing on the Internet each month, one recent example is the International Federation of Pharmaceutical Manufacturers Associations (IFPMA) who developed a series of pages on PharmWeb and are providing ICH documents on-line as part of their sites.

Conclusions

The concept of computers and networks still dissuades many people from using the Internet. However, within the last three years, current computer software has transformed these technologies into user-friendly systems that allow transparent communication between Internet users all over the globe. Many people have not had the time or the opportunity to digest these events. The Internet will undoubtedly change as technology makes further advances. Much of the information on the Internet is presently free, however, this is likely to change as secure and transparent payment technologies are implemented. Provided the above issues are addressed, the Internet will become a routinely used communications resource, and this period of history will surely be looked back on as the 'Communications and Information Revolution'. The development of the Internet is probably the most important breakthrough in communications since the telephone.

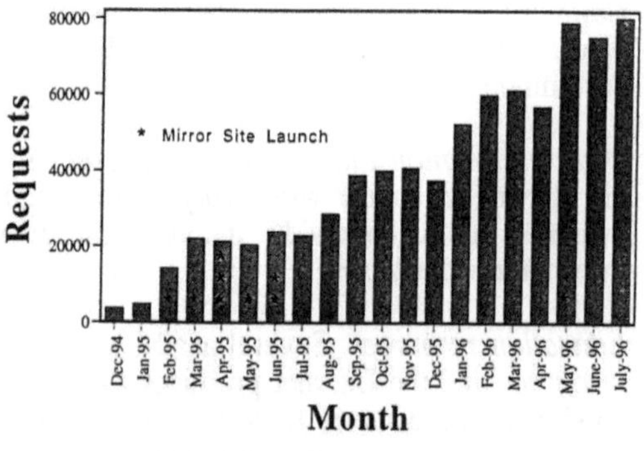

Figure 3. Number of page requests per month from the UK PharmWeb mirror site.

HOW MIGHT TECHNOLOGY HELP THE FLOW OF MEDICAL INFORMATION TO AND FROM DEVELOPING COUNTRIES

Jean G. Shaw, SatelLife, UK

Summary

Does a European association such as EAHIL need to be concerned with health information outside Europe?

Quite apart from any moral concern, international trade and travel made the world a much smaller place and there is no room for complacency about health problems in any part of the world. Also strategies for improving the two way flow of information between developing and developed countries might be adapted to improve health information to rural communities or the less well developed parts of our own continent.

Within this general context, the presentation concentrated on the work of SatelLife UK. Through its twinning programme SatelLife UK aims to make use of the new technology to improve communications between medical libraries in the UK and, at present, Africa. It is stressed that this needs to be a two way process. Active participation by European colleagues is welcomed.

S. Bakker (ed.), Health Information Management: What Strategies?, 223.

HEALTH INFORMATION, HEALTH RIGHTS AND THE EUROPEAN CITIZEN

Robert Gann, The Help for Health Trust, Highcroft, Winchester, UK

Introduction

This paper examines the development of health rights and health information in the European context and the contribution which libraries can make. It concentrates on Europe wide initiatives and on national developments in the UK and the Netherlands.

European health trends and challenges

Throughout Europe some common trends are emerging which create a fertile environment for health care consumerism. The European population is getting older with disproportionately heavy demands being made on health care services. As we tackle many communicable and acute diseases, lifestyle related and chronic illnesses become more prominent. It is in these areas that patients are experts in their own right. We have an increasingly mobile workforce with the health problems associated with migrant workers and new demands for information on unfamiliar health care systems. Health care expectations are rising, fuelled by new technologies and media coverage of medical miracles. At the same time health costs are rising. Ironically the healthier we are, the longer we live and the more we end up costing the health care system. All European nations are experiencing budgetary constraints and in countries including the UK and Portugal health care reforms have been introduced which separate the commissioning of health care from its provision. Health care consumerism is encouraged as part of this market approach to health care, but the trend is more deep seated than this. Consumer power is one of the megatrends of the late Twentieth Century.

European citizens' rights and health

Although official encouragement for greater patient involvement can be traced back to the World Health Organization Health for All declarations of the 1980s, there has been a particularly strong emphasis over the past 2 or 3 years. In October 1995 a European Health AGORA was held at the European Parliament in Brussels, under the auspices of HOPE (Standing Committee of Hospitals of the European Union). The author attended the AGORA as the representative of EAHIL. The meeting reviewed

S. Bakker (ed.), Health Information Management: What Strategies?, 225-227.

developments in health rights in Europe, noting that the Maastricht Treaty Article 129 identifies a role for the European Union in the promotion and protection of public health.

Other recent developments include the WHO Declaration on the Promotion of Patients' Rights in Europe developed in Amsterdam in March 1994 and the Council of Europe Convention on Bioethics. The Patients' Rights Declaration covers general human rights (self determination, religious belief etc.) as they apply to health, information, consent, confidentiality, and quality and choice in care. The Convention on Bioethics produced a draft declaration also in 1994 and is currently considering rights in research, genetics and transplantation.

European associations and initiatives

We are now beginning to see the development of pan-European organisations devoted to the promotion of healthy individuals and communities. The European Public Health Alliance (EPHA) is a network of non-governmental health organisations throughout Europe, focusing on issues such as consumer protection, health & safety at work and environmental health. EPHA is active in campaigns including Europe Against Cancer, tobacco, drugs & HIV/AIDS. EPHA recognises the importance of healthy public policy and legislation and has been active in lobbying on tobacco advertising.

International Union For Health Promotion & Education (IUHPE)

The IUHPE, a global association with Regional offices, including a European Regional Office in the Netherlands, is engaged with WHO programmes, including Healthy Cities, Healthy Schools and Health Promoting Hospitals. In the information world, the IUHPE Regional Office in Woerden, Netherlands is leading an EU funded Multilingual Health Promotion Thesaurus Project. A Dutch Health Promotion Thesaurus, first established by NIGZ (the Netherlands Institute for Health Promotion and Disease Prevention) is being developed into English, French and German versions by working groups of librarians and documentalists. Italian & Spanish versions will be next languages to be incorporated.

Pharmaceutical partners for better healthcare

One of the most intriguing recent trends has been the interest of the pharmaceutical industry in patients' rights and patient information. The pharmaceutical company umbrella the European Federation of Pharmaceutical Industry Associations (EFPIA) has been working with umbrella patient groups, including the UK Long Term Medical Conditions Alliance and the Dutch association for chronic diseases, WOCZ, to set up a series of activities under the heading of Pharmaceutical Partners for Better Health Care. A conference, Patient Empowerment: New Partnerships in Europe, took place in Brussels in November 1995 and a *Patients' Network* newsletter has been published. There is a commitment to further patient publications, conferences etc.

One might ask what is the motivation for this new interest? There is no doubt that there is a realisation on the part of the industry that patient empowerment is here to stay and some positive public relations benefits can accrue from association with it. It would also be fair to recognise a genuine philanthropic support for patient groups by some pharmaceutical companies. More subtly, the origins may lie in the benefits, and risks, of evidence based health care. A major objective of an evidence based approach to health is a reduction in irrational prescribing, with moves in some countries towards a restricted list of prescribable drugs of proven effectiveness. For the pharmaceutical industry there is a threat to sales; for patients there is a perceived threat to patient choice as medication which patients have found to work for them may no longer be available. This shared interest in having a wide variety of treatment options available has created a new alliance between some drug companies and patient organisations.

The industry is keen to find ways of communicating information on medicines to patients. Although European Union Directive 92/28 bans advertising of prescription drugs to public, we are seeing a growth in drug industry helplines, leaflets & newsletters, and drug company Internet sites.

European Commission programmes

A number of health information projects have been funded as part of the European Telematics Programme (DGXIII), in particular under the TIDE (Telematics for Integration of Disabled & Elderly people) initiative. The HELIOS/HANDYNET programme has seen the development of Europe wide information systems on disability equipment and we are looking forward to new opportunities under the new European Union Libraries Programme from December 1996.

National developments: United Kingdom & Netherlands

In the UK a national Patients Charter was published in 1991 leading to the establishment in 1992 of a national freephone Health Information Service (HIS) for the public. A single national freephone number (0800 66 55 44) routes callers automatically to the nearest of 23 local HIS centres. The Help for Health Trust provides a Central Support Unit for HIS, supplying training, networking and development.

In the Netherlands, 1995 saw new patients rights legislation, while NIGZ has developed its Patienten/Consumenten databases of self help groups and publications. At a local level there are networks of Gezondheidswijzers (health information shops) and Dental Information Points.

Working together

There are new opportunities to work together in Europe to promote the development of health rights and health information. We have:

Legislation	- at a European level and within member states
Libraries	- who are recognising their key role in consumer health information
Links	- through associations, including EAHIL, and via the Internet
Language	- development of multilingual tools
£££££	- funding opportunities through the European Union

THE SICK PERSON FROM PATIENT TO HEALTH CONSUMER: FROM INFORMED TO INFORMER

*Gaetana Cognetti and Adriana Dracos**, *Istituto Regina Elena, **Istituto Superiore di Sanità, Rome, Italy

"It is difficult to remain an emperor in presence of a physician: and difficult even to keep one's essential quality as man. The professional eye saw in me only a mass of humors, a sorry mixture of blood and lymph" Marguerite Yourcenar
Memoirs of Hadrian

Historical overview

For centuries the physician's main attitude towards patients was one of examining with cold scientific determination ever smaller parts of the human body, without considering the patient as a person. Nowadays the patient is considered as a whole, psyche and body together, in a developing relation with the environment and other beings. Historically, this approach is in accordance with the holistic Hippocratic view that man cannot be considered only as a sum of anatomical parts. Because the patient is no longer a passive object of studies and therapies the relationship between physician and patient has changed accordingly. In the 70s, the prevailing attitude of the phycisian towards the seriously ill patients was to conceal the truth. Gradually modified to the opposite, there is today a growing concern towards the patient's rights to information according to his/her potentiality to understand it.

The informed patient

A rise in the average cultural level together with the availability of health information resources on different media such as books, journals, television programs, etc. have triggered an irreversible process of self-information on diseases and their up-to-date therapies by the patients themselves.

In the USA, the moral need for granting the access to available information resources has been sanctioned by the President's Commission on Ethical Practices in Medicine and resolved by the most important librarian associations by essential acts stating free access to health information to all people, regardless of ethical, social or religious reasons.[1-2] This led to open hospital libraries to patients and to create a number of user-oriented information services. Previously, the user had to ask his/her physician's authorization to access the hospital library.[3-4]

Furthermore, the dissemination of new advanced information media, such as CD-ROM, CD-I, etc..., together with high-speed low-cost networks, have boosted

S. Bakker (ed.), Health Information Management: What Strategies?, 228-230.

information offer for the patient, too. To know something more on his/her disease and therefore to try to set up an informed consent, the patient can choose among a large number of information tools, even multimedial, on different topics such as health education, symptomatology, prevention, diagnosis, diet, nutrition, first aid, description of treatments and diagnostic procedures.[5]

At present, also in Europe, the patient's right to information has made great strides, thanks to the endorsement of informed consent by European countries. In Italy, the National Bioethics Committee and the Medical Ethics Codex stress the importance of the duty to inform the patient by medical or non-medical staff.[6-7] The duty is called for and is at the roots of a correct practice. Moreover, a large number of toll-free telephone lines for inquiring on different pathologies are available to the patients or their relatives; e.g. it is possible to get information on cancer at the Istituto Regina Elena and on AIDS at the Istituto Superiore di Sanità. By the latter, there are psychologists, physicians, sociologists and social workers who are available to answer all questions about AIDS in English, French, Spanish and Portuguese. There are, of course, many other activities organized by different institutions, associations of patients, relatives and volunteers, documentation centers on health education, even if at present these resources are not coordinated yet at a national level all together. This means that, unfortunately, a network of Italian patient-oriented documentation centers and libraries, able to in-depth disseminate information, is still lacking.

In other countries, such as the USA, exists a better coordination and a larger number of facilities for the patient, some of which internationally accessible. The most widespread information facilities for patients are hospital libraries, largely disseminated in the USA which are patient-oriented and differ from medical-staff libraries, that are shaped exclusively for physicians or allied health personnel. In a field where the information need of patients and their relatives is more urging, such as oncology, it is worth mentioning the following services:

The Physician Data Query (PDQ), the well known data bank produced by the National Cancer Institute and created also on the advice of a cancer patient who, in 1981, wrote to Vincent De Vita, Director of the National Cancer Institute, and suggested the introduction of a factual tool to help patients to acquire or improve their knowledge on their disease, state-of-the-art therapies, clinical protocols, institutions and clinicians involved in cancer care.[8] The data bank is addressed to both hospital staff (physicians, nurses, psychologists....) and patients. As regards patients, information is written by a group of experts in communication and do not include survival statistics. Since 1991, some of the PDQ information is free-of-charge accessible at an international level through an automatic procedure, by fax or by the Internet. Information is available in English but can be obtained also in Spanish, thanks to an automatic translation revised by mother-tongue experts in oncology.

The Cancer Information Service (CIS), founded in 1975 by the National Cancer Institute, operates through about a thousand telephone numbers and supplies information and documentation upon request by patients or their relatives, in addition to health workers. The service is staffed by experts in information.[9]

Patient-oriented documentation should include information on possible treatments or on the best way to prevent and/or face the disease. It should also give suggestions on the best way to reduce the adverse effects of therapies, and indications on diet, psychological support and exercise. The documentation should be accessible to all age brackets, including adolescents and children and be oriented to the various sections of readers, taking into account the different cultural levels.

From patient to health consumer and informer

The recognition of the patient as a person, the ever-increasing patient's need for information and the acknowledgement of information as a civil right to be protected gave rise to the concept of informed consent. This procedure is now obligatory for any professional practice, either diagnostic or therapeutic, which may result in injury, loss or damage to the patient. The above mentioned information tools are available to help patients to reach a more informed consent to different medical procedures.

The patient-physician relationship is strongly unbalanced as regards technical expertise. Only objective information can let the patient gain a large part of that autonomy on decision making. The issue of consent is therefore inseparably linked to that of information. In addition, the appearance of the patient on the scene of information has side aspects from two points of view:

1. Patients, once involved in the decision-making process on therapies, have better psychological resources and play a more active role in the fight against their disease. The search for information is a valid therapy itself, because it gives the patient the impression of keeping the situation under control.

2. The patient, whose search for information is only oriented to his/her personal case, may sometimes find out new therapies which the physician missed at first. The latter, in fact, following a number of patients suffering from different diseases, may find it difficult to keep abreast of updatings on different pathologies. Surveys underlined that in some cases the physician takes advantage of searches carried out by the patient and encourages him/her to find material useful for a better decision on therapy.[10] In other cases the search for information carried out by the patient enabled the physician to identify new therapies and to save human lives.[11]

In the global village where information is now at hand for anyone, individuals, even if not experienced in the field, can be personally and deeply involved in finding the solution and the right treatment for their own diseases or for their relatives' ones; take for example the case of "Lorenzo's oil", which inspired the homonymous movie.

Being no longer a passive subject the term 'patient' is substituted by 'health consumer'. It is indeed the access of new consumers to the scientific information that charges the librarians with new tasks. A new philosophy is required in the training of the information specialists in order to offer the right information in a form people can understand. This means high technological skills linked with high capacity to match the new ethical aspects the progress raises.

References

1 Aghemo A. Etica professionale e servizio di informazione. Biblioteche oggi 1993;Feb:30-33

2 La Rocco A. The role of the medical schoolbased consumer health information service. Bull Med Libr Assoc 1994;82:46-51

3 Hafner AW. Introduction: Patient access to medical information. Bull Med Libr Assoc 1994;82:44-45

4 Hafner AW . A survey of patient access to hospital and medical school libraries. Bull Med Libr Assoc 1994;82:64-66

5 Jimson HB, Sher PP. Consumer Health Informatics: health information technology for consumers. J Am Soc Inf Sci 1995;46:783-790

6 Comitato Nazionale per la Bioetica. Informazione e consenso all'atto medico. Roma: Presidenza del Consiglio dei Ministri. Dipartimento per l'informazione ed editoria, 1992

7 Federazione Nazionale degli Ordini dei Medici Chirurghi e degli Odontoiatri. Codice di deontologia Medica. 1995

8 Hubbard SM, De Vita jr VT. PDQ: an innovating informing dissemination linking cancer research and clinical practice. Important Advances in Oncology 1987;263-77

9 Manfredi C, Czaja R, Buis M, Derk D. Patient use of treatment-related information service. Cancer 1993;71:1326-1337

10 Lindner K. A piece of my mind. Encourage information therapy. JAMA 1992;267:2592

11 Thalenberg M. I saved my own life using Medline. Gratefully yours 1995;Sept./Oct:1-2

DEVELOPING A CRITICAL APPRAISAL SKILLS PROGRAMME FOR CONSUMER HEALTH INFORMATION SERVICES

Ruairidh Milne, Sandy Oliver and Gill Needham, Institute of Health Sciences, Oxford, UK

Critical Appraisal Skills Programme

The Critical Appraisal Skills Programme (CASP) is for people making decisions about health care, whether they are planning services, making clinical decisions or deciding which treatment, if any, they would like for themselves.

The ideas behind CASP are not new. The principles and practice of evidence-based medicine were developed at McMaster University and are being adopted and adapted world-wide. CASP's fundamental achievement has been take these principles and use them to develop a practical and accessible programme geared to the specific needs of decision-makers in the National Health Service.

The original CASP workshops in 1993, were developed in partnership with purchasers responsible for purchasing health services for their local population. Since then workshops have been adapted and run for hospital clinicians, public health doctors, managers, audit staff, general practitioners and their colleagues and patients, librarians, NHS committees, Consumer Health Information Services and self help groups. This has been done through a network of CASP co-ordinators who, between them, have run nearly 150 workshops across the UK, attended by nearly 3,000 people.

CASP's aim is to help decision-makers develop skills in the critical appraisal of evidence about effectiveness, in order to promote the delivery of evidence-based health care and encourage evidence-based patient choice.

CASP for Consumer Health Information Services

The need for the project was recognised because treatment outcomes information is an important part of the work of Consumer Health Information Services but they find it difficult. In 1994 the Kings Fund, a charity which funds innovative work in the health service, asked Bob Gann and Sarah Buckland to find out how well CHIS were coping with this responsibility. They found that "approximately half of local services and a third of regional services felt unable to answer these question satisfactorily, and few used MEDLINE or medical libraries".[1]

Responding to these findings the Kings Fund then commissioned five parallel projects to explore and develop the provision of treatments outcomes information by Consumer Health Information Services. This CASP project was one of those five.

S. Bakker (ed.), Health Information Management: What Strategies?, 231-233.

The aims of this project were "to help people who give health information to the public develop the skills they need to make sense of the evidence of effectiveness".

Our first task was to find as many Consumer Health Information Services as possible, to invite them to take part in the programme. There is no official comprehensive register and we found services through their own loose networks, by attending one of their meetings, advertising in a newsletter and through individual contacts.

At the same time we were working with maternity self help groups. The largest of these, the National Childbirth Trust, had already shown an interest and, at their request had hosted two CASP workshops the year before.

Backgrounds of staff at Consumer Health Information Services vary widely. Some of them are librarians and some have worked in the health service but many come with no professional training. Within the maternity self help groups are lay antenatal teachers, breastfeeding counsellors, mothers offering peer support and women who are lay members of NHS committees that co-ordinate maternity services.

We invited some of these people to cooperate in planning workshops for them and their peers. Planning meetings help us understand their interests and working practices so that the workshops could be tailored to their needs. We ran 4 pairs of workshops and at the end we supported these groups in taking this work forward.

We discussed the purpose of the workshops and the opportunities which might arise from them in planning meetings. The Consumer Health Information Service staff had two main objectives for this work. They wanted to be confident that they could understand and explain the importance of evidence-based consumer information, and see how Consumer Health Information Service staff and medical librarians can share their interest, skills, and resources to find and explain information for the public.

In the first workshop of each pair, we critically appraised a randomised controlled trial (topics were a fitness programme for arthritis, a drug treatment for Alzheimer's disease, aspirin to prevent migraine and a support programme for pregnant women), in the second, a systematic review from the Cochrane database (topics were family interventions for schizophrenia, aspirin to prevent secondary stroke and iron supplementation in pregnancy). The topics were chosen in discussion with the planning teams to reflect typical questions that the public bring: questions about long term conditions, questions about social support and questions about self care.

We ran three pairs of workshops for consumer health information services and one pair for maternity self help groups. These were attended by people from local and regional information services, telephone help lines, drop in centres, libraries, self help groups and health service committees. Some of these people hosted and co-led their workshops.

Overall participants said that they enjoyed the workshops and found them good or excellent use of their time. They also felt that they learnt something that was relevant:

"I feel much more confident now about using research literature"

"This... made me much more aware of what was and what wasn't being said in papers. Made me much less willing to accept what was being said at face value"

"I find it interesting and relevant but still rather difficult... I wouldn't know how to apply it yet"

"My two jobs (Community Health Council member and journalist) both require appraisal skills"

"We now need to cascade this training down to front line workers"

But learning the skills is not enough. There are barriers to providing treatment outcomes information.

"We are not resourced to do this in practice"

"After the first workshop I felt that we're stepping into a minefield providing this information at all"
"I don't want to tell people this condition is fatal, go away and read a leaflet about it. I feel bad giving people information without any support".

After a second workshop reinforced and extended the learning at the first, there was some enthusiasm for accepting the challenge.
"I don't see why we should sit there passing on dodgy information, abdicating responsibility".
"We should be campaigning for research to be done better. There are questions of funding and ethics. [We need] discussion of risk and uncertainty".

To take this work forward the National Childbirth Trust chose to run multi-disciplinary workshops for their members and midwives. NCT members were trained to lead workshops and were supported by CASP in the preparation of workshop materials. At a one day meeting following our series of workshops some of the participants returned to reflect on the workshops and discuss the implication for their work. From these discussions we developed recommendations about the work.

Information on outcomes

The quality of outcomes information for the public is very variable. There is a need to develop quality criteria. This is now being done as part of a British Library funded project, DISCERN. This will provide a valuable tool for producing good evidence-based information for the public, for vetting information already available and possibly to develop a database of high quality outcomes information.

Having information available is only part of the way forward. Giving information about their own treatment to vulnerable people is difficult. Training should include finding and appraising information and how to support members of the public. Giving information about outcomes of care is more difficult than giving information about service availability, and this needs to be addressed in planning and directing services. There is also an urgent need to debate the ethical and legal aspects of communicating outcomes information to the public, and librarians need to be involved in this.

Finally, taking outcomes information to the public opens up opportunities to listen to their informed responses and this can be important for directing what research is undertaken, how research is undertaken and how the findings are reported. So, when librarians are asked to find the evidence to answer patients' questions, if a thorough search reveals there is no evidence, then patients and librarians together can be instrumental in highlighting the need for new research.

The implications for librarians are:

- they may receive more enquiries about outcomes of care from consumer health information services
- the reports librarians find may help individuals to make decisions about their own care
- librarians' searches may find that information about the effects of care is missing and this may initiate new research.

Reference

[1] Gann R, Buckland S. Dissemination of information on treatment outcomes by consumer health information services. London: Kings Fund, 1994

FOCUS PDCA QUALITY IMPROVEMENT TOOL USED FOR CREATING FAMILY AND PATIENT LIBRARY

Kay Cimpl Wagner, Gundersen Lutheran Health Sciences Library, La Crosse, Wisconsin, USA

Introduction to Gundersen Lutheran

Gundersen Lutheran (GL) includes Lutheran Hospital, a 402-bed regional referral and specialty teaching hospital, and Gundersen Clinic with a medical staff of over 300 that provides specialty and primary care through over 712,000 patient visits annually. GL includes five hospitals, 10 health-related corporations, 34 branch clinics throughout a 19 county Tri-State Area of Iowa, Minnesota and Wisconsin, and a Health Maintenance Organization (HMO). GL employees over 6,000 FTE.

The library, vital to GL's medical education and residency programs, occupies 4,433 square feet in a central location within Lutheran Hospital. Expansion of the library has paralleled GL growth. The non-salaried budget expenses have grown nearly 350% in the past ten years. The library subscribes to nearly 800 journal titles which are retained for 20 years. Staff has increased from four to six FTE in the past two years including a second Masters in Library Science (MLS) position.

Background Information

As a result of six patient focus groups conducted by Lutheran Hospital Quality Customer Service Committee in 1993 each hospital Department was asked to develop a plan for improving patient relations. The library staff drafted a proposal to establish a Family and Patient Library as a response to the Committee's challenge. An existing library area housing older journals provided a good location across from the visitor's coffee shop. A library staff member could relocate there to help patients and families with their information needs.

In February 1994 I called together a multi-disciplinary group of health professionals to identify and propose how consumer information could be provided system-wide. On March 4th, this Task Force met and I led a focus session on the following question: "What would a successful family and patient information program look like at GL?" The following components were identified:

- Supported by physicians
- Customer-focused
- Supported by administration
- A gateway to other system resources
- Based on customer needs

It was evident that divisive issues could defeat this program. In an effort to find a systematic planning process that would address the variety of views and concerns to

S. Bakker (ed.), *Health Information Management: What Strategies?*, 234-238.

bring about a successful program proposal I talked to our QIS Coordinator and decided to use the FOCUS-PDCA Quality Tool.

FOCUS-PDCA

FOCUS-PDCA, created by the Hospital Corporation of America (HCA), is a systematic process improvement method. Through FOCUS-PDCA, a knowledge of how a process is currently performing to meet customer needs and expectations is used to plan and test process changes. FOCUS-PDCA is an extension of the Deming or Shewhart Cycle which includes Plan-Do-Check-Act. The HCA FOCUS piece precedes the PDCA with a five part plan: 1) Find a process to improve; 2) Organize to improve the process; 3) Clarify current knowledge of the process; 4) Understand the source of process variation; and 5) Select the process improvement. Based on the focus session and meetings as referenced above, the following focus statement was drafted:

F FIND A FOCUS TO IMPROVE

An opportunity exists to improve our patient and family information process beginning with evaluation of the need for information and ending with delivery of appropriate information. This effort should improve delivery of health information for the patients and families who utilize the Gundersen Lutheran (GL) Health System. The process is important to work on now because:
- There have been requests to consolidate information of this type.
- As a system, we don't know where this type of information is kept or if it exists.
- Patients and their families are asking for information.

O ORGANIZE A TEAM THAT KNOWS THE PROCESS

I assembled an initial multi-disciplinary Team consisting of three RNs, two MDs, one dentist, one pharmacist, a chaplain and two librarians. In the April 1994 Library Newsletter I asked for others interested in serving on the Team to contact me and at a June meeting six MDs, seven RNs, one chaplain, one administrator and two librarians attended and continue to meet quarterly. Everyone on the Team had an interest in patient information, although not necessarily *providing* information. Some of the issues we did agree on were:
- This library should be apart from the medical and nursing libraries, if possible.
- To investigate how the Public Library handles information requests of this kind.
- A lower level library, currently not staffed that houses older journals, is in "prime" space and could be a possibility for this usage.
- The program proposal might fail if money and staffing are sought.
- The library should be a gateway to system resources, people and programs.

C CLARIFY THE CURRENT KNOWLEDGE OF THE PROCESS:

We know that information is being shared with patients and families system-wide in a decentralized fashion. In 1993, six focus groups of approximately 60 patients discharged from Lutheran Hospital were conducted. The top desire of patients and their families was education. We also know that patients and their families are asking for information. The Medical and Nursing Libraries are located by Surgery and the Intensive Care Unit (ICU) so there is alot of traffic in our area and patients and families stop by now for information. Team members logged number and type of questions from patients in their areas June-September 1994.

Members of the Team visited Patient Libraries at Mayo Clinic and the Veteran's Administration (VA) Hospital in Tomah. Key observations were that most patient libraries are recently established, well-used and that location is a critical factor in usage. A visit with the La Crosse Public Library Reference Coordinator found that the typical Public Library visitor also wants to be a more knowledgeable consumer. This visitor very often holds a library card and is from the immediate area. The Public Library generally does not see people from GL's 19 county Tri-State Region of Wisconsin, Minnesota and Iowa which is a large percentage of GL's patient-base. This was a strong justification for establishing an information center on-site at GL.

According to the literature interest in offering medical information to patients has increased in recent years as a result of social, demographic and political changes as well as research documenting the benefits. Patients believe they have a right to understand their health care and participate in treatment decisions. If patients can convey their needs in clear and forthright manners, they are more likely to receive better care with more successful outcomes.

U UNDERSTAND CAUSES OF PROCESS VARIATION

Information at GL is given out in a decentralized manner without any formal policies or procedures. Reaching Team consensus on offering information was sometimes difficult. The following reasons were identified:

- Decentralized information exists within our system and there is no roadmap to follow.
- Our health care environment is uncertain due to impending mergers.
- Funding or space requests for a new service or facility might hurt the proposal.
- The Team had differing opinions on the value and nature of providing information to consumers.
- Administration did not unanimously agree on such a service.

S SELECT THE PROCESS IMPROVEMENT

Possible courses of measurable action to improve our patient and family information process might be:

- Widely provide and advertise access to the Information Access Company's (IAC) product, Health Reference Center on Compact Disk (CD). This product is already on the library network and used now for patient information requests.
- Organize and publicize what is already here institutionally and how to get to it.
- Monitor patient and family information needs.
- Establish a Family and Patient Library

P PLAN THE IMPROVEMENT AND CONTINUED DATA COLLECTION

On January 4, 1995 I met with administration to share the above FOCUS and gather future direction. Administration agreed we should begin planning the PFL. On January 17th the Team met and put together the beginning planning pieces:

Name: The name of the facility will be the Family and Patient Library.

Location: The lower level storage library across the Patio Coffee Shop will be used.

Opening: The Library will open April 1, 1995.

Resources: The Health Reference Center on CD, plus other hard copy materials evaluated by two Team physicians, will provide information. There is a photocopy machine available. Materials will be purchased out of the existing library budget. Leisurely reading material will also be provided. Other collections, such as bereavement and hospice materials, may be part of the collection. Team members will investigate locations of other GL patient information collections. An intern will create a database containing this information.

Staffing & hours: The Library will be open from 1-4 p.m. Monday-Friday and staffed by current library staff.

Advertising: GL's in-house newsletter, Bridges, will initially be used for promotion. A brochure will be created to advertise the library.

Cosmetics: The new library space was painted. Furniture was rearranged and computers were installed and networked. A CD player was installed.

Evaluation: A log-in form was developed.

Meetings: The Team will meet quarterly.

Grants: The Team will solicit potential grant funding, when appropriate.

D DO THE IMPROVEMENT, DATA COLLECTION AND ANALYSIS

The library opened, as planned, April 1st. A library staff member, temp or intern has staffed it daily from 1-4 P.M.

Collection: A small "starter" book collection was purchased prior to April 1st. Several special interest collections also found a home:

- The Bereavement cart.
- Advanced directives brochures.
- Sports Medicine newsletters.
- GL affiliate clinics information brochures.
- Hospice and pain management.

From June-October 1995 an intern surveyed campus departments to see what other patient information materials were available system-wide and identified nine departments:

- Anesthesiology
- Dermatology
- Family Practice
- Internal Medicine
- Hospice
- Otolaryngology
- Plastic and Reconstructive Surgery
- Teen Health
- X Ray

This information was entered on a database software program.

Facilities: In addition to air handling, painting, and lighting a partition is being made to conceal the older medical journals while still allowing retrieval. A new work station was assembled mid-April 1996. Other proposed remodeling changes could not be made due to either fire or safety codes. Softer furniture was included and approved in the 1996 capital budget.

Information requests: Our request log from April 1995-April 1996 showed that in one years' time we had **85** requests for information. Of the 85 requests, **66** were directly from outside customers (i.e. patient, family member). Nineteen were either medical staff, employees, or students. Common themes were Lyme disease, AIDS, multiple sclerosis (MS) and cancer. We have not created an input form.

Marketing: We met with Marketing Communications in January 1996 to design an advertising flyer.

Patient center: I am involved in an institution-wide committee established early in 1996 that is looking at a Patient Center for access, appointments *and* information.

C CHECK THE RESULTS AND LESSONS LEARNED

Staffing: From June 1995-June 1996 we did not have the Family and Patient Library coordinator position filled. At times it was difficult to dedicate staff every afternoon from 1-4 pm but we managed to do it either with the existing full-time staff, an intern and/or a Kelly Girl temp.

Collection: The hard cover collection was used to answer customers' needs but Health Reference Center on CD was the first source for information. Full-text could be printed and given to the customer to take with them.

Grants: The La Crosse Foundation awarded us $500.00 for diabetes education materials. A GL Vested Interest Partners (VIP) grant bought a skeleton and anatomical charts.

Computers: A second PC workstation was added for customer searching and three laptops with access to the World Wide Web were added.

Marketing: We received 500 flyers on April 23rd. Marketing agreed to let us place the flyers around the institution, including the Intensive Care Unit (ICU) waiting room. Exposure should create more business.

A ACT TO HOLD THE GAIN AND TO CONTINUE TO IMPROVE

I see the Family and Patient Library becoming part of the Patient Center. A proposal for the patient center is being drafted and will be presented to administration early June 1996. A library will definitely be a part of this Center and we will commit a half-time librarian to staff it. The Center will likely be in the adjacent Gundersen Clinic. Preliminary proposed estimates for furniture, equipment, computers and the collection (non-salaried expenses) will be about $100,000.00. The experience and exposure gained this past year will prove invaluable as we become part of a larger information center for our customers.

Bibliography

Kahn G. Computer-based patient education: A progress report. MD Comput 1993;10:93-99
Lindner K. Encourage information therapy. JAMA 1992;267:2592
Rees A. Communication in the physician-patient relationship. Bull Med Libr Assoc 1993;81:1-10

A HEALTH LIBRARY IN A HEALTH CENTRE

José Vasco Costa de Sousa, Centro de Saúde da Venda Nova, Amadora, Portugal

Staff Venda Nova Health Centre

PROFESSION	NUMBER
Doctors	61
Nurses	34
Social workers	1
Radiology technicians	1
Public functionaries	56
TOTAL	**153**

Working in a suburban Health Centre and providing Primary Health Care of good quality to the population living inside its area, is not an easy task. From the pregnant woman to the dying patient, there is a large array of medical, social, family and individual problems which look for solutions in the Health Centre. To answer them all, we must be prepared with both scientific and technical knowledge of good quality and lots of common sense.

Our Health Centre of Venda Nova is located in Amadora city nearby Lisboa. The population assisted by our staff is about 78599 persons, including people coming from the rural areas of Portugal, but also from Africa (Cabo Verde). Many of these are now growing older.

During the year of 1995 the total amount of medical consultations of any kind (including Children's and Women's Health consultations) was 126643. The quality of our work must go side by side with the Continuous Education of all professionals concerned. One of the ways to achieve this is the development of a Health Library.

Our library collection is small: 95 monographs on varies subjects, ranging from "pure" clinical books to legislation concerning Primary Health Care, and from Preventive Health to Palliative Care.

Several problems must be solved:

In the first place we must attract more readers and their suggestions to the Health Library. Readers are the soul of any kind of Library, even if it is a small one. Our target readers are now the workers of the Health Centre, but in a near future we hope to open our library to Community key persons, such as local government staff, elderly people organisations, parents associations, schools and teachers, sports associations, local enterprises, etc.

Secondly we need to improve the quality of our "librarian" work. Doing so will open doors to the co-operation with other Health Libraries of a higher level. This shall include the installation of computer data bases, and on line services available to the staff members of Venda Nova Health Centre, or other people or organisations concerned with health matters.

Our aim and our hope are to create in our health library a small "knowledge centre" which will be useful to different kinds of people.

References

Weston WW, Dunikowski IG. A library for family physicians. Can Fam Physician 1992;38:1051-70

S. Bakker (ed.), Health Information Management: What Strategies?, 239.

HEALTH PROMOTION STRATEGIES FOR THE GENERAL PUBLIC

Vilma Alberani and Paola de Castro Pietrangeli, Istituto Superiore di Sanità, Rome, Italy

National health authorities have an important role in developing strategies for the promotion of public health through the diffusion of information to the general public. "Information for all", in fact, is the first step to prevent and control the diffusion of diseases and reach the objectives stated by the "Health for all" program of the WHO. The channels of communication used by researchers and decision-makers in the scientific community are well known, but health promotion includes also strategies for the development of messages and materials to reach the most general public. Such materials may be presented in different forms (paper, visual and/or audio-visual) and may be spread through different channels of communication (e. g. institutional networks, mass media) to different target audiences (groups, individuals, etc.). This should permit to influence the behaviour of people changing wrong attitudes (alcohol, tobacco and drug abuse), prevent the diffusion of widespread diseases, reduce the effects of environmental pollution, etc.

The Istituto Superiore di Sanità, the technical scientific body of the Italian national health service, has recently developed some information channels for the general public: audiovisuals, leaflets, posters, spots, etc. Some example of the ISS realisations are given.

The Institute is graphically represented as a large tree with many leaves (reproduced as slides) and various kinds of fruit; people of different ages and social status can pick up the fruit of this tree and thus receive the messages proposed by the ISS for health promotion in order to: spread information, develop cooperation, change wrong attitudes. Among the information tools (leaflets, posters, videos, spots, CD-ROMs, hot lines, slides, reports, etc.) appearing on the branches of the tree, a special emphasis is given to the issues included in the research projects of the ISS receiving financial support by the Italian national health fund. In the last years, the health promotion activities for the general public were mainly related to infectious diseases (AIDS, influenza, viral hepatitis, pertussis, tuberculosis, malaria, etc.), organ transplantation (to increase the number of donors), drug addiction, etc. More recently, part of this information is also available through the Internet, thus overcoming the national boundaries.

The results of the promotion activity should be carefully monitored in order to focus on and develop the most appropriate strategies. By the moment, it is possible to state that all the ISS initiatives were welcome and that the requests for diffusion of the information material are continuously growing, mainly through the local health units. The next steps in the promotion activity should mostly concentrate on the channels of diffusion of the information material and on the financial support required to carry on a relevant health promotion program.

S. Bakker (ed.), Health Information Management: What Strategies?, 240-241.

Health Promotion Strategies for the General Public

Vilma Alberani, Paola De Castro Pietrangeli
Istituto Superiore di Sanità
Viale Regina Elena, 299 - Rome (Italy)

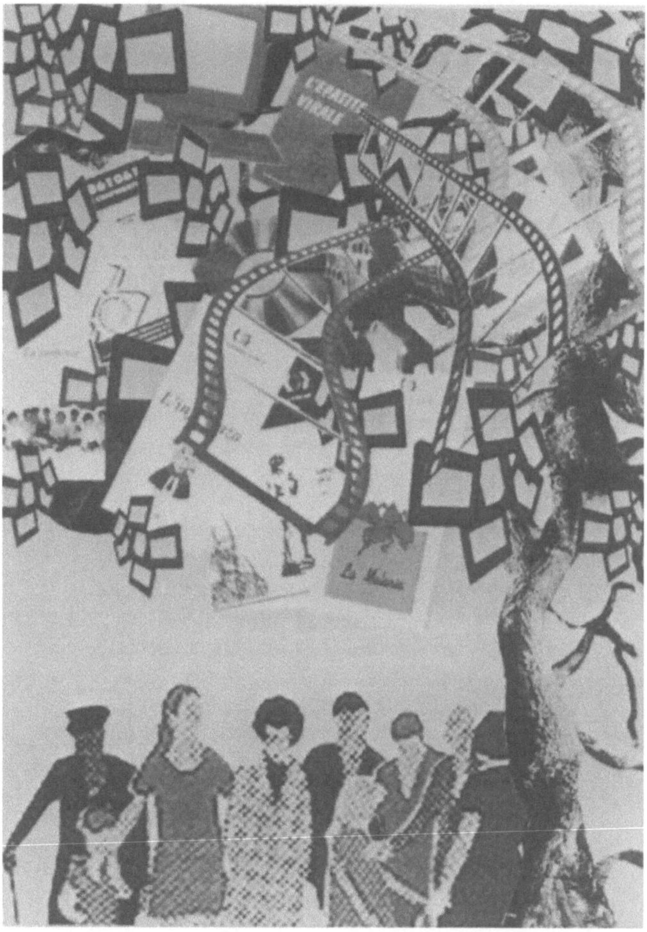

Graphic Design by Cosimo Marino Curianò

Health promotion tools are represented as fruit of a large tree... Everybody can pick up a fruit, receive a message, get informed, change wrong attitudes

A NEW PROFESSIONALISM FOR THE ELECTRONIC AGE?

*Tony McSeán and Derek Law**, *British Medical Association; **Kings College, London, UK

Scholarly communication

Ten years ago <50% of academics used a personal computer. Now they are assumed to be almost universal. Ten years ago the Internet did not exist. Now it demonstrates the fastest growth rate known for any technology. The number of Internet users was 39,000,000 in October 1995 and 42,000,000 in January 1996. Ten million computer nodes are linked to the Internet, each with its sub-network. At current growth rates computers will outnumber people by 2003. They will contain information of hugely varying quality as well as information which is simply wrong.

At the same time the paradigm of scholarly communication is changing. Over the last five years the number of multi-authored papers with trans-national authorship has risen from 10% to 25% of those listed in SCI. Working methods are changing. In physics, mathematics, computing and some areas of medical research the game has shifted. Papers are written, circulated, discussed and modified and the discipline moves on. Only later is there archival publication. And who is to do that archiving in an electronic world? Publishers — who have been incapable of doing it for the last 500 years.

Yet in that new research paradigm our role remains very uncertain. In 1995, British academic librarians were asked to predict when electronic journals would overtake the printed. The consensus was 2020 but already that prediction looks as though it is conservative by more than ten years. But not all is well on the Internet. It is the sheer volume and low quality of the available resources which will allow us, information professionals, to redefine our role.

Information management skills

Our core professional competences are selection, storage and support.

SELECTION

Although the decision to acquire or access information is mostly independent of the medium, electronic texts raise new issues. How do we define the original and uncorrupted text? How do we define the status of the latest and intermediate texts? Misinformation on the Internet is a literally deadly problem for us. Do we distinguish

S. Bakker (ed.), Health Information Management: What Strategies?, 243-245.

between supported resources and unsupported resources? It is now commonly accepted that we shall move from holdings to access strategies. How? Do we catalogue the things we don't have rather than the things we do? Do we really believe that Web crawlers can replace our judgement?

Making Internet resources accessible is a huge professional challenge which there is very little sign of our profession taking up. Quality assurance is an implicit but rarely stated part of stock selection, for we acquire only what is perceived as relevant and valuable. Electronic publications are much more susceptible to corruption since it is quite difficult to tell whence they originate and whether and when they have been changed, accidentally or by design. But there are other problems too. Conventional publication has markers. "Oxford University Press" implies something about quality. The network address OXFORD.AC.UK implies anything from a university press to a student bedroom. When everything is available without these markers, selection by the user becomes more of a problem.

STORAGE

We rely on a system where libraries form networks to retain and store the documents we consider of value. Very little thought has yet been given to how this will be managed in an electronic era. In archiving and preservation the range of issues is enormous. There are obvious issues related to databases and texts, but what about patient records or to CAT Scans? The record of research has tended to be preserved in the papers of researchers donated or bequeathed to archives. Who is consistently collecting the e-mail of Nobel prizewinners or the debates on bulletin boards which is where the scientific debate now takes place. We need to consider revivifying the University Presses and Learned Society Presses as a means of making scholarship properly available. We need to consider whether the creators of intellectual capital should set up a Copyright Licensing Agency in which we licence limited rights to commercial publishers on our terms. We need to look at how we preserve the intellectual record of the academy. And I would argue that the responsibility is ours. Some 35 institutions have survived largely unchanged since the fourteenth century, the Papacy, the parliament of Iceland, the Tynwald of the Isle of Man and 32 universities. Here again we neglect our roots at our peril.

Implicit in storage is another classic information skill, the organisation of knowledge. It is only when one watches others struggling to reinvent what are effectively classification schemes that we realise our skills. We should maintain and develop our heritage for electronic resources.

SUPPORT

The third area of skills lies in the general area of training in information skills. Although we have long talked about empowering end users, it is equally clear that users need help to take advantage of that freedom. One of the dangers facing information professionals is the complacency of the satisfied inept. Most student users have no learning curve since they are with us so briefly. Some of the trends in education suggest that we will see much greater emphasis on distance learning where support and instruction becomes critical. The same is true of telemedicine. There is a lot of experience which shows that the acquisition costs are trivial compared with the ownership costs. It is the support, the instruction and the documentation which makes a difference.

I am reluctant to use phrases for this such as "the library without walls" if only because a library without walls will find that the roof falls in. So let me settle for the conventional phrase of the virtual library. The future is going to be difficult, demanding and different, but the surest and best way of attacking and enjoying it is through the extension, development and renewal of our professional disciplines and training.

Having considered the threats and opportunities facing us, we can then articulate a strategy which will set information professionals at the heart of the information age. This strategy is based on the draft vision statement of the UK's Libraries and Information Commission.

A strategy for health libraries

Libraries and librarians will concentrate on three core concerns: connectivity - providing universal access to knowledge; content - creating a digital library of materials for health professionals; competences - equipping individuals and organisations to operate in the information society.

CORE VALUES

These grow from a restatement of the core values of librarians, who:

- work with *knowledge*; add value by evaluating, making accessible, mediating, packaging and promoting knowledge

- are the *memory of society* through collecting and preserving knowledge

- form a *substantial* and *growing sector* of the economy

- are necessary to the *well-being* of individuals, communities and society

- reach into *people's lives* in many ways; people use a range of LIS throughout their lives and often use several different "libraries" at any one point in their lives

- provide access to opportunities for *lifelong learning*; the knowledge which underpins all successful economic activity; the information which is central to a healthy and democratic society;

- empower the individual by *providing resources and information* for particular user groups and the information skills which are the essential coping skills for modern-day living

- embody the value of *collective activity*; engender a sense of community within places and organisations; and provide a space where people can feel secure within a shared value system

These will be achieved through redefining the core professional skills of selection, storage and support.

FROM TEA PARTY TO GLOBAL NETWORKING; EXPERIENCES FROM 40 YEARS OF EVOLUTION

Elisabeth Akre, Patricia Flor and Elisabeth Husem, Norwegian Library Association, Oslo, Norway

The very idea of a conference is to get together to share and exchange knowledge, experience and contacts. We would like to share with you the story of our association, the Norwegian Library Association. Section for Medicine and Health Sciences (SMH).

History

It was only after the Second World War that Norwegian hospitals and universities started engaging medical librarians. They soon understood that in order to develop their libraries they needed to cooperate and create a professional and personal network in their special field. The national library associations and the national bibliographic sources were not yet developed enough to meet their specific needs.

In 1953 medical librarians in the Oslo area started a «tea club» in order to discuss common problems and challenges. The discussions soon led to concrete fields of cooperation, such as:

- Cooperation between medical libraries in general
- Mutual reports on new journal subscriptions and cancellations
- Updating of the national union catalogue
- Exchange of duplicate journal copies
- Interlibrary loans

Among the results of the cooperation was more money for the national union catalogue, medical bibliography as a subject at the college for library education, and university courses in anatomy and physiology for medical librarians.

The number of medical librarians increased and so did the interest for the «tea parties». This led to structured meetings with educational programmes such as Medline, consumer education and computer courses.

In 1976 the «tea club» became part of the Norwegian Library Association as «Section for Medical Librarianship» (SMB) with the object: «- to take care of and promote medical librarianship». With small modifications this is still the main object of our association.

In 1992 the name was changed to «Section for Medicine and Health Sciences» (SMH), thus expanding the concept «medical librarianship».

Today SMH has close on 200 members, mostly in Norway, but also some in the other Nordic countries.

S. Bakker (ed.), Health Information Management: What Strategies?, 246-248.

Activities today

Norway is a long, thin country with a small and widely spread population. It is difficult for members from different parts of the country to participate in meetings and courses because the journey is long and expensive. Many work alone in small libraries.

One of the most imporant tasks for SMH is to find ways of facilitating communication between the members in all parts of the country.

For practical reasons the main part of the activities take place in the south east part of Norway, mainly the Oslo area, but we try to take care of all the members by giving travel grants for participation in seminars and meetings, editing a newsletter and arranging seminars and meetings outside of the central area, at least once a year. SMH's plan of activities for 1996 includes:

* 4 members meetings, at least one outside of Oslo.
* Continuing education courses, minimum 2
* Nordic and international cooperation
* Newsletter, 3 issues per year

The Nordic and international engagement

The Norwegian medical and health librarians soon understood the importance of participating in international conferences and workshops, as well as the importance of cooperation between the countries in general.

When the 1st International Congress on Medical Librarianship was arranged in London in 1953 almost all the Norwegian medical librarians attended. Maybe this was the inspiration to start the tea-club soon after.

When EAHIL was established as an organisation in 1987, a Norwegian medical librarian became a member of the first board. SMH works closely with EAHIL, and is an institutional member of the organisation.

In medical and health sciences librarianship cooperation and networking on an international level has always been necessary to find and procure medical knowledge and information. It will be even more so in the future, and SMH encourages its members to participate in international conferences by giving them as much economic support as possible.

From the 1960's there has been a close contact and cooperation with «sister» associations in the Nordic countries. In 1995 the «Nordic Association for Health Information and Libraries» was founded. A Nordic conference is held every fourth year - the next one is planned in Iceland in 1999. A common Nordic newsletter is published once a year, with contributions from the five Nordic countries.

EAHIL is working to establish and develop cooperation with the countries in Eastern Europe. The Nordic associations feel especially close to the Baltic countries, and cooperation programmes are being established. For practical reasons each Nordic association has its special partner country.

SMH is working with medical libraries in Lithuania, especially Kaunas Medical Academy Library. Up to now we have concentrated on integrating our Lithuanian partners into the international network by supporting participation at conferences. In the future we hope to expand our contacts and co-operation projects. The SMH's Baltic committee visited Kaunas and Vilnius in June 1996 in order to develop this.

In 1994 SMH hosted the 4th European conference for medical and health libraries in Oslo in cooperation with EAHIL.

Views for the future

Due to data security regulations there are still members, especially in hospitals, who do not yet have access to Internet. But we believe it is only a question of time before they get it. One of our most important tasks in the near future will be to create a better Internet communication for our members, and as a link to all of you. We have recently established a home page. The next step will be a SMH mailbox.

The net possibilities is a unique opportunity to fullfil the association's role as a link between individual members, between the members and other associations and to the professional international world.

Conclusion

The world is getting smaller and closer every day. Electronic communication is providing all the possibilities needed for professional updating. Our challenge is no longer to get access to sources, but to sort out from the overflow of information and possibilities what we really need for our work and our users, and how to define the role of information officers under the changing circumstances.

The role of library associations is changing accordingly. The changing structure of the information world does not make a national library association less needed. It is more important than ever for several reasons:

* we can achieve more professional development together than alone
* the association is a link between the individual members and the global electronic network
* the association is a link to personal networks
* the association should take care of the interests of its members in library politics

The third aspect is not the least important. The net can never make up for personal contacts and what they mean for the challenges we face in our everyday work. Maybe the title of this paper should be: not «*from* teaparty *to* global networking», but «*both* teaparty *and* global networking».

Reference

Hvardal M. Det begynte over en kopp te. SMH-Nytt 1993;18(3):2-4
Norwegian Library Association. Section for Medicine and Health. Plan of activities 1996

AN INTERNATIONAL JOB EXCHANGE: AN EXPERIENCE WHICH CAN CHANGE YOUR LIFE

Donna Flake, Coastal Area Health Education Center, Wilmington, NC, USA

International exchange programs

International job exchanges usually result in long term benefits for all persons involved. My paper covers different types of international job exchanges, some funding mechanisms, and a case study of my own job exchange.

Most job exchanges are arranged entirely by the *two persons* involved. This type of job swap is fairly commonplace, as is evidenced by the literature.

Another type is an exchange of librarians between *two libraries* in different countries, which have decided to exchange librarians over a period of time. This is easy for individual librarians, because the Library Directors have already organized the program. Sometimes this arrangement is between two universities in different countries.

Still another type of exchange involves working with *agencies* which organize job exchanges or help to facilitate job exchanges. Two examples offering international work to librarians are:

1) The Library Fellows Program of the *American Library Association* which places librarians in foreign libraries for up to a year and

2) the *Council for International Exchange of Scholars* which administers the Fulbright Awards.

Also, *library associations* try to foster international exchanges. The International Federation of Library Associations & Institutions Secretariat publishes lists of librarians seeking job exchanges. The Medical Library Association's Job Exchange Committee has developed a database of librarians seeking international exchanges. The database was published in the EAHIL Newsletter, as well as on MEDLIB-L. The database continues to be updated on the Internet.[1] Also, the American Library Association's International Relations Round Table fosters job exchanges, and they also have a database on the Internet of libraries willing to support international exchanges.[2] Also, the American Library Fellows Program of the American Library Association sponsors work programs for approximately 20 foreign librarians to work in the United States annually. Each librarian earns about $32,000 during his or her stay in the United States.

S. Bakker (ed.), Health Information Management: What Strategies?, 249-251.

Case Study of a Job Exchange

For six months in 1984 I participated in a job exchange. I swapped jobs with Oren Stone, a cataloger, from the Wessex Medical Library at the University of Southampton, England. At the time, I was working as Head of Reference at the Health Sciences Library at East Carolina University in Greenville, North Carolina, USA. The two libraries are similar in size, both being medical school libraries. Arranging such a work experience was no small feat.

HOW I ARRANGED THE EXCHANGE

My exchange was preceded by substantial planning. First, I searched the literature.

Then I wrote to 35 British medical libraries as well as several agencies but unfortunately, this did not produce an exchange partner.

Finally I advertised in the Library Association Record: Vacancies Supplement. This was the best approach because I received responses from four potential exchange partners. After much correspondence, I selected my exchange partner. My job exchange was organized solely by me and my exchange partner, and no outside agency provided funding nor support.

Many issues had to be resolved before the exchange could proceed. I had to verify that Oren and I had the same educational credentials, and after some investigation, I found we did. We decided on the exact job duties to be performed.

We further decided to keep our own salaries from our home libraries. We also decided to retain the vacation earned from our home libraries, and to take the vacation days during the exchange.

There were financial arrangements to make. I arranged for my salary to be deposited into my bank account in America. I calculated the amount that should remain in the American bank account, and arranged for the remainder to be sent to me in England.

Long Term Effects of a Job Exchange

First of all, I feel a tremendous sense of accomplishment for having been able to arrange the job exchange.

Another effect was my ability to travel. In 1986, in 1988, and in 1992, I visited England- to present papers or poster sessions at medical library meetings. I am sure these invitations are a result of working in England and getting to know many of the English librarians. Also, I presented the keynote address at the Second Annual CD-ROM Conference in Tokyo in 1991. Presenting papers in England helped me to receive this invitation to Tokyo.

Another change is that I published several papers on job exchanges. One of my papers on job exchanges was published in Health Libraries Review in 1985.

As a result of the publications, when I applied for membership in the Medical Library Association's Academy of Health Information Professionals, I was granted "Distinguished" member status.

Another important result has been in my work with the Medical Library Association. I served on several international MLA committees, twice I served on the Cunningham Fellow Selection Jury, and have held several offices in the International Cooperation Section of the Medical Library Association. In 1993, in 1995, and in 1996 I chair the Job Exchange Committee of the International Cooperation Section of the Medical Library Association. During 1996 and 1997, I am chairing the Cunningham Fellow Coordinating Committee which will plan the travels and working schedule for our next Cunningham Fellow, Ioana Gabriela Robu, from Romania.

My greatest honor since the job exchange has been my appointment as the Medical Library Association's representative to EAHIL. I feel this happened as a result of my job exchange, my subsequent international speaking engagements, and my persistent interest and involvement in the International Cooperation Section of the Medical Library Association. Now an entire new set of opportunities for international cooperation and travel have opened up for me. In 1995 I attended the EAHIL meeting in Prague. Now I have colleagues and friends in Europe too! I am full of enthusiasm for EAHIL, Europe, and my new European colleagues!

My resume which naturally enumerates the accomplishments just mentioned, is more impressive as the result of these international activities. In January, 1992 I changed jobs, and am now the Library Director for the Coastal Area Health Education Center, in Wilmington, North Carolina. My current employer was impressed with my international activities.

The job exchange allowed me to significantly broaden my horizons. Just before my English work experience, I felt very sheltered, and narrow in terms of my experience. Having that eye opening experience helped me to have the courage and gumption to apply for higher level library jobs, and I was hired for those jobs. I felt if I could be successful working in England, I could be successful in anything I tried to do.

The friends I made will always be a part of my life. I feel a part of me is still in England. I feel much closer to England than before the experience. I know exactly what many of the cities and villages look like. Foreigners working in other countries bring countries much closer together.

My job exchange had a profound impact on my professional and personal life. It was one of the happiest and most fulfilling times of my life. I will always treasure this very special time because it opened up a whole new world for me.

I strongly encourage other medical librarians thinking of a job exchange to turn their thoughts and dreams into a reality.

References

[1] Using Internet, select **http://ahsc.arizona.edu/~lei/mla/jobs.htm**

[2] Using Internet, select **http://www.ala.org**
then select ALA gopher site,
then select ALA Round Tables,
then select International Relations Round Tables,
then select International Exchange

EDUCATING INFORMATION PROFESSIONALS: THE CASE FOR A HEALTH INFORMATION MODULE

Susan Hornby, Manchester Metropolitan University, UK

Background

The BA (Honours) Information and Library Management course taught in the department was due for review. It was apparent from student feedback that they felt unsure of applying for appropriate work in health information. National Health Services information professionals indicated that while graduates had a good general grounding within information organisation, access and retrieval more subject specific knowledge would be advantageous for students taking up their first professional post.

In consultation with current students, recent graduates and practitioners within the health information field I designed a module, intended as an introduction and an overview to key issues in health information, for inclusion in the new BA/BSc Information and Library Management Course.

Methodology/Course design

The intention was that the student would be able to draw upon knowledge, ideas and information from other taught modules and from their own professional and personal experiences and relate them to specific health information areas.

Research by Noel Entwistle on student learning has developed the features of deep, surface and strategic learning.[1] The deep approach is characterised by an intention to understand the subject, to interact vigorously and critically with the content. The student will relate the ideas to previous knowledge and experience, will relate the evidence to conclusions and examine the logic of the argument.

It was decided, therefore, that the methods of assessment would be integral to the module and would be both summative and formative. Therefor assessed group presentations on specific health related issues would be part of the course delivery.

Challenges

There were three main challenges to the introduction of the module: time constraints, content of the module, module delivery and assessment.

S. Bakker (ed.), Health Information Management: What Strategies?, 252-254.

THE TIME CONSTRAINTS

The new BA/BSc course was modular in design and ran over two 15 week semesters. Each module was designed to last for one semester. The fifteen weeks included three weeks of assessments and/or examinations. In such a brief module it was necessary to utilise the time to its most effective. By involving a large amount of practitioner input both in the design and delivery of the course it was felt that current concerns would be addressed and students would gain a wider experience of practical as well as theoretical issues within health information.

THE CONTENT OF THE MODULE

Consulting widely with practitioners on the areas of current concern resulted in the initial programme of lectures and visiting speakers running as follows:
Introduction and overview: politics, economics and the role of information. (week 1)
The *National Health Service* as an organisation. Management in the National Health Service. The continuing changes within the organisational structure of the Health Service. (week 2)
Information for clinicians. Post Graduate Medical Centres. Funding. The effects of trust status. Access and costs. The role of the information. (week 3)
Information for nurse education. Project 2000. Post Registration Education and Practice. Current changes - links with Higher Education. Funding. The role of the information worker. (week 4)
Information for managers. The role of National Health Service manager. Information needs. Access points. Cost of information. Confidentiality. (week 5)
Information for purchasers/providers. Who are the purchasers. Who are the providers. The effects of the purchaser/provider divide. The role of the information worker. Accuracy and objectivity? (week 6)
The effects of trust status on *hospital wide information*. Sources of information in hospitals. The historic development of information sources. Duplication. Information overload. (week 7)
Information needs of patients. What are they? How are they accessed? Restrictions on access. Access to medical records. The psychology of limiting access. Problems of 'inappropriate' information. (week 8)
An introduction to *health informatics*. (week 9)
Information for professions associated with medicine. (week 10)
Student led seminars. (weeks 11 & 12)

It was a very intensive course. Of the ten weeks of the taught sessions four were presented by practitioners. The taught element engendered lively debate and very positive feedback from the students.

THE MODULE DELIVERY AND ASSESSMENT

Again Professor Entwistle has studied which factors in the learning environment influence the approach that students adopt (deep or surface).[2] He has argued that the assessment procedure can influence student approaches to learning. Students who rely on a surface approach tend to prefer lectures that are directed and lecturer led, those students that elect a deep approach prefer lectures that are challenging. Surface approaches to learning can be influenced by methods of assessment that emphasise the elementary aspects of the subject taught.

As Gibbs contends "Co-operative learning in teams offers tremendous scope for independent learning of quality with more students and reduced resources."[3] Using student experiences and knowledge part of the course was developed for assessed group presentations.By using the assessment as part of the course delivery students were encouraged to develop areas of specific interest and present them as part of small group to the other students on the course.It was necessary to give extensive guidelines and tutorial support for the students.

Problems had been expected with the content and accuracy of some of the presentations this, in the event, did not happen. However it was ensured that those assessing the presentations were available to correct any errors of fact and/or interpretation should they arise. The tutorial sessions given prior to the presentations also allowed monitoring of the direction the presentation was taking.

FEEDBACK

The impact of the course was assessed by asking feedback at the end of the course, before students were given their overall marks.

The results were positive as shown:

1. The delivery was clear and understandable
   14% Strongly agreed 86% Agreed
2. The content was appropriate
   28% Strongly agreed 71% Agreed
3. The unit was well organized
   43% Strongly agreed 43% Agreed 14% Agreed with reservations
4. I needed to do a lot of work in my own time.
   14% Strongly agreed 71% Agreed 14% Agreed with reservations
5. The unit was interesting and stimulating.
   86% Strongly agreed 14% Agreed
6. The assessment was a useful learning experience.
   86% Strongly agreed 14% Agreed
7. There was good supporting material (handouts, reading lists, workbooks, etc)
   29% Strongly agreed 43% Agreed 14% Agreed with reservations
   14% Disagreed

The students made the following comments:

Major strengths: (a) Visits from people employed in health were very interesting. (b) The course was well rounded and very enjoyable. (c) The usage of multiple speakers from outside gave a varied and interesting flavour to the course.

Other comments: A few visits would have provided added interest.

77% of students responded. Overall the course went well. It was obvious from the comments that students would have liked to have had time for visits to some of the health information centres locally. This was taken in to account and visits were incorporated into the course the following year. The student presentations were uniformly well done. The research and commitment shown by the students was excellent.

References

[1] Entwistle N. Recent research on student learning and the learning environment.

[2] Entwistle N. Approaches to learning and perceptions of the learning environment. Higher education. 1991;(22.3):201-4

[3] Gibbs G. Independent learning with more students. PCFC 1992:17

USER EDUCATION AS A CHALLENGE FOR PROFESSIONAL DEVELOPMENT

Maurella Della Seta, Gabriella Poppi and Adriana Dracos, Istituto Superiore di Sanità, Rome, Italy

Introduction

In this paper the authors consider user training-programmes as a vehicle to improve the role of the library and of the information professionals within their own institution. The professional prestige of librarians is usually low in most countries,[1] for many reasons, but there is no doubt that a way to improve the professional status and the image of the library is to raise the quality of the services offered, and at the same time to make them more user-oriented. In recent years the library and the documentation service of the Istituto Superiore di Sanità (ISS) have developed a global education strategy which takes into account two strictly related aspects - professional growth and end-user training - with a double aim: improving the image of the information professionals within their organisation and increasing the use of the services. This marketing operation is carried out through the analysis of the different factors involved: (1) library staff training and updating, necessitated by the spread of new products and services and by new approaches in accessing online resources; (2) evaluation of needs and typology of end-users. The objectives of the programme are on one side to achieve the awareness among end-users of the existence of new products and of new media available in the library, on the other to improve search effectiveness and to obtain independence from continual assistance by librarians.

End-users oriented professional education

PROFESSIONAL ACTIVITIES

The need for a substantive updating of the basic range of knowledge is motivated in any professional activity, and this is especially true in the field of information science and documentation. Education and training of the information professional, which in the past could be sometimes performed in a non-systematic way, has now become an important task in the context of daily activities. In our institution training of library staff was necessitated by the acquisition of products on different media - e.g. online databases and CD-ROM - and by the developments of technology which caused and causes changes in the way of accessing information. Requalification of personnel was achieved by attending national and international meetings, workshops and exhibitions organised by producers and distributors of information services; through the study of

S. Bakker (ed.), Health Information Management: What Strategies?, 255-257.

factsheets and manuals prepared by online database producers or enclosed with CD-ROM products; through the study of professional literature. In-house courses were provided by experienced librarians and included training in techniques of searching both CD-ROM and Internet resources.

END-USERS PROFILE

The following step of our programme was the analysis of end-users profile and of their present status of knowledge in the field of information retrieval. As emerges from recent studies the move from the paper library to the electronic library is not painless for users, which sometimes complain about negative factors as information overload.[2] End-users information needs must be taken into account in conceiving an educational strategy, which may be effective only if the information professional is motivated towards a user-oriented instruction.

In this perspective our programme included as an important step the preparation of guides and leaflets to be distributed to end-users during training sessions. As well known, users often refuse to read instruction provided by database producers, since this kind of documentation is too much detailed and the language used is not immediately understandable. Simplified handout guides have been therefore prepared by the staff of the library and of the documentation service: these guides deal with different topics such as databases available on disk or online and the use of the online catalogue set up in the library using DOBIS/LIBIS system. Moreover, a guide to reference sources to documents produced by World Health Organisation can be mentioned. In addition, one-page cards have also been prepared for all databases available, outlining contents of database, types of primary documents indexed, searchable fields and main function keys. Users were also encouraged to make use of computer assisted instructions, help screen and tutorials supplied by producers.

END-USER TRAINING

Following this preliminary approach collective training courses aimed at end-users were organised in the form of workshops to which a maximum of forty participants was admitted. Lessons included lectures held with the help of liquid crystal display screen linked to the workstation and hands-on experience on the basis of demonstrations prepared by the teachers. From the evaluation forms distributed at the end of each course it resulted clearly that there was a request, by users, for more practical experiences of searching online and CD-ROM databases: individualized training sessions were appointed consequently.

Another aspect of the marketing operation performed by the library and the documentation service was the dissemination of information through local and international networks. Home pages were prepared and spread through Internet, providing news about opening hours and the organisation of the library, scheduled training courses, new documents available, and so on.

PRODUCT EVALUATION

At present the user's attitude towards information retrieval is oriented not only to exploit CD-ROMs but also commercial online information systems.

Therefore, to meet the user's needs the information professional is asked for a thorough examination of the products available on the market. He is spurred on studying the characteristics of information retrieval products in order to select, among them, those directly accessible by the end-user, those requiring a short training and those conceived only for the experienced online users.[3]

Since the eigthies, in order to ease online searching, different interfaces such as form-filling, graphical or menu ones were introduced in addition to the already well-known command systems. This trend has been so successfully that a large number of ever more flexible interfaces have been developed and are now essential tools to improve and facilitate the online approach mainly by end-users.

The information professional is well acquainted with command searching languages of the major files he uses on a routine basis and tends to neglect the latest products in the field. It is the user's request to become self-sufficient that spurs the information professional on keeping up to date with new interfaces. These can be so flexible and user-friendly that even the information professional may use them to optimize a bibliographic search or to work with files he doesn't know in depth. Among the different interfaces the user has at his disposal one of the most intuitive and easy-to-use is certainly the natural language interface, which allows translation from natural language terms introduced by end-user to controlled vocabulary specific to the system being searched. By the spread of this kind of online search interfaces, the user may perform simple bibliographic searches, while the librarian may concentrate his efforts on more complex queries. After an initial period of user training, which might cause an increase in librarian engagement, there could be a trend towards a deeper concern, on librarian side, to activities related to organization and study.

Conclusions

The results of our programme emphasized to staff the importance of end-user feedback, since a close contact with user needs improved both the quality of the service offered and the image of the library. The end-user, through promotional and educational initiatives proposed by the library, is gradually introduced to paths which were previously unknown to him, and the awareness of new possibilities stimulates him towards a deeper study of this field. This is demonstrated by figures indicating an increasing number of users attending the library, performing bibliographic searches, and requesting all kinds of tools and media available. In addition this represents an opportunity for the library to reconsider its objectives and role: the great reward in terms of professional growth makes the effort in this direction worthwhile.

References

1 Prins H, de Gier W. The image of the library and information profession: how we see ourselves - an investigation. (IFLA publications; 71). Munchen: Saur, 1995

2 Barry CA, Squires D. Why the move from traditional information-seeking to the electronic library is not straightforward for academic users: some surprising findings. In: Online Information Proceedings. London: Learned Information, 1995, pp.177-187

3 Fisher J, Bjorner S. Enabling online end-user searching: an expanding role for librarians. Spec Libr 1994;85:281-287

KNOWLEDGE AND THE CONTAINER

Lucretia W. McClure, Librarian Emerita, University of Rochester Medical Center, Rochester, NY, USA

Introduction

Librarians have always been interested in format, in the container of information and knowledge. We are fascinated by the clay tablet or the parchment scroll, by the illuminated manuscripts of earlier times. Computer technology brings with it an entirely different kind of container. No one is likely to stand and gaze at a CD-ROM for its elegance or extol the beauty of a green screen, but there is a breathtaking quality in the concepts of these new modes of information transfer. Just imagine your thoughts winging through the air, to find a home in the computer of a far-off colleague! There is one other container of knowledge and that is the librarian. I would argue that the librarian is one container that cannot be replaced in this ever-changing information/knowledge world in which we live. The purpose of my paper is to consider the value of content vs. the container. Has the container become more important than the content? Are we learning better? Are students doing better? Is the material better, more accurate? I believe that knowledge rather than the format or container should drive our work.

Knowledge and the container

There is an old saying: "Don't judge a book by its cover." But, of course we do. We are greatly impressed by the beautifully-bound book, by the illuminated manuscript. Locked in our library vaults are those special containers, finely-tooled leather bindings, covers made of ivory, volumes of parchment decorated with marbled papers and encrusted with precious metals and gems. Whether or not we are interested (or can even read) the contents of these treasures, we collect and protect them because of their containers.

These volumes are artifacts as well as writing and for those scholars who can study and appreciate the contents, they are worth the care and attention given by countless generations of librarians. One wonders if future historical collections will contain floppy disks or magnetic tapes as the artifacts of the late 20th century. Interesting they may be, but there is no comparable beauty such as we find so appealing in handling a Vesalius or a Jenner. The book format has been the most common and acknowledged container of the library. Ever since the printing press produced books for everyman, people have taken to the book (and I include in that

S. Bakker (ed.), Health Information Management: What Strategies?, 258-260.

term the bound journal). It is a marvelous container--easy to carry. A book can be transported wherever you go, on a plane, in the park, or in the comfort of your bed. The book is not only a convenient package, it has the advantages of fixed print. The book, as published, remains true to its origins. Whether true or false, beautifully written or downright dreadful, it is frozen on its pages. It has not been manipulated or changed. Despite all the electronic devices available today, one has only to visit a library or book store to see the throngs of people who are browsing and reading. This container is too satisfying to fade away.

Librarians know how to deal with print containers. They can acquire, catalog, store and preserve the traditional book and journal. After all, they have been doing this for ages. Speaking on our work with the "container," Robert Braude says that the "greatest impediment to the continued development of librarianship has been the traditional view that librarians manage the containers of information rather than the contents."[1]

MEDICAL KNOWLEDGE

I would suggest that there are two facets to this container vs knowledge discussion. First, in the days before the electronic database, librarians were often very knowledgeable about medicine and its literature. Searching for information in printed indexes and abstracts was tedious, but it also required that one read the articles to determine relevance. Today that has become the function of the search structure. But in reading to find information, librarians became educated in the discipline of medicine. The speed and accuracy of database searching has eliminated the need to read dozens of articles to select the most relevant. The librarian who has always had the support of a computer and a myriad of databases at hand has different skills and interests. The computer has become the "container" of today. There is no doubt that the electronic capabilities of today will change our world and our work. We can link our libraries and users to all manner of databases, knowledge bases, libraries and institutions. The challenge and the burden for librarians is how to harness this mass of information.

LEARNING PROCESS

In which direction will we go? The answer to this question, and to my concern about the container vs knowledge, will be determined by the extent that librarians establish their place in the realm of learning. This becomes the second facet of the question. Where are librarians in the continuum of container-knowledge-learning? Learning, from whatever method or format, is of the utmost importance to our users and to the librarian in his or her own development The ability to find large amounts of information on the Internet or to print out extensive bibliographies from databases does not signal that learning has taken place. Providing a great array of electronic resources is satisfying to the librarian, but represents only one kind of resource. Too often the staff may assume that students can utilize the access provided by databases and knowledge bases and successfully extract what is of high quality and what is accurate. It is no more true of electronic resources than it is certain that a reader can pick out the most relevant book or journal.

We need more research on how students learn, how faculty and researchers keep up to date, and how scientists absorb and communicate ideas. We need to know much more about how the computer has changed and detracted from or enhanced learning. How to compare this correlation with examination results and a study of use of

Internet sources would be a logical next target for research. Another useful topic for research is the quality of a variety of sources used by students and faculty. Edmund Pellegrino makes this observation about some electronic sources saying they primarily deal in processed information, information that is "predigested, preselected, and preordered to satisfy some special purpose." He goes on with this dire comment: "Today's scholarship already shows the result of overdependence on processed information. To be able to select what to read calls for knowledge that only self-directed reading can supply. We seem to be entering a state of infinite regression--key words of key words, abstracts of abstracts, summations of summations." Pellegrino suggests that books and computers can have peaceful coexistence, but cautions that book based literacy is necessary if coexistence is not to undermine the most human of our cognitive capabilities.[2]

KNOWLEDGE PURSUIT

We need people who can read and study; people who explore the ideas of others, involving their own thoughts along with the thoughts of the author. That must never stop if we are to have educated, thinking, and open-minded physicians and scientists. More than a quarter century ago Jesse Shera wrote: "The object of the library is to bring together human beings and recorded knowledge in as fruitful a relationship as is humanly possible to be."[3] If that is true, and I believe it is, then we can make that relationship happen only if we have librarians, users, and recorded knowledge. Any container can be utilized. What really matters is what happens to the contents. Will new knowledge be developed? Will a learner's ability be enhanced?

Pursuit of knowledge must be the cornerstone of science. And we, as partners in the scientific endeavor, must take part in it. More than ever it means that librarians must promote scholarship and creativity, must provide content and interpretation as well as information. Our purpose is to foster learning, to be concerned with the quality of knowledge, and to seek ways to enhance the learning that is so vital to the discipline of medicine.

References

[1] Braude RM. Impact of Information Technology on the Role of Health Sciences Librarians. Bull Med Libr Assoc 1993;81:409

[2] Pellegrino ED. The Computer and the book; the perils of Coexistence. In: Cole JY (ed) Books in Our Future; Perspectives and Proposals. Washington, DC: Library of Congress, 1987:86

[3] Shera J. In: Sociological Foundations of Librarianship. 1st ed. New York: Asia Publishing House, 1970:30

CO-ORDINATING THE DEVELOPMENT OF LIBRARY AND INFORMATION SERVICE SUPPORT IN THE NEW NHS

Margaret Haines, NHS Library Adviser, London, UK

The New National Health Service

The National Health Service has undergone massive change in the last ten years. Whilst the overall aim remains the same - to secure the greatest possible health gain for the population in the most cost effective way - the focus has shifted to a primary care led NHS. There has been a dramatic downsizing and reorganisation of the NHS Executive as well as more devolution of responsibility to an internal market of local health care purchasers and providers.

There have also been changes to the education of clinical professionals, including a shift towards a problem-based, self-directed learning approach in undergraduate teaching and a a consolidation of all undergraduate training in higher education institutions. Moreover, the organisational and educational changes have been accompanied by fundamental culture shifts towards patient participation in health decision making and evidence-based practice.

These changes are reflected in the Priorities and Planning Guidance issued by the NHS Executive[1] and in a variety of national policies and strategies such as the R & D Strategy, the Patient Partnership Strategy and the Promoting Clinical Effectiveness Initiative.

Information Challenges

The impact of these changes has been to create needs for:
- mechanisms for efficient information transfer between NHS staff and organisations
- sources of information about clinical effectiveness at point of care
- information resources suitable for patients and their families
- quality filters to assist rapid retrieval from Internet and other networks
- better indexing and coverage of grey literature in existing databases
- understanding of the needs of new NHS staff such as GP Fundholders

Roles for Librarians

Even if these needs were met, it has been suggested that most NHS staff would still experience problems in handling information due to lack of time and lack of skills in information retrieval, appraisal and organisation.[2,3] These problems could be partly

S. Bakker (ed.), Health Information Management: What Strategies?, 261-263.

resolved with the services of health librarians: information organisation, retrieval, indexing, abstracting, current awareness, end-user training, document delivery, etc.

However, there have been concerns that despite the apparent opportunities to demonstrate their value in solving some of the information challenges in the new NHS, NHS librarians are not making as effective a contribution as possible. This is reflected primarily in duplication of effort and lack of co-ordination but also in the lack of visibility for the profession with the wider NHS.

A series of national seminars in the early 1990's, chaired by the Parliamentary Under-Secretary of State (Lords), Baroness Cumberlege, explored these issues in the context of managing the knowledge base of health care.[4,5] Reasons given for the failure of NHS librarians to meet their potential were: inadequate and complex funding mechanisms, lack of integration with IT networks in parent organisations, lack of up-to-date guidance on libraries from the NHS Executive, lack of adequate training for new roles in supporting evidence-based health care, etc.

What Should be Done?

The debate begun at the Cumberlege seminars resulted in four strategic objectives. The first two suggested that the knowledge base needed to be improved and more widely disseminated using new technologies such as the Internet and the NHS's Intranet. The second two suggested that good library and information practice needed to be promoted and that local organisation and access to libraries and thus to the knowledge base needed to be improved.

WORK OF THE NHS LIBRARY ADVISER

Following the Cumberlege Seminars, the Department of Health and the NHS Executive agreed to appoint an NHS Library Adviser to ensure that library and information issues were on their agenda. Specific tasks included:
- encouraging local library co-operative initiatives,
- facilitating the development of national co-ordination strategies,
- considering and promoting standards and good practice,
- encouraging initiatives to signpost the knowledge base of health care,
- strengthening links between government and the health library community.

The priorities established by the NHS Library Adviser when she took office in 1995 included:
- simplifying and clarifying library funding,
- encouraging multidisciplinary library services,
- encouraging co-operation with other sectors,
- developing library accreditation systems,
- facilitating continuing professional development for librarians,
- ensuring NHS libraries were linked into the NHSnet and the Internet,
- encouraging library support for primary and community care staff.

It is important to note that the NHS Library Adviser does not work in isolation but works closely with the NHS Regional Librarians Group and with key policy makers in the NHS Executive.

What is Being Done?

Much progress has been made since the Cumberlege seminars largely due to the enthusiasm and hard work of the library community itself with support from the NHS Executive. Training for librarians to support evidence-based practice has been initiated in many regions, led by the innovative Librarian of the 21st Century project which was funded by the R & D programme in Anglia and Oxford Region.[6] The R & D programme and the British Library have funded research into primary care information needs and into the role of libraries in supporting the NHS. Librarians have helped develop new resources such as the Cochrane Library, and new guides to Evidence-Based Medicine. Finally, a new professional body, the LINC Health Panel has been created to co-ordinate work on cross-sectoral issues, such as library accreditation and library support to the nursing profession.

The NHS Library Adviser has been involved in some of these initiatives such as the accreditation project and others such as a CPD Training Kit for NHS Regional Librarians. Most of her work has focussed on encouraging better co-ordination at local level through the creation of NHS Regional Library Adviser posts and there will soon be at least one full-time Regional Library Adviser in every region. She has also been encouraging new policy from the NHS Executive and to that end, an NHS Executive Working Party on Libraries has just been established which will be issuing the first guidance on NHS libraries since 1970.

What Remains to be Done?

Whilst progress towards the Cumberlege objectives is good, much remains to be done. There are still many NHS staff working in primary and community care who do not have access to library support and the issue of funding this support will need to be addressed. Even if funding can be found, these staff have problems in finding time to visit libraries and therefore libraries will need to develop innovative outreach programmes. Accreditation should help to improve and develop libraries but standards of information support should be identified for all staff working in the NHS. Finally, there is still a need to encourage NHS managers, not just librarians, to be involved in making the knowledge base of health care accessible for all NHS staff.

References

1 Priorities and Planning Guidance for the NHS: 1997/98. Leeds: NHS Executive, 1996

2 Rosenberg W, Donald A. Evidence-based medicine: an approach to clinical problem-solving. BMJ;310:1122-6

3 MacDougall J. Information for health: access to healthcare information services in Ireland; a research report on the information needs of healthcare professionals and the public. Dublin: Library Association of Ireland, 1995

4 Health Care Information in the UK. Report of a Seminar Held on 1 July 1992 at the King's Fund Centre, London. British Library R&D Report 6089. London: The British Library, 1992

5 Managing the Knowledge Base of Healthcare. Report of a Seminar Held on 22 October 1993 at the King's Fund Centre, London. British Library R&D Report 6133. London: The British Library, 1994

6 Palmer J, Streatfield D. Good diagnosis for the twenty-first century. Libr Assoc Rec 1995;97:153-4

EDUCATION FOR A NEW HEALTH INFORMATION PROFESSION

Jane Farmer, The Robert Gordon University Aberdeen, Scotland, UK

Introduction

These are tremendously exciting times for the health information community. Several exciting initiatives and concepts are moving health information professionals out of the perceived confines of traditional libraries into new and challenging areas of work. For example, health information professionals are learning the skills of critical and economic appraisal, high precision searching techniques and research design, as well as the interactive skills required to work optimally with subject-based practitioners. Committed health information professionals are leading the way forward for fellow professionals in other sectors of information work by extending the base and enhancing the status of their skills.

Poster presentation

The presentation aimed to examine the role Library and Information Schools can play in providing students with the knowledge and skills they require to work in the developing health information environment. More specifically:

* the areas which could/should be covered

* how new skills can learn to live with the existing curriculum

* how health information management can be introduced and marketed to students

* how students can transfer these skills to various information settings

* the ways in which the new skills being used by health information professionals have the potential to revolutionise the curriculum and product of LIS schools

S. Bakker (ed.), Health Information Management: What Strategies?, 264.

STRATEGIES OF CHOICE OF AD HOC CLASSIFICATION NUMBERS

Elisabetta Poltronieri, Istituto Superiore di Sanità, Rome, Italy

Introduction

The main purpose of classification practice is both to meet user needs and to reflect document contents. In a multidisciplinary context a single concept is likely to pertain to different subject areas. The library of the Istituto Superiore di Sanità, (ISS) - the Italian National Institute of Health - uses both the *National Library of Medicine* (*NLM*) schedules for medicine and related areas and the *Library of Congress Classification* (*LCC*) for other subject fields (e.g. Agriculture, Geography, Science, Technology).

Strategies of choice

Assigning a notation drawn from classification schemes requires:
- selection of appropriate classification numbers for unambiguous access to documents;
- observance of the logical sequence if classification numbers are used for shelving;
- updating of classification numbers when new notations are provided.

EXAMPLES

1) item: *Encyclopedia of nuclear magnetic resonance: contributor list.* Grant DM, Norris RK (eds). Chicester: Wiley, 1996

QC 762	(LC)	Physics. As a magnetic phenomenon
QD 96.N8	(LC)	Chemistry. As a special method of spectrum analysis
QH 324.9.N8	(LC)	Biology. As a method of research of biological systems
WN 440	(NLM)	Radiology. Diagnostic imaging. As a technique of radioimaging in nuclear medicine

ISS library choice: **QC 762** motivation: in such a reference tool (encyclopedia) the topic (nuclear magnetic resonance) is treated as pertaining to physical phenomena.

S. Bakker (ed.), Health Information Management: What Strategies?, 265-266.

2) item: *Cytoskeleton proteins: a purification manual.* Berlin; Heidelberg: Springer Verlag, 1995

QP 552.C96 (LC) Physiology. As special proteins included into the organic substances
QU 55 (LC) Biochemistry. As a class of proteins

ISS library choice: **QU 55** motivation: the index to LC Classification prescribes the above notation for this class of proteins (cytoskeleton proteins)

3) item: *Drug abuse in the modern World: a perspective for the eighties.* New York: Pergamon Press, 1981

HV 5801 (LC) Social pathology. Drug abuse and drug habits as a social aspect of drug dependence
WM 270 (NLM) Psychiatry. Substance dependence. Substance abuse as a cause of mental disorders

ISS library choice: **HV 5801** motivation: the focus of studies involves a social perspective

Conclusions

The experience gained in the ISS library shows that:
- decisional process leading to the suitable choice must be discussed and shared with users
- contacts with users and knowledge of their searching paths are essential for determining the right choice of classification number.
- well trained personnel of indexing departments must be able to involve library users in working out problems related to classification of documents.

Bibliography

Library of Congress classification: H, Social Sciences. Washington: Library of Congress, 1994
Library of Congress classification schedules combined with additions and changes through 1991: class Q, Science. Detroit: Gale Research, 1992
National Library of Medicine. National Library of Medicine classification: a scheme for the shelf arrangement of library materials in the field of medicine and its related sciences. 5 ed. Bethesda: U.S. Department of Health and Human Services, Public Health Service, National Institutes of Health, National Library of Medicine, 1994
Kao ML. Cataloging and classification for library technicians. New York: the Haworth Press, 1995

PHARMACEUTICAL INFORMATION ASSOCIATIONS ACTIVE IN EUROPE

Vincent Maes, Pfizer, Bruxelles, Belgium

Introduction

We all know the importance of belonging to an Association. As Dr Lyders stated: "I don't see how a health sciences library can function effectively without the services of a library association. How to run your library, what are the current issues, how to improve your library, and meet and discuss library issues with other colleagues. How can a library not belong to *an association* ?"

The purposes of this paper are: (1) to investigate the activities of pharmaceutical information associations; (b) to find what is (are) the association(s) which best fit(s) our needs? As Secretary of the Pharmaceutical Information Group, I will also assess if there is room or a need for an additional body.

The criteria I will take into account are the scope, the status (standalone or subgroup), the objectives and the members. Lack of time and place prevents me from presenting the results of the analysis on the structure and the services of these associations. Full results will be published later.

Identified associations

International scope

Standalone:
- Association of Information Officers from the Pharmaceutical Industry (AIOPI),
- Pharma-Documentation Ring (PDR),
- Drug Information Association (DIA).

Subgroups:
- Medical Library Association / Drug & Pharmacology Section (MLA/PDI),
- Special Libraries Association / Pharmaceutical Division (SLA/PD),
- European Association for Health Information and Libraries / Pharmaceutical Information Group (EAHIL/PhInfG).

National Scope:
- Information Managers from the Pharmaceutical Industry (IMPI), UK;
- Pharmaceutical Information Librarians (PILS), UK;

S. Bakker (ed.), Health Information Management: What Strategies?, 267-270.

- Gruppo Italiano Documentalisti dell'Industria Farmaceutica e degli Istituti di Ricerca Biomedica (GIDIF-RBM), Italy;
- Läkemedelsindusrtins samarbetsgrupp för I & D-Fragor (LIDOK), Sweden;
- Belgian Information Officers of the Pharmaceutical Industry Club (BIOPIC), Belgium,
- Association des professionnels de l'information et de la documentation, Groupe Santé, Médecine, Pharmacie, Biologie / Business & Marketing (ADBS/SMPB/BM); France.

OBJECTIVES

These associations have all roughly the same global objectives:
- to enhance the knowledge of their members
- to provide a forum for the exchange of experiences and views
- to encourage the development of professional skills
- to encourage the use of professional standards
- to initiate better information products
- to defend the interests of their members
- to represent their members in relevant bodies

But some specificities are found regarding their mission, the members they serve, and the means used to achieve their objectives.

MISSION

AIOPI: "To assist members in the execution of their professional duties"

PDR: "To attain improved access and coverage and to achieve better distribution and optimum use of the chemical, biomedical, pharmaceutical, scientific and patent literature for the common benefit"

DIA: "To provide a worldwide forum for the exchange and dissemination of information that is intended to advance the discovery, development, evaluation and use of medicines and related health care technologies"

MLA/PDI: "To foster excellence in the professional achievement and leadership of health sciences library and information professionals to enhance the quality of health care, education and research"

SLA/PD: "It provides a forum for exchange of information and ideas among individuals interested in *the management* of knowledge in all aspects of the [health care devices], and other health care fields [...]". As a subgroup, it also subscribes to SLA objectives: "To advance the leadership role of special librarians in putting knowledge to work for the benefit of the general public and decision-makers in industry, government, the profession"; and "To shape the destiny of our information society".

IMPI ".. provides an informal forum for discussion of issues relevant to information handling as well as a focal point of contact with suppliers of information products, services and software"

The following groups have no formal mission statement, but have leading principles:

EAHIL/PhInfG: "with all respect of copyright and other intellectual property rights". EAHIL has also a particular focus: "...in European countries and on other continents, in particular in less developed parts of the world"

PILS: academic pharmaceutical information group

GIDIF-RBM: "fundamental spirit: a practical approach to help members solve the problems they meet in their daily work"

LIDOK asks for active participation by the members, generous information exchange between members, and minimal management and no bureaucracy

BIOPIC. A priority is the informal nature of meetings, where the important point is to know each other. They focus on discussion on concrete daily concerns.

ADBS/SMPB/BM exchanges best practical solutions for business and market information, evaluate services, and is open to everyone interested. The ADBS specificity is clearly the dissemination of information by issuing many publications.

MEMBERS

AIOPI gathers individuals engaged in scientific, medical, technical or business information work within the pharmaceutical industry

PDR is limited to Scientific Information & Documentation Depts of Research and Development pharmaceutical companies

DIA tries to involve all people engaged in the drug information process

MLA/PDI members are people or institutions working or interested in a health or in an information sciences environment

SLA/PD: Information professionals, people or institutions interested in specialised settings, especially health care fields.

EAHIL/PhInfG: Professionals and institutions interested in pharmaceutical information

IMPI: Scientific Information and Documentation Depts of UK R & D pharmaceutical companies (kind of national PDR)

PILS are librarians from UK university schools of pharmacy, but is open to everyone interested.

GIDIF-RBM are information people and institutions from Italian pharmaceutical industry or from biomedical research institutes

LIDOK: Scientific Information and Documentation Depts of Swedish R & D pharmaceutical companies

BIOPIC: information people working for the Belgian pharmaceutical and health care industries

ADBS/SMPB/BM: information professionals or information depts of pharmaceutical companies, including consulancy firms or anyone interested.

We can distinguish two tendencies:
- to gather as much information professionals as possible (which is the case for most associations);
- to limit membership in order to work more effectively (PDR, IMPI, LIDOK)

MEMBERSHIP TYPES

The *"Formal"* groups, with different membership types (AIOPI, DIA, MLA, SLA, EAHIL, EAHIL/PhInfG, GIDIF-RBM, ADBS). It corresponds to international scope, except the PDR, but including EAHIL/PhInfG, GIDIF-RBM, and ADBS

The *"Informal"* group (PDR, MLA/PDI, SLA/PD, IMPI, PILS, LIDOK, BIOPIC, ADBS/SMBP/BM). It corresponds to the subgroups, minus EAHIL/PhInfG, National scope (minus GIDIF-RBM, ADBS), including the PDR

Except EAHIL/PhInfG, all subgroups have only one membership type.

Conclusions

About the choice, here are some general rules:
- join a national scope association if it exists... otherwise create one !
- to broaden your views, join an international scope association.
- if you are a R & D information manager: choose PDR. If not choose AIOPI, but most activities are organised in the UK.
- if you don't want to be limited to Europe and to pharmaceutical information only, choose the EAHIL/PhInfG, or the SLA/PD. The latter deals with special libraries, and has a strong focus on USA.
- MLA/PDI is more US academic dedicated, but is a classic in health information !
- keep an eye at DIA activities (meetings and publications), although workshops are quite expensive.

But the key word must be COMPLEMENTARITY !

By the way, we can regret a lack of collaboration. It could be beneficial for all in some areas such as "lobby" initiatives or common projects.

Anyway, all groups should make their findings and publications more widely available !

We also suggest to make more use of Internet, especially of discussion lists.

THE SECOND INTERNATIONAL CONFERENCE OF ANIMAL HEALTH INFORMATION SPECIALISTS

Anna Eslau Larsen, Danish Veterinary and Agricultural Library,
Frederiksberg C., Denmark

Animal Health Information: Structuring and Sharing, Global and Local

THE FIRST CONFERENCE

In July 1992, the First International Conference of Animal Health Information Specialists, under the theme of "Animal Health Information, Planning for the 21st Century", was held at the University of Reading, England. It was organized by members of the Veterinary Medical Libraries Section of the Medical Library Association (VMLS/MLA), and English colleagues. It was a conference designed to enhance the flow - as well as facilitate international communication of animal health information worldwide. The conference was directed to librarians and other information professionals working in

- Veterinary Medicine
- Laboratory Animal Science
- Primatology
- Zootechny
- Zoological and Wildlife Medicine and Biology

The conference was attended by 81 delegates from 18 countries with 14 contributed papers and three invited speakers. The topics of the papers ranged widely from managing a small library to facilitating global availability of animal health information, and from animal welfare issues to the services if the U.S. National Agricultural Library. Several papers focused on technological advances in the field, and suggested ways for improved utilization of technology. The conference was a great success and the participants strongly supported the idea of a second conference.

National/regional groups. As a result of the first conference a group called Animal Health Information Specialists- United Kingdom (AHIS-UK) was formed. In 1995, an European group, called The European Veterinary Libraries Group (EVLG), was founded. The EVLG exists inside the European Association for Health Information and Libraries (EAHIL). Also in 1995, the First Conference of African Health Information Workers, was held at the University of Pretoria in South Africa.

S. Bakker (ed.), Health Information Management: What Strategies?, 271-272.

THE SECOND CONFERENCE

The Second International Conference of Animal Health Information Specialists will be held at the Danish Veterinary and Agricultural Library, 1-4 July 1997, organized by the Danish library staff in cooperation with colleagues from Sweden, Finland and Norway.

The aim of the second conference is to enhance the structuring and sharing of information, global as well as local. International networks like The Internet has given us the possibility to fulfil the goal of international sharing of information in our daily work, through facilities like the mailing list of veterinary librarians, the VETLIB-L, homepages with links to library catalogues (OPACS) and other sites with important animal health information. Communication via E-mail, fast and relatively reliable, makes it possible to solve problems that normally took days or weeks. This conference is again an attempt to gather colleagues from all over the world for an intensified discussion and understanding of each other's daily work and research. Even using networks as the Internet as common connection, it is still a matter of great value for international cooperation when colleagues meet. This can be realised by the formation of an international organization, to take care of the global communication between colleagues working in animal health information. As mentioned earlier, the first conference resulted in the formation of three regional groups of animal health information specialists, one covering the United Kingdom, one covering Africa and one covering Europe as a whole. And then there is of course the group covering the United States. If these groups supported the formation of a worldwide organization, one of the goals could be to take the responsibility for the arrangement of the Third International Conference of Animal Health Information Specialists.

To improve the local sharing of information, another aim of the second conference is to aquire and share experiences between animal health information specialists from both university libraries and private company libraries. Therefore, the second conference is also directed to information specialists working in

- Veterinary Pharmacology
- Food Hygiene

Topics appropriate to the second conference include:

International cooperation; Exchange of information, experience and research by Organization of regional groups cross borders, Network communication, Improving access to local information sites, International projects

Management and marketing of library services by Improving contact to university/company staff, Consultative activities, Advertising

User education; Evaluating needs and demands, Teaching as a part of curriculum, Specialised courses directed towards researchers, Technical tools

Animal health specialities within fields like Biotechnology, Patents, Pharmacology, Alternative Medicine, Zoonoses, Ethology, Feeding Science, Food Hygiene, Laboratory Animal Science

We look forward to welcome you to the new surroundings of the Royal Veterinary and Agricultural University as well as our new Veterinary and Agricultural Library in Copenhagen, Denmark 1-4 July 1997.

INFORMATION FOR HEALTH: ACCESS TO HEALTHCARE INFORMATION SERVICES IN IRELAND

Beatrice M. Doran and Jennifer MacDougall, Royal College of Surgeons in Ireland, Dublin, Ireland

Introduction

In 1994 the Irish Department of Health published its first national health strategy,[1] which set out objectives for the reorientation of the health service. Also in 1994 An Bord Altranais (the Nursing Board) published a report on the future of nurse education,[2] which presented recommendations for fundamental changes in nursing organisation and education.

These publications signalled changes which, together with other reforms such as an increasing requirement for continuing medical education for doctors, will have far-reaching implications for all Irish healthcare information services. A set of basic standards for healthcare libraries had recently been formulated by the Library Association of Ireland (LAI),[3] but it was apparent that the general lack of primary data on information needs in the health service, together with inconsistency and unevenness in healthcare library services, should be addressed.

The LAI therefore embarked on a review of information needs and services, with a view to making recommendations for their development. Funding was made available by the Department of Health with money raised from the National Lottery. In April 1994 an experienced research officer was appointed and the project began. This paper presents a summary of the project's findings and recommendations. The full report was presented to the Secretary of the Department of Health in September 1995.[4]

Objectives and methods

The principal objectives were to determine information needs and access levels for the whole range of healthcare practitioners as well as for patients and their carers; to determine best practice internationally; to make recommendations for the development of healthcare information services in Ireland.

The methods employed included literature searches; interviews with senior managers of a wide range of healthcare organisations; a questionnaire survey of the information needs of health service staff; a telephone survey of all City and County Librarians in Ireland; follow-up interviews and consultations around the country; a review of international best practice.

S. Bakker (ed.), Health Information Management: What Strategies?, 273-275.

Results

SAMPLE AND RESPONSE

A sample of 1,087 health services staff was included in the survey. Categories surveyed included medical, nursing and paramedical staff, environmental health officers and senior managers. The overall response rate was 46%.

INFORMATION NEEDS

The most frequently cited reasons for seeking information were to keep up to date, to help with patient care, and for continuing education. 70% of doctors regularly needed information within 24 hours. A third of respondents needed to access information out of normal office hours.

SOURCES OF INFORMATION

The most frequently used information sources were colleagues at work, followed by journals. About half the staff surveyed seldom or never consulted a librarian or used an electronic system such as MEDLINE or CINAHL. Hospital doctors were the highest users of libraries amongst the medical and nursing professions, and were the most likely to have relevant libraries easily accessible to them.

A general lack of awareness of library services was evident. Only 22% of respondents indicated that they used inter-library loans, while less than a third had ever had any training in information handling skills. Yet almost 50% of respondents reported that they were successful in satisfying their information needs.

Many barriers to access were identified, including lack of time, lack of facilities and geographical location. Those in rural practices or hospitals without libraries experienced particular problems, and the lack of facilities for nurses, paramedical staff and especially environmental health officers was commented on. Also reported were restricted access to libraries, lack of qualified librarians and lack of computer systems and networking facilities.

Suggestions on improving access to library and information services were most frequently concerned with increasing the amount of computers, networks and CD-ROMs, and with improving awareness of information resources. Better education in the use of libraries and information services was seen as important by many respondents. Those who had experienced a professional library service were aware of the benefits.

CONSUMER HEALTH INFORMATION

The interviews revealed a high level of concern at the lack of sufficient resources for consumer health information. There has been some improvement in recent years, with an increasing range of leaflets, television and radio programmes devoted to health matters. But there were gaps in coverage, and the problems of rural areas were once again highlighted.

The vital role of the public libraries in providing consumer health information was identified by the health service staff. Public libraries are experiencing an increasing demand for health information. All public libraries said they tried to maintain a core stock of material, but it was difficult to keep track of leaflets coming from a wide variety of sources.

Conclusions and recommendations

Although many health science libraries and librarians were praised and obviously well used, the research identified serious deficiencies in access, awareness and availability of healthcare information both for staff and for the public. Overall, the research revealed an unsystematic and uneven approach to the provision of library and information services. The lack of appropriate resourcing and recognition from central government has meant that the development of healthcare information services in Ireland has been restricted.

The recommendations place the emphasis on a structured review of library and information services. A government commitment to the importance of information for healthcare is vital, as is recognition of the value of professional library and information specialists.

A number of initiatives were recommended, including the development of library and information skills training courses for healthcare staff; major improvements in networking; the provision of a library service by all health boards, including official recognition of the professional status of librarians with appropriate grading and career structures. Services to nurses were singled out as a special case, especially in need of improvement. Emphasis was also placed on the need for good communications with voluntary organisations.

Perhaps the most important recommendation concerns the involvement of central government agencies and health boards. It is essential that attention to the important issue of health information is given at the macro level. Without this, Ireland will lose an opportunity to be at the forefront of healthcare information development, and the resources already invested will be less effective.

One final proposal was that further research should be conducted on consumer health information provision in Ireland, and this has now formed the basis for a new LAI research project.

References

[1] Department of Health (Ireland). Shaping a healthier future: a strategy for effective healthcare in the 1990s. Dublin: Department of Health, 1994

[2] An Bord Altranais. The future of nurse education and training in Ireland. Dublin: An Bord Altranais, 1994

[3] Health Sciences Libraries Section of the Library Association of Ireland. Standards for Irish health care libraries. Dublin: Library Association of Ireland, 1993

[4] MacDougall J. Information for health: access to healthcare information services in Ireland; a research report on the information needs of healthcare professionals and the public. Dublin: Library Association of Ireland, 1995

PORTUGUESE LIBRARIES AND INFORMATION CENTRES IN HEALTH CARE

Ana Miguéis, Centro Hospitalar de Coimbra, Portugal

Institutions in Portugal having libraries related to health care facilities are:
(1) General and Specialised hospitals; (2) Universities, technical schools and training centres; (3) Central and (4) Local health administration centres; (5) Mental health facilities; Pharmaceutical industry; Associations; Non-profit institutions.
To get a better knowledge of the profile of these libraries a survey was conducted by the Associação Portuguesa de Documentação e Informação de Saúde (APDIS) on 232 previously selected, most important institutions. The published results have been analysed and some conclusions are now presented.[1]

Data were obtained from 114 libraries, i.e., 49%; reasons for not responding were absence of a library or a complete lack of human resources. In the 114 libraries considered, almost 500,000 monographs and 30,000 periodicals are registered. Even when resources are limited, periodicals are in favour; 11,000 titles of periodicals are still subscribed to and almost all libraries possess them (98% versus 94% for monographs). The results of the survey show that only 55 responding libraries (52%) make use of databases and process their information automatically, which is certainly related to lack of financial resources. Most libraries afford technical services, such as cataloguing (89%), indexing (62%) and classification (60%). The majority uses either national or international rules for cataloguing (Portuguese Cataloguing Rules 71% or International Standardized Bibliographic Description 44%); for indexing (Bireme Health Sciences Descriptors 27% or Medical Subjects Headings 13%) and for classifying (Universal Decimal Classification 42% or National Library of Medicine classification 13%).

Conclusions

* Human resources should be improved and specific technical training should be taken into account in order to face all professional requirements
* Library automation is the most significant drawback
* In spite of limited technical, financial and human resources, a substantial effort is made to provide a wide set of library services to the users
* Most libraries provide technical services and use national and international standards
* Portuguese health administration managers must become aware that medical and health libraries are important and crucial to provide documentation and information, and constitute an essential support for clinical decision making.

S. Bakker (ed.), Health Information Management: What Strategies?, 276-277.

Reference

[1] Associação Portuguesa de Documentação e Informação de Saúde. Repertório das bibliotecas e serviços de informação em saúde. Lisboa: APDIS, 1993

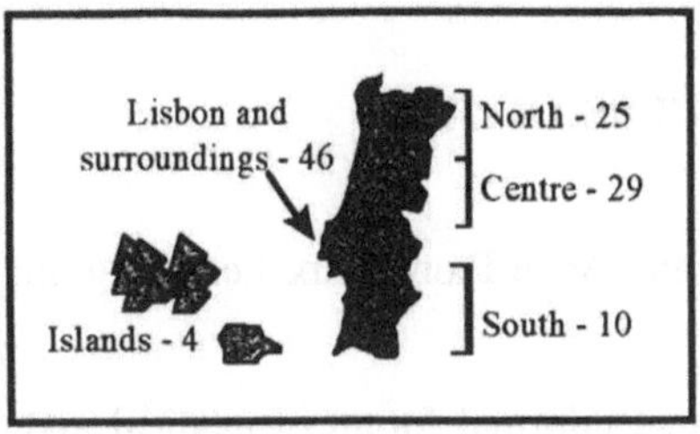

Figure 1 - Geographic distribution of the number of respondent libraries.

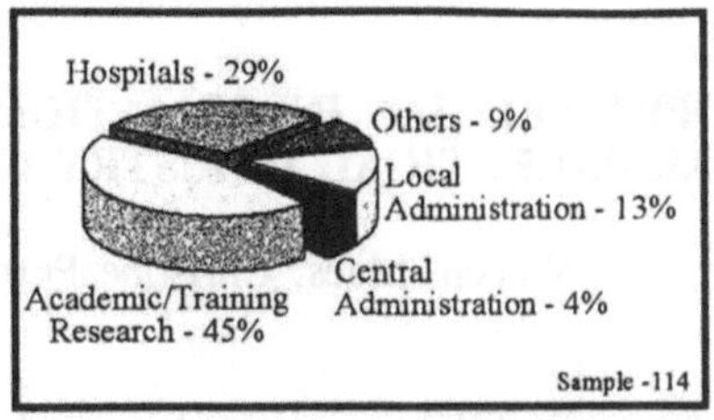

Figure 2 - Percentage distribution of respondent health libraries according to the type of institution.

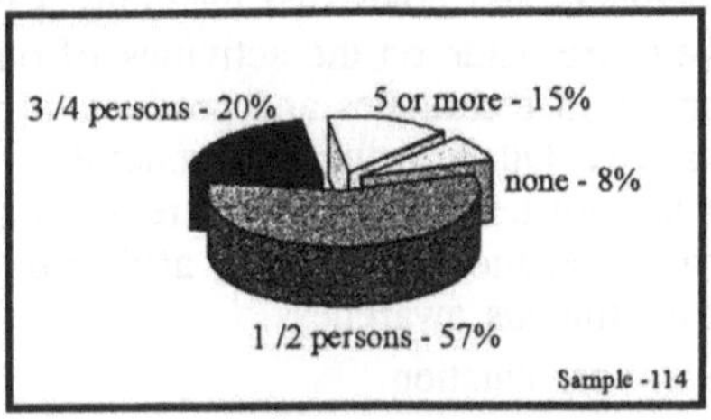

Figure 3 - Percentage distribution of respondent health libraries according to the number of human resources.

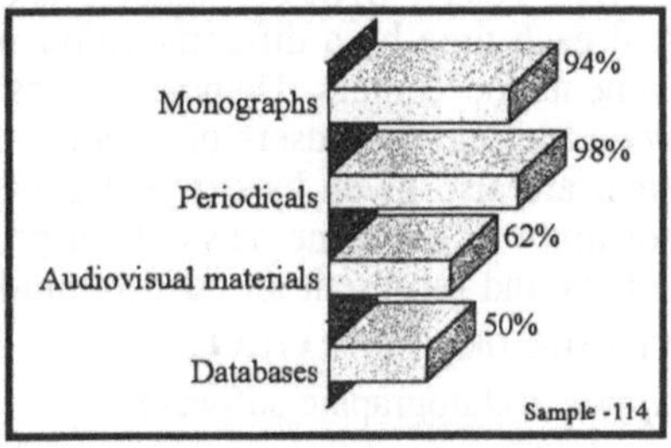

Figure 4 - Presentation of the percentage of respondent libraries using each one of the information resources.

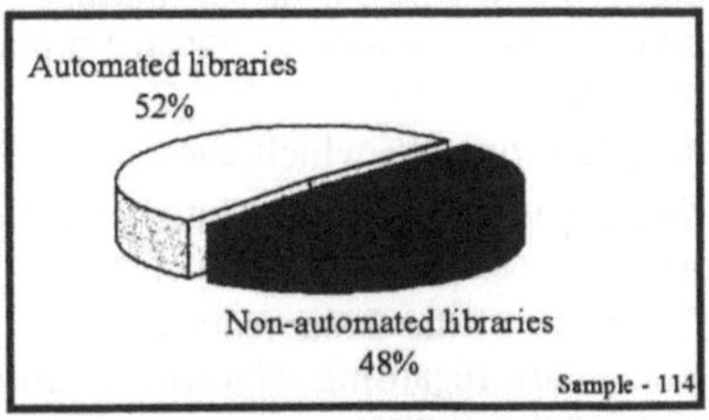

Figure 5 - Percentage distribution of respondent libraries according to automatic data processing.

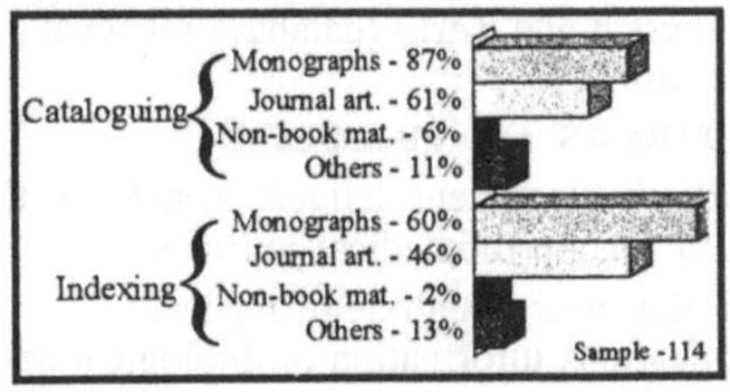

Figure 6 - Percentage of respondent libraries cataloguing and indexing the different information materials.

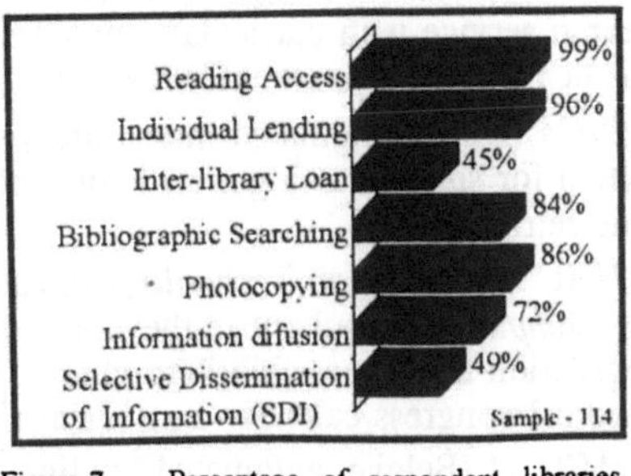

Figure 7 - Percentage of respondent libraries providing each one of the library services.

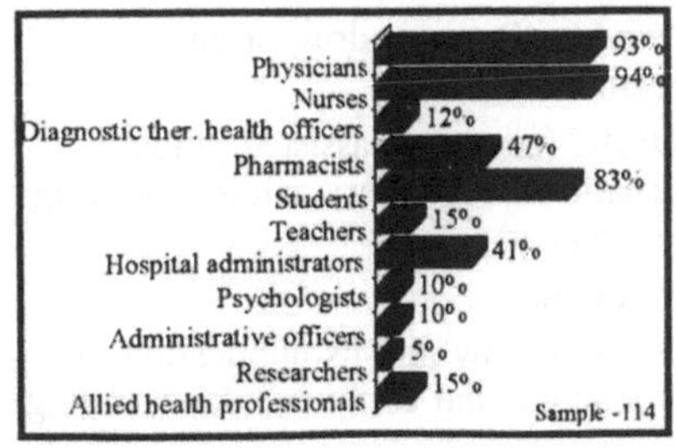

Figure 8 - Percentage of respondent libraries indicating each one of the different professional categories

BIOPIC: BELGIAN INFORMATION OFFICERS OF THE PHARMACEUTICAL INDUSTRY CLUB

Vincent Maes, Christine Permentier and Anne Pion, Bruxelles, Belgium

Abstract. BIOPIC was created in april 1988 as an informal forum of medical and health care documentalists from the private sector. Our initial aim was to know each other, to share experience, tricks and addresses and to discuss about concrete daily concerns. Today, BIOPIC numbers about 20 members and holds two meetings a year, hosted each time by a different company. Surveys are made on the activities of our documentation centers. Demonstrations of information techniques and products are provided by member users or vendor representatives. Other lectures of general interest are also given by external guests. Last but not least, gatherings are a good opportunity to get some news about professional associations from their affiliated members and represent an open round-table of continuous awareness.

SOFTWARE DEMONSTRATIONS:

- *Papyrus* (bibliographic software)
- *Trisoft* (document management system)
- *Knight-Ridder Probase* (interface to the *DataStar* databases in *Windows*)
- *Assassin* and *Texto* (database retrieval software)

DATABASES AND PRODUCTS:

- *Adonis* (document delivery system on CD-ROM for top biomedical journals)
- *Biobusiness* (database of business applications information on biological and biomedical research)
- *Medline* (Silver Platter CD-ROM version)
- *Adis* (drug intelligence literature monitoring services)
- *Ringdoc* (*Derwent* drug-oriented specialised database)
- *IDRAC* (computer-assisted guide to international regulatory affairs and drug development)

LECTURES:

- *Copyright* law and its application to reproduction and computer downloading
- Introduction to *patent* literature
- *IBES - Institut Belge de l'Economie de la Santé*: presentation
- Initiation to *programming*
- *Internet:* history, tools and resources

REVIEWS:

- *Management* of our libraries/ documentation centres: tasks, holdings, computer tools, outside contacts, permanent education
- Outside *suppliers*: which choice?
- *Photocopy survey*: two-months statistics of reprint requests, delivery and costs
- The *status* of the documentalist: questionnaire regarding education, carrier, professional activities

SERVICES:

- *BRS Information Technologies* (on-line search service with particular emphasis on medical and healthcare information)
- *PICA* (Dutch automated inter-library sytem for shared cataloguing, loans and on-line retrieval)
- *ITAC - Information Technology assisted by Computer* (consultant in the fields of EC legislation and issues, bibliographies, medical congress calendar and visual aids)
- *IMPALA* (Belgian automated lending system)

S. Bakker (ed.), Health Information Management: What Strategies?, 278.

BIBLIOMETRIC METHODS AS SUPPORT FOR HEALTH MANAGEMENT DECISIONS

Ingegerd Rabow and Lennart Rabow, Lund University, Sweden

Introduction

Health administrators and politicians are generally not aware of the existence of bibliometric methods and that these may be used as support for decisions regarding resource allocations to clinical disciplines. The background of this paper is the widespread experience that imprecise disciplinary boundaries may lead to decisions that are neither cost-beneficial nor scientifically well-grounded.

Several diagnoses are treated by two or more disciplines, which may result in doubling of resources. Decision-makers must consider whether it is more cost-beneficial to allocate resources to multiple specialties treating the same diagnoses than to concentrate those resources to one specific field. This decision has to rely on the expected quality of the clinical treatment, taking into account:

- Clinical results - difficult to compare especially in surgical cases;
- Efficiency evaluated by number of patients treated and average length of stay;
- Selection of patients for treatment;
- Total costs for treatment including outpatient service, radiological examinations etc.;
- Published clinical research.

Since it can be supposed that clinical research reflects interest and competence in the field, and that these two factors are important for the overall quality of a medical institution, we have decided to test the use of a simple bibliographic model for decision support.

In this pilot study we have chosen to examine surgical treatment of intervertebral disk displacement as this operation traditionally is divided between neurosurgeons and orthopaedic surgeons. Practice varies between countries with neurosurgeons dominating in the US and orthopaedic surgeons in Scandinavia. Low back pain is common and has an enormous effect on health care utilization and on costs. The lifetime prevalence of low back pain ranges from 60% to 90% and the annual incidence is 5%.

Methods

1. Articles on disk surgery during two five-year periods 1985-1989 and 1990-1994 were searched in Medline. We used the MeSH main heading INTERVERTEBRAL-DISK-DISPLACEMENT in combination with the subheading SURGERY.

S. Bakker (ed.), Health Information Management: What Strategies?, 279-281.

2. Institutional affiliations were checked using synonyms for neurosurgery and orhopaedic surgery.
3. The source journals were classified as Orthopaedic (O), Neurosurgical (N) or others according to List of Journals Indexed for Index Medicus.
4. We then checked the distribution of papers during period II by neurosurgons and orthopaedic surgeons respectively in journals classified as O, N or others. The search results for O- and N-papers respectively were ranked according to source publication.
5. Scisearch[R] was used to find all citations in ten randomized papers from the O- and N-group respectively. The cited journals were manually classified as above. Period II was chosen to find the most modern results.

Results

For period I were found 142 papers on disc surgery from neurosurgical and 88 from orthopaedic institutions and 209 resp. 164 for period II.

During period II 29% of the papers from neurosurgical institutions were published in non-neurosurgical journals, compared to 9% of "orthopaedic" papers in non-orthopaedic journals.

Using major subject aspect we found 14% of papers from N-institutions published in O-journals and no O-institution papers at all in N-journals (Table 1).

Of the citations in "neurosurgical" papers 22% were to orthopaedic journals, while 4% of the citations in "orthopaedic" papers were to neurosurgical journals.

Discussion

It is necessary to note some possible sources of error with the methods we have used.
1. Papers emanating from institutions with no subject specific name or an unexpected subject synonym are excluded and also papers with no address.
2. Medline supplies institutional affiliation only for the first author and cases of collaboration between neurosurgeons and orthopaedic surgeons may be missed. A randomized test indicated this was of no importance for our results.

We have shown that more papers on disk surgery emanate from N- than from O-institutions and conclude that they do more research on this subject. We have not tried to evaluate the quality of the research as reported in the published papers.

The use of Impact Factors (IF) was not considered in this context because of the well-known fact that the highest IFs have a tendency to follow the size of the presumed readership. The leading journals of a large discipline, in this case orthopaedics, will usually have higher IF than those of a smaller discipline.

The fact that neurosurgeons publish outside their own specialty journals to a much higher extent - more than 3 to 1 - than orthopaedic surgeons may indicate a higher quality. It is commonly believed that it is more difficult for a paper to be accepted for publication outside its own specialty. As mentioned earlier we cannot guarantee that we have found all the papers from N- or O-institutions. This could affect the exact numbers, but very unlikely the tendency, i.e. the different publication patterns between neurosurgeons and orthopaedic surgeons.

Neurosurgical researchers cite orthopaedic journals to a larger extent than vice versa. In fact, orthopaedic surgeons hardly cite neurosurgical journals.

Since there is no reason to believe that disk surgery research published in neurosurgical journals is less worth citing, it seems as if orthopaedic surgeons find that these papers reflect another school of thought or that these journals do not belong to the traditional reading matter of orthopaedic surgeons, i.e. their scientific worlds do not overlap, although neurosurgeons traffic the roads between the two worlds significantly more than orthopaedic surgeons. This probably has some qualitative implications.

We have not proved that doing research increases a surgeon's operative skills, as we have studied institutions, not individual doctors but we find it likely that surgeons working in institutions with active and good research will be more up-to-date and more critical regarding surgical indications, techniques and equipment, and thus will be better prepared to do highly qualitative surgery.[1,2]

Conclusion

Using bibliometric methods we have demonstrated that:
1) More scientific papers on disc surgery are published from neurosurgical than from orthopaedic institutions.
2) Significantly more neurosurgical papers have been accepted for publication in papers outside the specialty.
3) Neurosurgical researchers cite orthopaedic ones to a significantly larger extent than vice versa.
4) Points 1-3 indicate that neurosurgical research and accordingly clinical competence would rank higher.
5) The bibliometric results suggest that resources for disk surgery should be allocated to the neurosurgical rather than to the orthopedic specialty or only to those hospitals where general conditions for a close collaboration between the two specialties are good.
6) Bibliometric methods can be used as one of several factors for health management decisions.

References

[1] Does research make for better doctors? [editorial]. Lancet 1993;342(8879):58
[2] McCormick J. The contribution of science to medicine. Persp Biol Med 1993;36:315-22

Table 1. Number of highest ranked journals for each specialty. 1990-1994

Disk papers from N-institutions.			Disk papers from O-institutions.		
R1	26	ACTA-NEUROCHIR	R1	39	SPINE
R2	14	ZENTRALBL-NEUROCHIR	R2	8	Z-ORTHOP-IHRE-GRENZGEB
R3	12	NEUROCHIRURGIA	R3	7	J-SPINAL-DISORD
R4	11	SPINE	R4	7	ACTA-ORTHOP-SCAND-SUPPL
R5	10	AKTUELLE-PROBL-CHIR-ORTHOP	R5	5	CLIN-ORTHOP
R6	8	NEUROSURGERY	R6	3	CHIRURGIE
R7	8	NEUROSURG-CLIN-N-AM	R7	2	ORTHOPEDICS
R8	6	J-NEUROSURG	R8	2	J-BONE-JOINT-SURG-AM
R9	6	NEUROSURG-REV	R9	2	AKTUELLE-PROBL-CHIR- ORTHOP
R10	5	MT-SINAI-J-MED	R10	1	J-CHIR
etc			etc		

QUANTITATIVE ASPECTS OF THE MANAGEMENT OF HEALTH INFORMATION

Leo Egghe, LUC and UIA, Diepenbeek, Belgium

Introduction

Nowadays, services must continuously prove themselves: prove that one is still needed and even that one performs better with shrinking budgets. This is the more true for medical libraries, being services that are not money making but, on the contrary, cost (lots of) money, with users who are in general not very "library minded". We must be able to convince subsidising leading bodies that libraries play an increasingly important role in modern scientific life. This "proof" can be given by establishing public relations (PR) and public awareness (PA) activities. By PR is meant: making libraries and their services attractive ("sell" the services) and publicising the library; by PA is meant: informing directors, making them aware of activities and needs of the library and make sure that libraries are in their minds when they have to make (budgettary) decisions.

The physical form of PR and PA actions include diverse reports of several types: for PR: informative brochures, guides, folders, WWW pages in an attractive form, press releases (via the organisation or press conferences); for PA: special reports prepared for discussions in meetings, annual reports. Of course, in some cases annual reports do also serve as PR tools, especially in the case of company information.

All these PR and PA actions do not only serve the goal of informing the subsidising leading bodies: they are also needed to inform the library users. Giving them good information leads to an understanding of certain rules or to the acceptance of the fact that one is obliged to ask a fee for certain services.

Last but not least, reports are also needed for the library management itself: only by producing professional reports the librarian and his/her staff are able to fully "understand" what is going on in the library and to predict future uses and problems.

Reports can only be produced in a professional way by collecting concrete and sufficient "hard" correct **data**. Collecting such data is very well possible in the everyday life of a library but its complexity is sometimes underestimated. Important in this matter is knowing the **context** (universe) to report about and the exact **definition** of the property under study.

It is clear that all the techniques mentioned above are applicable in the general area of information science and hence in any library.

S. Bakker (ed.), Health Information Management: What Strategies?, 282-289.

Data

CONTEXT OF DATA

First one has to know and decide from which "universe" (total population) to extract data and on what to report. Some examples:

PROPERTY	UNIVERSE
- number of circulations	library (I)
- prices of books	library (I or NI) at a bookseller (NI) worldwide (NI)
- OPAC use	library (I) network (I)
- delivery times of books at a bookseller or of interlibrary material by a library	bookseller (NI) used library (NI)
- users' satisfaction	users of the library (NI)
- number of authors of medical books	library (I or NI) worldwide (NI)
- thickness of medical books	library (NI)

Integral counts (I) means that every single element in the universe can be checked and exact conclusions on the property can be given; non-integral counts (NI) means that not every single element in the investigated universe can or will be checked and hence a sample will be taken. With NI counts we cannot draw 100% sure conclusions for the investigated property in this universe.

DEFINITION OF THE INVESTIGATED PROPERTY

Investigated properties must be clearly defined and must be the same for all library staff members otherwise they will report differently on the same topics, hence making the outcome useless. Two examples of possible confusions:
"Money spent for books" is ambiguous unless specified: are we interested in the budgetted amount, the amount of money appearing in the orderings, the total price of the delivered books, the total amount of the invoiced books or the total amount paid for books in a certain year? Is the definition of "book" clear (e.g. does it include serials)?
"Number of circulations" Are continuations included or interlibrary circulations?

A clear definition of the investigated properties is essential when common (or comparable) reports amongst similar libraries (e.g. in a library consortium) are to be made. Often many meetings of co-workers (or colleagues) are necessary in order to get a common view and understanding of the topics to report on. Common or comparable reports can be very useful to prove that a library is not receiving enough budgets/manpower.

ORGANISATION OF GATHERING DATA

Data are usually collected on a yearly basis, e.g. for the annual report. Collecting data needs a continuous effort throughout the year. Only when data will be generated by a computer, they can be produced in the beginning of the next year (e.g. number of circulations, number of books catalogued). In all other cases a kind of "logbook" (e.g. for counting the number of books reshelved or for counting the number of library visitors) or a file (e.g. of invoices) must be kept. From the above it is clear that, along with the dicussions on automating the library, the issue of the automatic generation of library statistics must be kept in mind.

It depends on the type of library and even of the local situation which topics are important to prove something or to support certain claims. It is better to collect few data in an accurate way than many inaccurately or unreliably. A good example are the statistics of the American Research Libaries, collecting only 33 "basic" statistics.[1]

Very important is the "added value" when one collects the same data are collected over a long time period (i.e. several years). From these "derived results" such as time analyses (e.g. regression lines predicting trends in time) can be produced. It is therefore strongly advisable, once an agreement on the definition of a topic is reached, to keep this definition fixed. Otherwise time series are worthless. Notwithstanding the need to introduce new statistical data e.g. on new technologies (CD-ROM, Internet use).

The building of a good data collection takes a long time. It is clear that if one decides in year **x** to report on a new topic, one can only start collecting in year **x+1**, hence reporting on this topic can only start in year **x+2**. Add to this several more years in order to have a time dimension in these data!

EXAMPLES OF DATA

The following list of examples is based on data that are collected in my library (a small university library, mainly consisting of literature in the exact and medical sciences and in applied economics).

Data on the collection:

- number of books ordered, catalogued, invoiced, possibly divided over several subjects, including the budgets spent. The same goes for journals, series, CD-ROM products, other multimedia publications and so on. Make clear if series are counted in the books data or not. Compare e.g. medicine with other subjects,
- binding issues (journals, restauration, ...).

Data on user services:

- on opening hours, giving also statistics on the use of the library in the different periods that the libary is open (e.g. in the evening);
- circulation data (incl. renewals, new borrowings, books returned or reserved) and all administration involved with this. Distinguish between the different types of borrowers and different types of lended material. This can e.g. prove that medical staff members or students do not use the library so often and then one can search for an explanation of this and propose possible solutions.
- interlibrary loan data, both on incoming or outgoing requests and both on lending (of books) or copying (of articles). Calculate the success rates, inform about the relative importance of each participating library and on response times.
- photocopy service, printing service;
- use of OPAC: total and average session time. These data can yield conclusions to what extent the OPAC is used as a bibliographic database,
- use of external databases online (commercial hosts or Internet) or on CD-ROM. Compare the use of similar databases (e.g. EMBASE versus MEDLINE) in order to decide on future use. Calculate all costs and try to make a distinction between different types of users.
- library facilities and maintenance: number of seats, number of books reshelved, number of stolen or misshelved books and so on.

Automation and catalogue:
- if this is done in a network, then briefly report on the profile of the partners and situate your library in this, and indicate the total use of the system.

Staff:
- describe the employment in persons and in FTEs, inluding the help of students,
- draw an organisational chart.

External relations:
- report on activities like interlibrary meetings, network activities, talks, conferences;
- report on research, incl. (contributions to) publications (in books, journals, conference proceedings).

Data on companies involved in the library's activities:
- measurements on the quality (speed, price, ...) of booksellers or journal intermediaries;
- quality of the binding company, companies involved with maintenance of PCs, photocopying machines, furniture, etc.

The use of the data

The "raw" data collected form the building blocks for later use: they need to be streamlined, summarised and described in a clear way, incl. conclusions and interpretations. These activities then form the basic ingredients for the diverse reports that are made.

THE USE OF COMPLETE DATA (OF INTEGRAL COUNTS)

Once the universe (the total population) is determined it is possible to investigate every member of this population and thereof our conclusions are 100% sure, but of course limited to this population. These data are summarised in *graphs*, such as bar diagrams (for discrete data) and histograms (for continuous data). Examples of *discrete data* are: the age (in years) of a book or the number of years that a book is in the library, number of authors of medical books, number of library users and so on. Examples of *continuous data* are: the thickness of medical books (e.g. in cm), retrieval times (in minutes or seconds) in an OPAC, CD-ROM or online system, delivery times (in days) of books that are ordered at a book seller. Note that the division between discrete data and continuous data is sometimes vague: delivery times are discrete data (i.e. entire numbers of days) but we are only interested in them in groups, say periods of 5 or 10 days in order to estimate the order of magnitude. Ages in years are clearly discrete while retrieval times in seconds are clearly continuous!

In reports the time dimension is very important. In order to visualise the "trend" in time we can calculate the so-called regression line: on the graph consisting of the different points (with the x-axis representing time t) we add a straight line, fitting the "cloud of points" in the best way. By doing so we can see the trend by visual inspection of the line and are able to make (short term) predictions (see fig. 1).
The question of "how to make or not to make" graphs is dealt with in the literature.[2]

"Summary statistics" are also needed to interpret data in a professional way. The basic ones are: the *mean* (average) denoted by $\bar{x}$, the *standard deviation* (dispersion) denoted by s and the so-called *percentiles*. The square of s is the *variance*.

The average gives an overall view of the data, e.g. the average price of books. The standard deviation and the percentiles yield information about the degree of irregularity of the data, the former (s) is mainly used with incomplete data, the latter (percentiles) with complete data. For instance answers can be given to questions such as: how long does it take to deliver 50 or 75% of the books ordered at a certain bookseller?

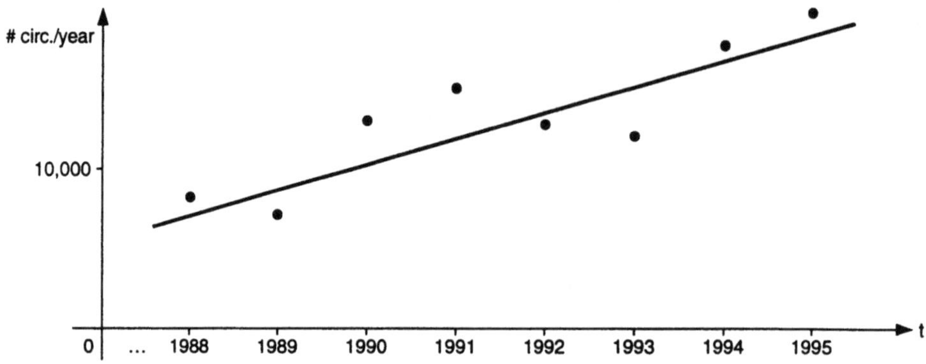

Figure 1. Scatterplot: Number of circulations/year in function of the year

THE USE OF INCOMPLETE DATA

The case of one data set

This case will be illustrated by an example. Suppose we sampled 100 books, delivered by a bookseller and the average delivery time was calculated (say 61 days). When making a complaint and requesting a faster delivery, the bookseller can question the validity of our data because we sampled only 100 books out of 2,000 deliveries. An estimate of the real average delivery time of this bookseller can be made by calculating the confidence interval as follows. With a sample size N (100 in our example), an average $\overline{x}$ and standard deviation s, we are 95% sure that the real "overall" average delivery time of this bookseller is in the interval

$$\left[\overline{x} - 1.96\frac{s}{\sqrt{N-1}}; \overline{x} + 1.96\frac{s}{\sqrt{N-1}}\right]$$

Example: N=100, $\overline{x}$=61 days and s=18 days. Then the real average delivery time is between the values 57.5 and 64.5 days (with 95% certainty).

Other applications could be: thickness of medical books, length of reference lists of medical articles, number of authors of medical books, or, in the area of user studies: fraction of certain types of users of the library, fraction of users who agree with a change of the opening hours, fraction of the loan transactions containing the maximum number of books that are allowed to check out at one occasion, fraction of books that are returned too late, fraction of lost/stolen books, fraction of users that are interested in an SDI-service on the acquisitions of the health library. Finally we mention another important application: measuring the overlap between two libraries or between two databases: O(B/A) = the overlap of database B w.r.t. A (i.e. the fraction of the articles in A that are also in B).

The case of two data sets
It is an interesting issue to compare two populations. For example to compare two libraries w.r.t. to their speed of delivery of interlibrary loan requests. As we will have here two incomplete data sets, what can we say about the difference? Techniques in statistics allow us to draw 95% or 99% conclusions about the possible different behaviour.

Examples of application: difference between the delivery times for books at two booksellers or of books coming from different countries (or, as mentioned above, of interlibrary loan material coming from different libraries), difference between the average thickness of medical books and of mathematics books, difference between their average number of authors, fraction of female users of library A versus the same in library B. Final general example: difference of use when we consider two different time periods (measuring changes in quality or in use of certain services).

THE ESTABLISHMENT OF INCOMPLETE DATA

How to collect incomplete data is a nontrivial problem. By the very definition of "incompleteness", we are faced with the problem: which elements of the population will be sampled? The main problem is the possible bias, the unequal chance for elements of the population to be picked.

Examples of bias: to give a questionnaire only to library users that are in the library (in this way you might miss the unsatisfied absent users), picking books in the library shelf by measuring lengths (this way thicker books have a higher chance to be picked), checking the length of services by sampling say every 30 minutes, and so on.

A perfect method to sample correctly is random sampling. Every element of the population has an equal chance to be picked. The method uses a computer generated list of random numbers and they determine the elements of the population that should be picked (for materials that are in the computer this random sampling can be executed in an automatic way). Executing random sampling in a manual way is time consuming; faster methods exist that are almost as good (e.g. the Fussler sampling technique). For more details, consult statistical or other literature.[3,4]

BIOMEDICAL EXERCISES

Research of a student in marine science librarianship
As part of a development project, funded by the Belgian government and executed by LUC[5] a study visit was executed in 1995 by one of the Kenian scientific assistants in the project. This person was interested, amongst several other things, in the special characteristics of medical books as compared to other scientific books, such as: the number of co-authors, the thickness and the age.

For the first problem he investigated a sample of 112 medical books from the LUC library and found an average number of co-authors of 1.88. With a little bit of more work he was able to draw conclusions about the total population of medical books (without investigating them all; in fact only the small sample is needed). He therefore calculated the standard deviation s and used the formula on page 286 in order to reach the conclusion that there are on average 1.88 +/- 0.28 authors per medical book (with 95% certainty) in the LUC library. He then did the same for the average thickness of medical books. He reached the answer that the average thickness of medical books in the LUC library is 36.96 mm +/- 3.25 mm. This type of conclusion is important to plan space and shelving in the library. Finally he did the same for the average age of medical books. Here he found the year 78.5 +/- 1.5.

The next question was: are these results different as compared with other disciplines or w.r.t. to the general library characteristics ? If so, then we have proof that special attention must be given to medical collections and, of course, the used methods yield a professional way to inform policy makers about it. As to the first characteristic we studied medical books versus mathematics books. For the latter we found on the average 1.64 co-authors per mathematics book and a test on the difference of two population averages revealed that the difference was indeed significant. The same conclusion could be drawn for the second characteristic (again the larger number for medical books) but not for the third one.

Results from common statistics in a library consortium

Other statistical aspects on the use of the biomedical literature in the LUC library can be found in the annual report of the LUC library.[6]

Last year a study was carried out by the VOWB (Flemish Council on Scientific Library Aspects), comprising all Flemish university libraries on the strength/weakness of the diverse library collections. The medical journal collection of my library turned out to be unacceptably small in the following sense. One had calculated - for each library - the percentage of the titles (appearing in the consortium of university libraries) that belong to this library. To my surprise the score of LUC was the lowest in medicine, even lower than in the human or applied sciences, directions in which LUC does not even offer teaching! It is clear that such reports are more influential than any series of data that I can derive from my library alone.[7]

Other bibliometric techniques, referring to the case of biomedical literature

The medical sciences are one of the best disciplines to evaluate the research output of scientists. The method is based on citation analysis: it measures the number of citations that an article (published in a so-called source journal) receives. The basic data can be found in the SCI (Science Citation Index), a product of ISI (Institute of Scientific Information) and in its side product, the JCR (Journal Citation Reports).

The vast majority of publications on "medical bibliometrics" found in the LISA (Library and Information Science Abstracts) and ISA (Information Science Abstracts) databases are in this "citation analysis" area (mainly published in Scientometrics but also in the Bulletin of the Medical Library Association). Medical scientists should know that their research is measured in this way (by their proper institution but also by several subsidising bodies such as National Science Foundations or governments).

Citation analysis yields a powerful tool for the health information manager to estimate the research degree of journals: the higher the impact factor (the relative number of times an article in this journal is cited by source journals in a 2 year period), the higher its use and its visibility and hence (to a large content) its research degree and research quality.

Citation analysis can also be used to estimate obsolescence (also called ageing) of literature in a research area. Ageing data on scientific journals can help the librarian in his/her acquisition policy. It is one of the elements (the price of a journal obviously is another element of course) in the decision on whether a journal should be bought or not (also in comparison with interlibrary loan requests for this journal, again incl. the age of the requested materials).[1]

Ageing is the diminishing use in time of literature. Growth is the increased production in time of literature. At first sight ageing and growth do not have any relationship nor influence on each other. This is not true. First of all, the techniques to study ageing and growth are exactly the same. In both cases one calculates a so-called "rate" function, being the amount in year t+1 divided by the amount in year t. Here "amount" means: "number of citations" for the ageing case or "number of publications" for the growth case. Secondly there is an influence of growth on obsolescence.[8-13]

We finally remark that many techniques used by scientometricians are based on multivariate statistics. This method consists of mapping a high dimensional space onto a "preferred" plane so that natural groupings and interrelationships between the points become clear. The points in this high dimensional plane are obtained by the formation of a matrix of data linking a set of objects to a set of variables (the number of objects determines the number of points; the number of variables determines the number of dimensions). Examples of these mapping techniques are:

- *Atlasses of disciplines:* both objects and variables are journals and the link between them is the number of times one journal cites another. A variant consists of linking two journal articles that are co-cited a certain number of times. The so constructed maps visualize a certain coherence of disciplines and subdisciplines.[14]
- *Scientific "schools":* both objects and variables are authors and the link between them is the number of times they are co-authors. Schools of collaborating scientists, or research groups, are taken into account in the evaluation of the scientific output.[15,16]
- *Journal clusters:* a reference is made to pharmacological journals.[17]

References

1 ARL Statistics 1993-94. A compilation of statistics from the one hundred and nineteen members of the Association of Research Libraries. Washington, DC: Assoc Res Libraries, 1995

2 Cleveland WS. The Elements of graphing Data. Monterey, CA: Wadsworth, 1985

3 Egghe L, Rousseau R. Introduction to Informetrics. Quantitative Methods in Library, Documentation and Information Science. Amsterdam: Elsevier, 1990

4 Egghe L, Rousseau R. Management of modern Libraries and multimedia Centres using elementary Statistics. [preprint], 1996

5 Egghe L, Pissierssens P. Managing marine science information in East-Africa: the RECOSCIX-WIO project. [preprint], 1996

6 Universiteitsbibliotheek LUC (1996), Jaarverslag 1995. Unpublished report

7 Muyldermans J, Braeckman J, Bosmans W. Eindrapport Sterkte/Zwakte-Analyse van lopende Tijdschriftencollecties in tien Vlaamse Wetenschappelijke Bibliotheken. Brussel: VOWB, 1996

8 Egghe L. On the influence of growth on obsolescence. Scientometrics 1993;27:195-214

9 Egghe L. A theory of continuous rates and applications to the theory of growth and obsolescence rates. Inf Proc Manag 1994;30:279-292

10 Egghe L, Rao IKR, Rousseau R. On the influence of production on utilization functions: obsolescence or increased use? Scientometrics 1995:34:285-315

11 Rao IKR, Meera BM. Growth and obsolescence of literature: an empirical study. In: Rao IKR (ed). Proceedings of the Third International Conference on Informetrics (Bangalore, India, August 1991), 1992. pp.377-394

12 Humphreys BL, McCutcheon DE. Growth patterns in the National Library of Medicine's serials collection and in Index Medicus journals, 1966-1985. Bull Med Libr Assoc 1994;82:18-24

13 Pratt GF. A decade of AIDS literature. Bull Med Libr Assoc 1992;80:380-381

14 Duplenko YK, Burchinsky SG. Computer-aided clustering of citation networks as a tool of mapping of research trends in biomedicine. Scientometrics 1995;32:247-258

15 Herbertz H. Does it pay to cooperate? A bibliometric case study in molecular biology. Scientometrics 1995;33:117-122

16 Logan EL, Shaw Jr WM. A bibliometric analysis of collaboration in a medical specialty. Scientometrics 1991;20:417-426

17 Rousseau R. Evolution d'importantes revues pharmacologiques. Rev Franç Bibliometr 1989;5:102-117

BARBER'S NOMOGRAM TO EVALUATE THE UTILIZATION OF DATA BANKS ON CD-ROM

Moreno Curti, Gabriella Gabutti, Andrea Zeccato, Cesare Carrà, Catherine Klersy, Carmine Tinelli, IRCCS Policlinico S. Matteo, Pavia, Italy

The development and the widespread of informatics technology have opened new perspectives of growth in the world of scientific documentation as well. The onset of new data banks on CD-ROM on one hand, but primarily the multiplication of personal computers and of networks allows an access to scientific information which is quick, direct and decentralized. These solutions obviously imply costs related to the purchase of users' licenses for data banks.

In this study, we plan to evaluate the efficiency of such a use of scientific information by means of Barber's nomogram (fig. 1). The latter was born and traditionally used as an instrument for evaluating the efficiency of hospital admissions. It allows to graphically represent and analyze data on a Cartesian diagram, by integrating the following variables: mean number of sessions by terminal and by time unit (UTY=Users/Terminal/Year); mean time of use (MTU) of data banks expressed in hours; mean time between each session (turnover interval - TI, in hours); and finally rate of occupancy of the workstations (RU=Rate of Use). By projecting one single point on the set of axes of the nomogram, a synthetical description is possible of the use of data banks, so to derive further indications for the evaluation of the system in terms of efficacy as well as of efficiency.

FIGURE 1
Barber's nomogram

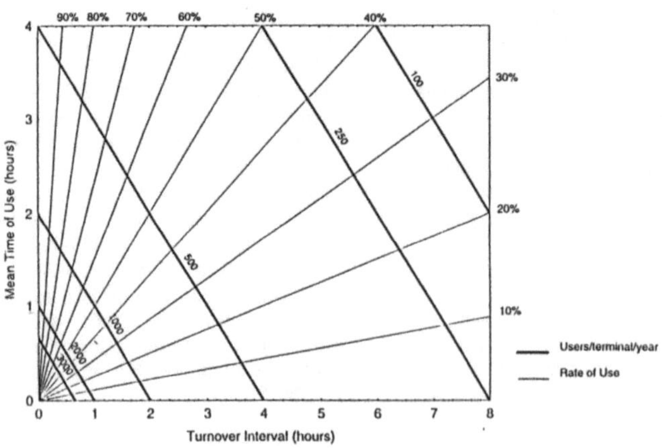

S. Bakker (ed.), Health Information Management: What Strategies?, 290.

A QUANTITATIVE ANALYSIS OF SPANISH BIOMEDICAL RESEARCH

Maria P. Barredo Sobrino, J. Burriel Bielza and F. Martínez García,
Universidad Autónoma de Madrid, Spain

Trends of English and Spanish language publications (1989-1994)

The biomedical scientific production (1989-1994) by Spanish authors or institutions, recovered from Medline on CD-ROM, was quantitatively analyzed to study its repercussion in the international scientific world. Of the whole scientific production from a country, the most known by foreign authors is the part that appears in international databases. Medline on CD-ROM is the most used in Spain. This database currently indexes about 4.100 worldwide journals, and contents more than 370.000 articles per year, approximately 80% in English language.

Articles of Spanish authors or institutions were recovered from Medline by searching *Spain, Espana, Espanha, Spanien, Espagne* and *Spagna* (with the **or** command) in the address field. *Port of Spain* addressed items recovered were discarded. The items recovered were divided in *English* and *Spanish* production from the language field. The search was done in November of 1995 (update code = 9511).

The Spanish production in English language showed a progressive increment from 2.505 articles (1989) to 4.316 (1994). As a whole, the Spanish production in English language among 1989-1994 was of 20.991 articles. In all years researched the increase was constant referred to the previous year. Regarding the total production in English language collection in Medline, the Spanish production in this language grew from 0,87% (1989) to 1,31% (1994). The Spanish production in Spanish language collected from Medline suffered a continuous falling, from 3.909 articles (1989) to 3.213 (1994). In percentages, this decrease was 4,1% in 1990 and 5,8% in 1994, in relation with the previous year. However, their representation in this database was the one that diminished the least, along with Chinese and Portuguese languages. The descent for the 1989-1994 period was of 18% for Spanish and Portuguese languages, and 10% for Chinese language.

A progressive tendency of Medline to exclude journals in non-English language was observed. This fact was highly significant for the production in Russian language, which went down in its representation a 58%, probably related to the break up of the Soviet Union. From this study come off that, on one hand, the Spanish production in English language is increasing quantitatively, although it's reaching a consequent balance because it can't grow limitless. Besides, on the other hand, the Spanish production in Spanish language, is holding the pressure that is produced by the scientific international production on that production written in non-English languages.

S. Bakker (ed.), Health Information Management: What Strategies?, 291.

A SIMPLE INSTRUMENT TO EXPLOIT CLINICAL AND SCIENTIFIC ACTIVITY

Laura Bianciardi and Maria Cristina Costantini, Università degli Studi, Siena, Italy

Linee di ricerca e pubblicazioni, 1987/1988--

The Siena University Medical Library produces, starting from 1989, a yearbook about the searchlines and the scientific production of the members of the Medical Schools. This book, edited by Dr. Deonilla Pizzi, has the Dean of the Faculty as publisher. The aim of the book is to collect systematically the data relating to the scientific activity of each Institute, Clinics and Department of the Faculty and to create an updated bibliography of their scientific production, in order to diffuse information about this activity and promote the knowledge and the cooperation with other Italian and foreign researchers. In this paper the authors outline the methods of collecting and processing data and the relevant data obtained. The book is divided in three parts: 1) Searchlines; 2) Publications; 3) Synthesis.

SEARCHLINES

The first part of the yearbook is divided according to the Institutes and Departments, each labelled by a letter; each section opens with the description of the staff and their function: Professors (and relative Teaching), non Regular Professors, Researchers, Technical Personnel, Health Services Physicians, etc...; the list of searchlines follows, divided into Financed Searchlines and non-Financed Searchlines. At the end of the First part, the lists of Medical Graduated Schools, Special Schools, "Masters" follow. Searchlines are described by: Title, Coordinator (or the Coordinators, if the Research is National or International), Participants of the Institute, eventual other Participants. If researchers of other institutions or countries are present, the corporate source is specified. If the research is financed, the fund of the financing is indicated.The last element of the citation is constituted by the type of the Research, that can be carried out in the same Institute or in collaboration with other Institutes, Universities, or Research Centers. Every citation is marked by a signature composed by the letter corresponding to the Institute, followed by the letter R (Ricerca) and a progressive number; these signatures are used as reference in the Indexes. For the collection of the data Professors are requested in May to communicate their searchlines to the Library by using a special form.

S. Bakker (ed.), Health Information Management: What Strategies?, 292-293.

PUBLICATIONS

The second part of the yearbook has the same structure as the first part and collects data on the scientific production of the single Institutes and Departments, constituted by bibliographic citations of articles and monographs (first group) published in the year preceding the publication year of the book, and meeting participations (second group). For the citation form the Index Medicus standards and the Italian Cataloguing Rules are followed. A signature, made with the same standards adopted in the first part, but marked by the letter P (Pubblicazione) is assigned to the citations. Professors are requested to send original off-prints of the publications to the library; the off-prints are catalogued in a separate file of the Siena Libraries Online Catalogue, in conformity with citation standards.

SYNTHESIS

The third part collects the data obtained from the processing of the professors' communications with the aim to exploit the Medical School activity; composed of four sections: keywords; funds; searchline-type; author index.
a) *English keywords* permit to searchers to individuate who is studying what. For the construction of this index, keywords suggested by the researchers are used and controlled through the Medline Thesaurus, the Embase Thesaurus and, for psychological terms, the PsycInfo Thesaurus. Every keyword is followed by the signatures of the corresponding searchlines.
b) data relating to the different *funds* used for searches; searches with specific funds and searches with more funds are counted; the total sum of the funds is analyzed by percentage and visualized by a graph to compare the proportion of the various funds.
c) This section points out the *cooperation* with other researchers and other institutions. Searchlines are divided by the type: *Institute / Department search; *search in collaboration with other Institutes / Departments of the Faculty; *search in collaboration with Institutes / Departments of other Faculties of the Siena University; *search in collaboration with other Italian Universities; *search in collaboration with foreign Universities / Research Centers. Also in this case a graph allows to visually confront the data.
d) The book closes with the *author index*, that shows the complete activity of each teacher in that year. Each name is followed by the signature that makes reference to the first part, which includes searchlines and/or to the second part, which includes publications.

This volume represents the necessary completion of "The Faculty Day", instituted just since 1989, at the beginning of each Academic Year: this meeting is an important occasion for researchers and professors to let know their own activity and to discuss subjects of common interest. Also the physicians of the Health Services of the neighbouring towns are invited to the "Faculty Day": in order to diffuse information and promote scientific activity, the book is sent not only to the Institutes and Departments of other Faculties of the University of Siena, but also to all Italian Medical Faculties and Research Centers.

Bibliography

[1] Uniform requirements for manuscripst submitted to biomedical journals. International Committee of Medical Journals Editors. JAMA 1993;269:2282-2286
[2] Visintin G. La citazione normalizzata. Biblioteche Oggi 1985;3(2):21-24

THE SCIENTIFIC PUBLICATIONS OF THE FACULTY OF VETERINARY SCIENCE ON SOME CD-ROM PRODUCTS

Mirella Mazzucchi, University of Bologna, Italy

Introduction

Over the past few years we have become accustomed to reading in professional journals something of the impact of the most recent technological innovations on library services. Whereas traditionaly bibliographic research was based on indexes and abstracts journals, nowadays we have the Internet and CD-ROM, on-line rather than card catalogues. The ready availability of and accessibility to information does not howewer guarantee exhaustiveness on a particular subject. When surfing the Internet, bear in mind that it is a veritable chest of information, both valuable and entirely useless.

This is also partially true for CD-ROM. As it is so easy to access the answers to ones queries, one tends not to consider how the database being used is formed. In a quasi-automatic manner the librarian suggests which database to use and how to make the search correctly with the result that the user may be convinced that the system being used is the only one available, the only place to search.

People who use CD-ROM in Faculties of Veterinary Science expect to find most of the world publications on veterinary science and animal health in the most common consulted databases. Some of these users actively hope not to find anything on a particular subject to thereby be the first to carry out research in that particular area. It is known that cd-rom improves the availability of scientific information, however it is important to point out which kind of information it includes and why.

Veterinary publications

The aim of this study is therefore to compare the entire scientific production of the researches of our Faculty with what is indexed in the more common CD-ROMs, such as CAB, FSTA and Medline, used in various faculties of Veterinary Science. Of the entire production of our Faculty of Veterinary Science, from 1988 to 1996, only 19% is present in the aforementioned databases. This is subdivided into 14% on CAB (Vet+Beast), 1% on Food Science and Technology Abstracts, and 4% on Medline.

At the beginning of this study it was suspected that most of the work of non-English speaking countries had not been indexed due to the language barrier but the above data sample does not support this view. The whole body of work produced between 1988 and 1996 by the Faculty of Veterinary Science of the University of

S. Bakker (ed.), Health Information Management: What Strategies?, 294-296.

Bologna constitutes 1513 articles, 33 % of which are written in English. The same percentage represents the articles in English indexed in the databases, whereas 66% are in Italian and 1 % in other languages. This is proof that the language question is not the primary cause of the lack of representation.

One of the departments of the Faculty of Veterinary Science publishes the majority of its work (62%) in English, perhaps due to the similarity between this department and the Science of Human Medicine, but only 27% of its articles are indexed (12% of the entire faculty).

If one is to examine the Journal selection for Index medicus /Medline page one finds stated that the criteria for selecting journals written in a foreign language should be the same as for those written in English. Other factors being equal, additional consideration should be given to the availability of adequate English-language abstracts which extend the accessibility of the content to a broader audience.

Discussion

There are two more possible reasons for the large number of non-indexed articles. The first is that the Italian researcher chooses the wrong journal to which to send his or her paper, sending it instead to less reputable or worthwhile journals.

The second is the wrong choise on the part of the database producers, who don't expand the lists of titles and who won't correct the lack of adequate coverage given to veterinary literature. In Medline the list of veterinary titles continues to decrease. This could be one of the reasons for the lack of Italian works in veterinary science in that database. There is a project to renew the list of veterinary journals and the veterinary librarians have been asked to check the 209 titles and to suggest the inclusion of some new titles.

The criteria for inclusion in Medline index are the following:

a) journals must contain articles predominantly on core biomedical subjects.

b) any journal whose content is predominantly on a subject peripheral or related to biomedicine will be brought to the attention of the Literature Selection Technical Review Committee who will then examine the quality of the content and the contribution that publication makes to the subject in question.

One of the most important criteria is the quality of editorial work. Journals should include features that contribute to objectivity and quality, information about the methods of selecting articles, especially on the explicit process of external peer review, timely correction of errata, and so on. Another limiting factor would be if the articles had been published for a local audience.

For inclusion in the CAB International databases the Impact Factors of the journals are not considered, completely international coverage is provided, including many titles from developing countries. Comprehensiveness is persued and any journal containing original refereed scientific research will be considered.

Covered by Medline there are 91 journal titles from Italy, but only 28 are on Veterinary Science and only 2 have the status of being currently indexed. Acknowledging the efforts of the National Library of Medicine to keep the database up to date, particularly difficult as they are now experiencing some support contractor problems, it is nonetheless true that the picture one has when making a search is not as complete as it seems. The scarcity of articles in Medline is understandable, where journals are in great part biomedical but the small number in the CAB database is not quite so comprehensible, where the journals are on veterinary science and animal health, animal production and dairy technology.

In parallel Italian authors must increase the number of their publications in English if they wish to see their papers circulate the world. There are some departements which publish a lot in English but are not well represented. The Veterinary Biochemical Department for instance publishes 62% of its work in English but represents only 3% of the database, as opposed to representing 12% of the output of the whole faculty. One of the reasons for this could be that the different areas in which the researchers of these departments work, are more closely related to other databases. The Zoothechnical Department, 15% of the Faculty, publishes 20% of its work in English, but on the databases only 19% of its work is present. The Veterinary Pathology Department publishes 12% of the output of the faculty, but it constitutes 27% of the CD-ROM and in English it publishes 38%. The Department of Infectious Veterinary Diseases is the best represented in the databases with 35% of its articles (14% of the whole faculty) and 18% written in English.

Conclusion

Data resulting from this research could be useful to the Faculty of Veterinary Science of the University of Bologna to keep its works circulating, being more selective in choosing where to publish, examining the Impact factors of the ISI (not used) and adding English abstracts in some Italian journals, which could be more readily included in Veterinary CD-ROMs. On the other hand foreign researchers would be more conversant with Italian projects heretofore not studied, and database producers should look to their guidelines and criteria with a mind to changing or modifying some.

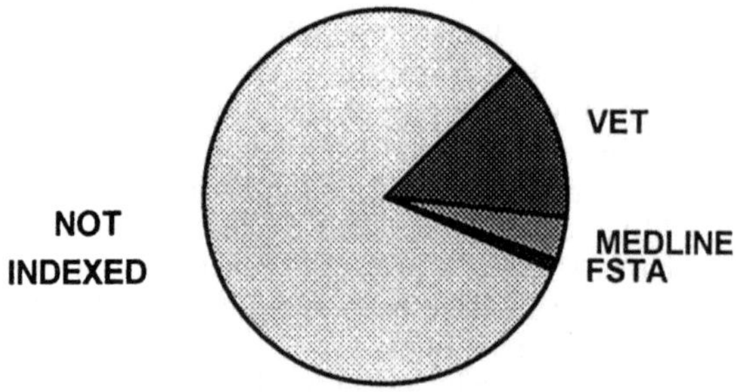

Figure 1. Bologna Faculty works 1989-1996 in databases

COOPERATIVE COLLECTION DEVELOPMENT AND DOCUMENT DELIVERY IN HUNGARY

Márta Virágos, Medical University, Debrecen, Hungary

Academic libraries in Hungary are changing tremendously due to technological developments world-wide, major political changes in the country from a centrally dictated educational system to an autonomous one, and a new higher educational law. Within the framework of the developmental project initiated by the Ministry of Culture and Education, a special sub-project is designated for current collection assessment and the elaboration of a new acquisition strategy at a national level.
The *Conspectus methodology*, developed by the Research Libraries Group (USA) and used in several European libraries was found the most suitable model for collection evaluation. Work groups were set up in each library field to adapt Conspectus in a national context.

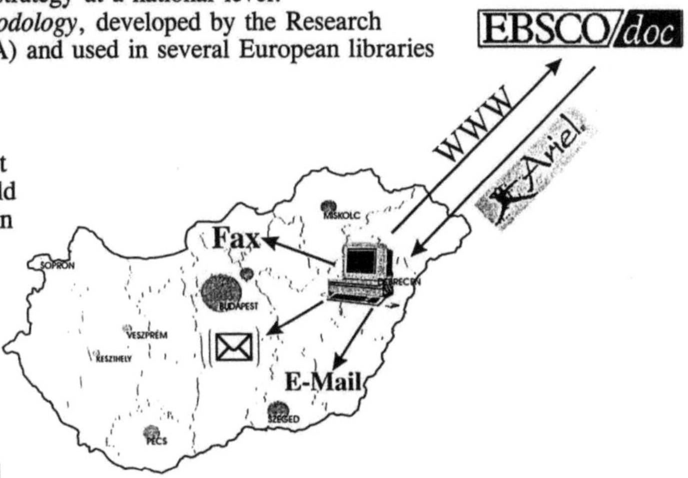

Recommendations
* Librarians should participate in curriculum planning and development in higher education, in particular for new graduate and doctoral programs.
* University librarians should develop standards for collection development.
* A national plan for the preservation of library collections should be developed including electronic preservation strategies.
* A distributed interlibrary loan system should be created based on a shared union database and cooperative cataloging system.
* The conceptual model should be based on the latest available technology.

New initiatives. By installing ARIEL, the Central Library of the Medical University, Debrecen has launched a program for the enhancement of the quality of document delivery for medical universities and hospital libraries. Documents received through ARIEL are distributed by the Library to the readers by E-mail, fax or mail.

S. Bakker (ed.), Health Information Management: What Strategies?, 297.

WHERE IS THE EVIDENCE - TEACHING HEALTH PROFESSIONALS HOW TO FIND THE EVIDENCE

Judith Palmer on behalf of the CASP-FEW Team*

Introduction

In the United Kingdom the NHS reforms have emphasised the importance of developing an evidence-based culture in which all health care interventions are clinically effective and increasingly scant resources are used for maximal health gain. Consequently, health professionals are being encouraged to seek evidence, to critically appraise it and to act on the findings.

Beginning in 1992 a series of workshops was held in the Anglia and Oxford Region of the NHS to introduce public health physicians and those working closely with them, to the techniques of critical appraisal and to the special importance of systematic reviews and meta-analysis.[1] Their success led to a new series of workshops - Critical Appraisal Skills for Purchasers (CASP) which was launched in 1994.

Finding the evidence

Since January 1994, 2600 people from all professional groups have attended CASP events throughout the UK and 8 events are being held every month. All have been well received. A number of participants expressed an interest in learning more about 'finding the evidence'. As a result, in May 1994, the CASP team and librarians in the Health Libraries and Information Network (HeLIN) began planning a workshop on 'Finding the Evidence'.[2]

In November 1994 a Pilot Workshop was held, and as a result of the feedback from this event, a revised version was designed which aimed:

1. to help participants improve their ability to find evidence systematically about clinical effectiveness, especially in reviews and other summaries;
2. to be aware of the range and quality of available sources of evidence about effectiveness, irrespective of format;
3. to be aware of how searching techniques and search strategies may affect outcome;
4. to share and learn from the experience of others.

S. Bakker (ed.), Health Information Management: What Strategies?, 299-301.

Programme

A Pre-Workshop task asked participants to find information either on a given topic or on a topic of their own choosing. At the Workshop, after a brief Introduction to the Critical Appraisal Skills Programme and the origins of the Workshop, participants were split up into small groups (8 or less) with a facilitator, to discuss the problems they had encountered when searching for information. Each group was asked to identify a rapporteur who would feedback to the whole group. This allowed all participants to share their experience.

The next part of the programme provided the opportunity for local librarians to talk about some of the services that they offered. This was followed by a session on sources and searching and a second, shorter period of group work in which participants revisited the problem they tackled before the workshop. Time was allocated at the end of the Workshop for evaluation forms to be completed.

Post-pilot activity

The CASP-FEW Team has worked together to produce a comprehensive Workshop Organiser. We see this as a key educational support tool for anyone who wishes to understand and run 'Finding the Evidence' workshops. We believe that it makes good sense for others to take advantage of our efforts rather than to duplicate them. We expected that anyone intending to run a 'Finding the Evidence' Workshop would wish to tailor the documents and slides as well as the structure of the workshop to the needs of their audience. This has indeed proved to be the case in subsequent workshops.

In the workshops that have followed, changes have been made in each, based on the feedback that has been received from the previous workshop, e.g., the pre-workshop task specified a scenario, rather than ask participants to provide a topic themselves; more 'hands-on' time was provided; the didactic session on sources and searching was integrated with the feedback session to avoid unnecessary repetition and to present the information in context.

Lessons learned

We originally planned to start the workshop with a short talk/discussion on the services that users might expect to obtain from their local libraries. We received very little positive feedback about this part of the programme and now incorporate this implicitly rather than explicitly.

From participant feedback, it was clear that there should be a move away from didactic sessions to a more interactive approach. This answers individual needs better, and creates a more effective learning environment. More time needs to be given to the formulation of questions, and to the design of search strategies. Our experience shows that users want:

1. hands-on most of all and priority given to practice;
2. help while doing it;
3. modelling of practical techniques - "show us how";
4. examples of "effective" searches on "owned" problems;
5. minimal theory, tied to, or arising from, practice;
6. something to take away - e.g.search results.

The greatest problems we have encountered have been in finding suitable accommodation in which there are sufficient terminals with access to databases on a network and where there is good local hardware/software support. We are also concerned that the workshop approach does not supersede nor diminish the importance of other forms of user education and training. Workshops are not meant to replace the need for all health professionals to learn general searching skills. The 'Finding the Evidence' workshops are designed with a specific context in mind - the need to help professionals find the best available evidence. They also offer librarians the opportunity to work closely with other health professionals in a multidisciplinary context.

Linked developments

We have provided workshops for particular professional groups such as dentists, general practitioners, clinical biochemists, occupational therapists, physiotherapists. Our experience has also been used to inform the development of other workshops for teaching information skills. A group of librarians in the Region together with some members of the CASP-FEW team have planned two out of three Search Clinics which are part of the International EBM Workshops held in the UK over the past two years. The most recent workshop was built around the formulation of a clinical question.[3] An introduction, outlining the aims and structure of day, was followed by hands-on searching; group work, more hands-on searching and a concluding session in which the days work was reviewed. Feedback was extremely positive.

Another linked development is the information skills module in the new Oxford University Certificate, Diploma and Masters Programme in Evidence-based Health Care, which began in 1996 and is supported by funds from the NHS. The Health Care Libraries Unit with the Cairns Library are planning the modules around the experience gained through CASP-FEW and the EBM Workshops as well as the user education programme in the Cairns Library.

Conclusion

We have found that an evidence-based culture can provide the opportunity for libraries to become Centres of Evidence and librarians to play a new, high-profile, pro-active role as educators and facilitators.

References

[1] Milne R, Chambers L. How to read a review article critically. Health Libr Rev 1993;10:39

[2] Palmer J. Finding the evidence. Health Libr Rev 1994;11:282-286

[3] Richardson WS, Wilson MC, Nishikawa J, Hayward RSA. The well-built clinical question: a key to evidence-based decisions. ACP J Club 1995;(Nov/Dec):A12-A13

*CASP-FEW Team: The Planning Group consisted of Ruairidh Milne, Martin Allaby, Bill Gutteridge and Nicholas Hicks (CASP) and Judy Palmer, Carol LeFebvre and Gill Needham (HeLIN). Subsequently Rosemary Stark, Steven Ashwell and Jane Holdsworth joined the Planning Team together with Dorothy Husband, Karen Henderson and Anne Brice. Sue Nayee, from North Thames also helped develop the pilot. Robin Snowball, Douglas Badenoch and Reinhart Wentz helped to develop and run the EBM Search Clinic

SUPPORT FOR EVIDENCE-BASED MEDICINE: COLLABORATIVE TEACHING BY INFORMATION PROFESSIONALS AND CLINICIANS

Richard L. Faraino and Dorice L. Vieira, New York University Medical Center, USA

The Environment

The confluence of information technology and the principals of Evidence Based Medicine (EBM) have fostered an environment for collaborative curriculum development among medical and library faculty. The rapid expansion of high speed networks that cross the globe provide easy access to a myriad of information providers. Many institutions have direct access to biomedical sources such as MEDLINE, other commercial biomedical databases, institutional information sources, and the Internet from their patient floors as well as from research departments. Internet sites seem to increase daily, and it has become difficult to fathom the amount of information available to a physician with a computer. According to Davidoff, to keep abreast of their field, general physicians must process 17 original articles per day, 365 days per year.[1] EBM began at McMaster University and is defined as "the ability to access, summarize, and apply information from the literature to day-to-day clinical problems."[2] To apply EBM techniques to daily practice physicians need to acquire the skills to frame the clinical question in such a way that lends itself to eliciting key terms and concepts to search and to develop effective strategies for literature searching. Additionally they need to understand the structure of information and be able to determine the quality of published research as it may be applied to clinical decision-making. Medical librarians are professionally trained in the development of sophisticated search strategies for rapidly locating clinical research, and in the use of a variety of search engines on different computer platforms. Medical librarians are able to incorporate the principals of EBM to searching the literature and can impart those skills to residents. Medical faculty are trained to instruct residents to use EBM in applying epidemiological principles to a clinical setting, critical appraisal of the literature, decision-making and decision analysis. It is in this environment that the medical and library faculty came together to develop a curriculum in Evidence-Based Medicine at New York University Medical Center/School of Medicine.

BACKGROUND

The sessions that are outlined here have evolved over the last 4 years and continue to be modified and adapted. This curriculum was developed with the director of medical education for the residency training program in Pediatrics and two faculty librarians in the Educational Services Department of the Library and is offered twice a year. It

S. Bakker (ed.), Health Information Management: What Strategies?, 302-305.

has been modified for use in training Primary Care residents and for several undergraduate components of the medical school curriculum. While the librarian-led sessions have been planned with the medical faculty and designed to complement the broader curriculum of EBM, the sessions described in this paper focus on informatics issues that involve the expertise of medical librarians.

Process

Planning begins a minimum of three months in advance of instruction. Medical and library faculty meet to discuss the overall goals and objectives of the course and the best methods available for achieving them. Proficiency in framing the clinical question, searching the literature and understanding the structure of information are frequently identified as the priority for librarian faculty. Critical appraisal and quality assessment can be a shared goal of all faculty, while epidemiological principals, decision-making and decision analysis remain in the realm of medical faculty to teach. Such issues as facility, number of teaching faculty needed, number of instruction modules, schedules, and means of evaluation are of highest priority for program implementation. Because faculty will undoubtedly have other commitments throughout the curriculum, measures must be taken to ensure continuity, such as team teaching. A minimum of two librarians is assigned to each module in which searching the literature takes place. This facilitates small group instruction and enables the instructors to devote more attention to individual needs of participants, which becomes increasingly important as participants bring in a variety of clinical questions from their own daily rounds.

APPLICATIONS TO CLINICAL PRACTICE

There are a variety of scenarios in which the librarian-led modules can be integrated into a larger EBM program. Typically the resident or student identifies a clinical question based on the patients seen on the floor. They perform a literature search online. By analyzing the search results several key studies are identified. The resident or student then has to locate the study and apply critical appraisal techniques to determine the scientific validity and applicability of the studies to the clinical decision-making process. Librarian faculty are consulted on search strategies and information resources. The resident or student then presents their findings to their department during grand rounds, journal club, or regular meetings. The medical faculty then leads a discussion of pertinent issues raised by the presentation. Other scenarios might involve searching the Internet for a practice guideline issued from an authoritative organization such as the Cochrane Collaboration, or finding cost analyses for diagnostic techniques, or a meta-analysis of patient outcomes. The goal is for physicians to use the rules of evidence in practice throughout their careers.

RESOURCES NEEDED

Facility: Hands-on experience using computers is essential for the success of an EBM program. At least 1 computer per 2/3 participants in a networked environment with access to MEDLINE and the Internet is adequate. Presentation software programs and Web Browsers are very useful. Other application programs for word-processing, email, database and bibliographic file management programs are also used.

Medical faculty: In addition to their leadership role, offer validity on the necessity of the course. They can bring in examples from daily practice and apply them to the course and are essential for evaluating resources. It is prerequisite that medical faculty recognize the importance of the information professional in teaching EBM.

Library faculty: Teaching skills and a good understanding of EBM and how it applies to information environment are basic requirements for librarians. They should also serve as consultants for not only accessing and searching information, but also for managing information.

Technical support staff: They are needed for the set up and maintenance of equipment and networks.

Curriculum director/committee/department chairs: Administrators are needed to provide the directive to offer the course and to provide support for the program.

HOW MODULES ARE ADAPTED FOR OTHER AREAS

Because the basic principles of EBM remain constant, it is easy to adapt the modules outlined here to meet the needs of incoming requests for EBM. Time factors, availability of faculty, facilities and the level of the participants are all variables which this program can accommodate. When a request for an EBM course comes to our library we are able to offer them any combination of the modules from the outline. Each module can be viewed as a template which can be expanded upon or scaled down to meet the individual needs of a course director. Lectures stored on presentation programs can be easily edited for any given audience and time table. Search strategies can be adapted to any user level without compromising the basic principals of EBM. The program described has been offered to medical students and residents and has also been adapted for attendings, nurses and allied health students.

Conclusion

To develop a successful EBM program, librarians must play an integral role in rounding out the faculty "team" providing instruction. While knowledge of Evidence-Based Medicine as it pertains to information science is an essential ingredient, the ability of librarians to adapt their skills to teaching in the clinical environment is another. Though we were fortunate to have our faculty body first seek us out, we have since taken advantage of opportunities to support our medical faculty and institution by seeking out those opportunities through our daily contacts and attending a variety of meetings throughout the institution.

References

[1] Davidoff F, Haynes B, Sackett D, Smith R. Evidence-based medicine. BMJ 1995;310:1085-1086
[2] Evidence-Based Medicine Working Group. Evidence-based medicine: a new approach to teaching the practice of medicine. JAMA 1992;268:2420-2425

Appendix - Curriculum Outline

COMPUTER PRE-COURSE - 3 ONE HOUR SESSIONS
Basic Computer Terminology, Mouse Manipulation, Introduction to Word-processing: This pre-course was designed for those with little or no computer experience. It was necessary to offer this in advance of the program so that all participants would have comparable computer skills throughout the course.

INFORMATION NEEDS OF AND RESOURCES FOR PHYSICIANS - 1 HOUR
An overview of library and information sources for the physician covering traditional resources and services and introducing new resources such as email, listservs, electronic full-text and the Internet.

INTEGRATING COMPUTERS INTO DAILY PRACTICE - 2 ONE HOUR SESSIONS
Participants use computer applications to set up a sample patient database. The exercises incorporate database management, word-processing and email applications.

INTRODUCTION TO INTERNET - 1 HOUR SESSION
The history and nature of the Internet, search engines and sample medical and EBM sites are examined. Guidelines for determining quality resources are also examined.

EVIDENCE BASED MEDICINE - 3 TWO HOUR SESSIONS
Basic Principals: "EBM is an approach to health care that promotes the collection, interpretation, and integration of valid, important and applicable patient-reported, clinician-observed, and research-derived evidence."[1]

Examining the Literature: tools that support EBM: ACP Journal Club: a digest of clinical research articles; Users' Guides to the Medical Literature: a series of articles published in The Journal of the American Medical Association devoted to using the literature for EBM.

How to Frame a Clinical Question: Participants redefine a clinical question in terms of EBM and for performing a literature search on MEDLINE.

Searching the Literature: Getting around MEDLINE: Focusing on the structure of MEDLINE database, Medical Subject Headings, categorical limits and publication types.

Searching the Literature: MEDLINE Strategies: Group and/or individual search exercises in the areas of diagnosis, etiology, therapeutic efficacy, or prognosis.

Critical Appraisal: Examining the search results based on the rules of evidence and includes types of studies and the structured abstract. Participants discuss clinical content with medical faculty.

Reference

[1] McKibbon KA, Wilczynski N, Hayword RS, Walker-Dilks CJ, Haynes RB. The medical literature as a resource for health care practice. J Am Soc Inf Sci 1995;46:737-742

WHO NEEDS EVIDENCE-BASED HEALTH CARE?

*Jenni Tsafrir and Miriam Grinberg**, *Chaim Sheba Medical Center and **Tel-Aviv University, Israel

Background and Definitions

The proliferation of published material in the clinical and biomedical sciences has made it difficult for clinicians to keep up-do-date with developments in specific fields, and conflicting results on diagnostic and therapeutic procedures may introduce doubts in decision-making for patient care. Physicians and health services researchers alike have had to develop their skills in retrieval and effective use of the literature, and in the selection and critical appraisal of published findings.

The concept of Evidence-Based Medicine (EBM), which has developed over the past 15 years reflects the change in approach which has taken place in medical practice. It involves the critical application of results of population-based studies or large clinical trials to clinical decision-making and patient care.

Scientific medicine has always implied both the theory and the practice that flow from objective data, in other words, the "evidence".[1] However, the nature of clinical evidence itself has changed, as regards the standards for gathering information, and the tools for analyzing it. The new standard for etiologic and diagnostic evidence is epidemiologic, while the Randomized Controlled Trial is the "gold standard" for therapeutic evidence.

EBM uses "value-added" strategies to complement the physicians' and experts' personal knowledge, in order to resolve clinical problems. It integrates individual clinical expertise, acquired through experience and practice, with the best available up-to-date external evidence from systematic research clinically relevant and applicable to the problem at hand.[2]

Sources of Evidence

Firstly, there are publications which select and distil other publications, sometimes adding comments or annotations by expert groups and covering a vastly greater amount of literature than any physician could hope to read and absorb, e.g. Journal Watch, ACP Journal Club, etc.

Secondly, there are factual databases, providing direct data from field studies, such as that produced by the International Cochrane Collaboration, which publishes systematic reviews on a variety of common clinical subjects and updates them each time an important new trial is reported.[3,4]

S. Bakker (ed.), Health Information Management: What Strategies?, 306-308.

Thirdly, some answers may be found in meta-analyses published in the medical literature, and finally, relevant guidance in specific clinical situations might be obtained from Clinical Practice Guidelines, based on randomized trials or meta-analyses.

Limitations of Evidence-Based Medicine

EBM offers little help in the many "grey zones" of practice, where the evidence about the risks and benefits of competing options is incomplete or contradictory.[5] Some studies giving negative results or results that are not statistically significant, may never be reported, as potential authors may be discouraged if their research results do not provide a breakthrough.[5,6] Some reports are published in journals not indexed in MEDLINE or other widely available biomedical databases, or in the "grey literature" such as research reports, policy documents, dissertations and conference abstracts.[7] There is also the "Tower of Babel" bias, whereby exclusion of non-English papers in meta-analyses or in Review journals may lead to erroneous conclusions.[8] All these result in a publication bias, which naturally affects the data collection for a systematic review.[7,9]

How Applicable is Evidence-Based Medicine?

In a small study conducted amongst physicians at our hospital, we found a significant correlation between the preference for original, specialized articles, for purposes of keeping up-to-date, research and writing for publication. This preference was also correlated with the number of years elapsed since completion of medical studies, and with a preference for mediated literature searches. There was a significant relationship between the preference for review articles, meta-analyses, etc., and the high priority set on reliability of information. In other words, this type of article was considered highly reliable. However, and this is meaningful in the context of EBM, there was no correlation between this preference and information-seeking for patient care. Thus, in combining this "evidence" with our personal "experience" as librarians, we have concluded that physicians in a dilemma concerning patient care will seek information most closely related to the patient in question, whether by consulting their peers or other experts, or in published case-reports or highly relevant reviews. Thus, the type of epidemiological evidence used in EBM does not as yet seem to be considered of high importance for daily decision-making related to patient care.

Role of Libraries and Information Centres in EBM

While the use of meta-analyses and randomized controlled trials may increase, the ability to formulate clinical problems into answerable questions, to retrieve the information efficiently from available resources, and to appraise critically publications of all types will remain an invaluable skill.[10] Our ability to impart these basic librarianship skills to physicians will be crucial in enabling them to make the best possible use of the available evidence.

Health care is viewed today as "a complex endeavour" that is highly dependent on information, considered an important resource to be efficiently managed to enable the practice of EBM.[11]

The involvement of librarians in various facets of this endeavour ranges from the attachment of clinical librarians to patient care teams, through active participation in research design and conduct,[12] to the more traditional information-gathering services provided. In all such services, librarians provide the "added value" to the expertise and knowledge of the in-house experts.[11] As information becomes more readily accessible electronically and delivered directly to the end-users, libraries will have to focus on materials that are more difficult to come by, or which are not found in traditional publications.

Finally, since the requirements of evidence-based health care may influence the attitudes of clinicians to the published literature and its evaluation, they are of importance to medical libraries and information centres. They may affect collections and their management, staffing, and the interaction between clinicians and information specialists.

References

[1] Davidoff F, Case K, Fried PW. Evidence-based medicine: Why all the fuss? Ann Intern Med 1995;122:727

[2] Sackett DL, Rosenberg WM, Gray JA, Haynes RB, Richardson WS. Evidence based medicine: What it is and what it isn't. BMJ 1996;312:71-2

[3] Sackett DL, Haynes RB. On the need for evidence-based medicine. Evid Based Med 1995;1:5-6

[4] Rafuse J. Evidence-based medicine means MDs must develop new skills, attitudes. Can Med Assoc J 1994;150:1479-81

[5] Dickersin K, Min YI. Publication bias: the problem that won't go away. Ann NY Acad Sci 1993;703:135-48

[6] Dickersin K, Scherer R, Lefebvre C. Identifying relevant studies for systematic reviews. BMJ 1994;309:1286-91

[7] Gregoire G, Derderian F, Le Lorier J. Selecting the language of the publications included in a meta-analysis: is there a Tower of Babel bias? J Clin Epidemiol 1995;48:159-63

[8] Buckley NA, Smith AJ. Evidence-based medicine in toxicology: where is the evidence? Lancet 1996;347:1167-9

[9] Rosenberg W, Donald A. Evidence based medicine: an approach to clinical problem-solving. BMJ 1995;310:1122-5

[10] Rees J. Where medical science and human behaviour meet. BMJ 1995;310:850-3

[11] Doyle JD. Knowledge-based information management: implications for information services. Med Ref Serv Q 1994;13:85-97

[12] Smith JT Jr, Smith MC, Stullenbarger E, Foote A. Integrative review and meta-analysis: an application. Med Ref Serv Q 1994;13:57-72

MISSING INFORMATION: SOME ISSUES MEDICAL LIBRARIANS SHOULD BE THINKING ABOUT AS THEY BRIDGE BETWEEN PUBLISHED INFORMATION AND DELIVERY OF HEALTH CARE

Barbara Aronson, World Health Organization, Geneva, Switzerland

Introduction

The aspects of scientific literature which are usually cited as being problematic for medical librarians are: volume, exponential growth, subject fragmentation, lack of clear borders between disciplines, timeliness, direct access by the end user via communications networks, and cost. Implicit in these analyses is the notion that all the information our library users need exists: that while some information may be difficult to identify, to access or to organize, given the appropriate tools, technology, training, and budget, the medical librarian should be able to locate any needed fact, study or commentary.

Is this indeed the case? Is all the biomedical information necessary for effective public health policy and medical practice available somewhere? Sufficient thought has perhaps not been given to the information which is missing: the information which simply does not exist, which is not published, or if published is not accessible for a variety of reasons.

Information is prevented from existing by many factors. This paper examines the categories of missing information, and proposes possible approaches for counteracting this problem.

What kinds of information are missing?

INFORMATION WHICH IT IS NOT PROFITABLE FOR THE AUTHOR OR PUBLISHER TO DISSEMINATE:

- Negative results
- Information viewed as private property
- Information distorted to change direction and force of impact

INFORMATION WHICH DOES NOT FOLLOW FASHION:

- Funding tied to research fashions
- Bias in peer review and publishing
- Pressure groups setting research priorities

S. Bakker (ed.), Health Information Management: What Strategies?, 309-310.

INFORMATION EXCLUDED BY CULTURAL AND LINGUISTIC HEGEMONIES:

- Non-English information
- Information originating outside the first world

ISSUES INVOLVING THE ACCOUNTABILITY OF JOURNALS:

- Scientific fraud
- The commercial basis and needs of journals

WHERE THERE IS NO EVIDENCE:

- Rare diseases and orphan drugs
- Under- and non-reporting of diseases

Can anything be done about this situation?

INNOVATIVE INFORMATION CATEGORIES, PACKAGES, PRACTITIONERS:

- Legitimize publishing of negative and non-significant results
- New reporting and information systems
- Evidence synthesizer: a new medical profession

WHAT CAN LIBRARIANS DO?

Awareness of these issues may make a critical difference in the quality of key functions in the medical library. Certainly the problem of missing information is something librarians should be keeping in mind and transmitting as they develop collections and catalogues, give reference services, and train students, doctors, researchers and other patrons to use information resources.

Copies of the full text of this paper, including an extensive bibliography, may be requested from the author by fax: +41-22-791-4150 or E-mail: aronsonb@who.ch

A CORE JOURNALS SELECTION FOR EVIDENCE-BASED MEDICINE

Rafael Bravo Toledo, Concepción Campos Asensio, Concepción Muñoz Tinoco and Elena Guardiola Pereira, Getafe; Madrid; Barcelona, Spain

Introduction, materials and methods

The present study was planned in order to identify the journals that publish more, and more sound, articles for the daily medical practice. To achieve this objective, bibliometric techniques were used. MEDLINE (SilverPlatter, SPIRS version 3.11) on CD-ROM was searched for the period 1993-1995. Search strategies were performed according to McMaster's University validated strategies to retrieve relevant articles dealing with diagnosis, treatment, prognosis and etiology, and based on the best single-term searches identified by that group (Tables 1a and 1b).[1-4] A database was created with all retrieved references, the Bradford's distribution was calculated.

for Etiology: Risk (tw)
for Diagnosis: Sensitivity (tw)
for Prognosis:
Explode cohort-studies (mesh)
for Therapy: pt= Clinical-trial
tw= title and abstract fields
mesh= medical subject heading field
pt= publication type field

Table 1a. Best single-term search

Results

The MEDLINE file for 1993-1995 contained 148,719 journal articles indexed under the search terms related with evidence-based medicine, published in 3,201 different serial titles. These journals were sorted in rank order according to the total number of articles identified in this topic in MEDLINE. A table was generated taking into account the cumulative number of serial titles (n) and the cumulative number of articles or frequency (An). Bradfod's distribution was then represented (Fig. 1).

The nucleus of the most productive journals was calculated by means of the adjustment method of Bradford's distribution proposed by Ferreiro Aláez.[5] As a result, Bradford's nucleus for evidence-based medicine was formed by the first 297 journals ranked, accounting for 50% of the total number of journal articles indexed.

Conclusions

This study is based solely on the quantity and percentage of evidence based journal articles published over a three-year period and no attempt was made to judge the quality of the articles or the journals that published them.

The list of journals obtained in this study, as a core collection of special interest for physicians in the process of solving clinical problems, can be helpful, by itself or

S. Bakker (ed.), Health Information Management: What Strategies?, 311-312.

as complement to the experts opinions, in the selection of journals to subscribe to in specialized clinical libraries, the creation of specific databases, the selection of articles to be abstracted or evaluated, etc..

More detailed classifications, taking into account the different medical specialties involved in this area, as well as other serial titles selection methods, are needed in order to obtain a more accurate core set of journals, where relative weights of journals that publish a big amount of articles are minimized, and to avoid the lack of specificity of the single-based term search strategy used.

#1	RISK
#2	RISK
#3	(#1 in TI) or (#2 in AB)
#4	SENSITIVITY
#5	SENSITIVITY
#6	(#4 in TI) or (#5 in AB)
#7	explode COHORT-STUDIES /ALL
#8	PT=CLINICAL-TRIAL
#9	**#3 or #6 or #7 or #8**
#10	PT=JOURNAL-ARTICLE
#11	TG=ANIMAL
#12	TG=ANIMAL
#13	TG=HUMAN
#14	#11 not (#12 and #13)
#15	#9 not #14
#16	**#15 and #10**

Table 1b. Search strategy

References

[1] McKibbon KA, Walker Dilks CJ. Beyond ACP Journal Club: how to harness MEDLINE for diagnostic problems [editorial]. ACP J Club 1994;121 Suppl 2:A10-2

[2] McKibbon KA, Walker Dilks CJ. Beyond ACP Journal Club: how to harness MEDLINE for therapy problems [editorial]. ACP J Club 1994;121 Suppl 1:A10-2

[3] Walker Dilks CJ, McKibbon KA, Haynes RB. Beyond ACP Journal Club: how to harness MEDLINE for etiology problems [editorial]. ACP J Club 1994;121(3):A10-1

[4] McKibbon KA, Walker Dilks C, Haynes RB, Wilczynski N. Beyond ACP Journal Club: how to harness MEDLINE for prognosis problems [editorial]. ACP J Club 1995;123(1):A12-4

[5] Ferreiro Aláez L. Leyes empíricas bibliométricas. in: Ferreiro Aláez L. Bibliometría. Análisis bivariante. Madrid: Eypasa, 1993. pp.403-423

Note: The complete list of journals, with their frequencies, the data used for the graphical display of Bradford's distribution, and all the mathematical calculations performed to find out the nucleus of the most productive journals is available upon request.

Figure1 Bradford distribution

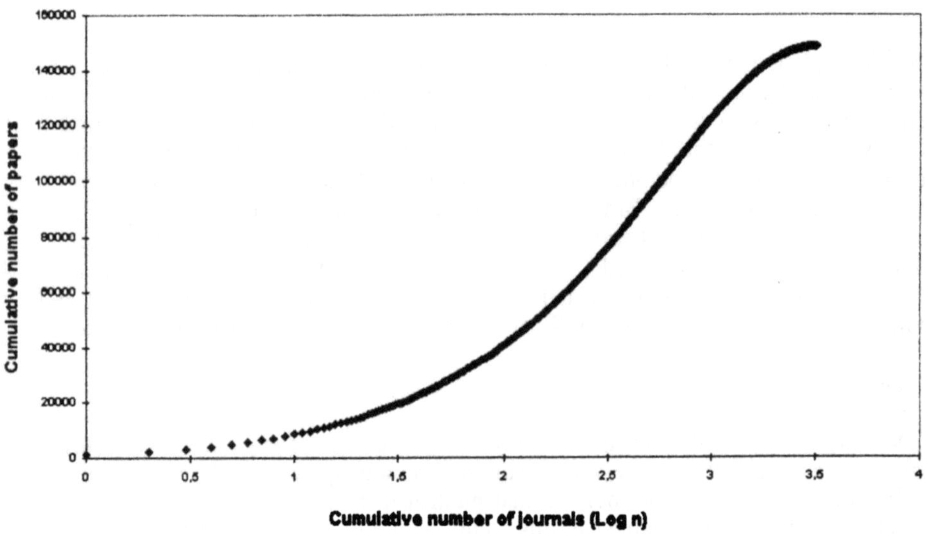

ETHICAL QUALITY AND PHARMACEUTICAL MANUFACTURER'S LITERATURE

Luisa Vercellesi, ZENECA S.p.A., Basiglio MI, Italy

Rationale

Pharmaceutical promotion with continuing education and independent information is worldwide a primary source of updating for health professions.[1] In view of the implications for health, pharmaceutical information is ruled by a European directive (92/28 EEC), from which Italy has derived a national law (D.Leg.541,1992), which are essentially consistent. Moreover the WHO has set ethical criteria for medicinal drug promotion. The drug industry associations at international, European and local levels, are applying their own codes; individual drug industries are adopting even more stringent guidelines, aiming to produce literature suitable for an objective and good taste promotion, with scrupulous regard for truth.

The Italian scenario

Continuing education. Local law provisions foresee postgraduate education for doctors contracting with the national health system, but no obligation is set for prescribers working on a private basis; in addition to that there is no public nationwide initiative in continuing education.

Independent information. Few sources are available and even the national datasheet compendium has been no longer published since 1992,[2] and in any case the inclusions of datasheets were not even compulsory earlier.[3] This is leading to an unbalance of informative sources available on drugs.

Information from pharmaceutical industries. In this country therefore it is important that pharmaceutical literature is providing reliable and quality information both for the implications for health and to regain a reputation to the drug industry.

Establishing a process

To assure that the legally required and company desired level of ethical quality is maintained, a process to improve the written information issued and consequently enhance the correct use of drugs could be established.

S. Bakker (ed.), Health Information Management: What Strategies?, 313-315.

EDITORIAL COMMITTEE

The appointment of an editorial committee could be an answer (fig. 1). Drug information professionals could have a role in securing updatedness, correctness and overall representative view of cited references; other key members of this committee obviously could be the marketing and medical functions, with conventional responsibilities. In particular the drug information professionals could ensure that the evidence used is the best available and well substantiated, that it is referred in an accurate way, that it is not misleading, still updated and reflecting the totality of current knowledge.

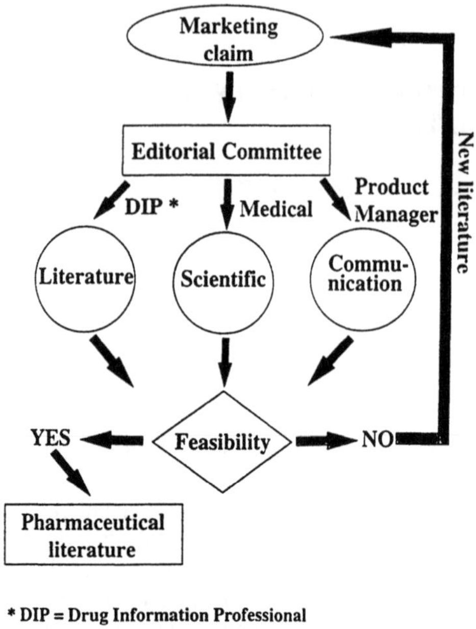

Figure 1. Responsibilities and process within the Editorial Committee

QUALITY ASSURANCE COMMITTEE

At a higher level a quality assurance committee (fig. 2) could secure the compliance to ethical codes issued locally and internationally by the company and the associations of pharmaceutical manufacturers as well as the adherence to national laws; this could provide an internal assessment of subsequent approval of promotional material by local regulatory authorities. The appoitnment of the quality assurance committee could take into account seniority and lack of hierarchical implications with the editing members. A reasonable deadline for revisions could be set.

TRAINING AND SUPPORT

A notebook for the editorial committee, summarising features of laws and codes could be provided, issued and revised by the quality committee. A checklist for revision and internal approval processes could help to support and speed up medical writing and approvals. Notebook, checklist, legislations and codes should be available to all those involved in the process (including external copywriters or medical writers); proper training in medical writing should be provided if necessary.

INFORMATION, PROMOTION OR EDUCATION?

All the information material used as a promotion, sponsored or issued by the drug company, addressed to health professionals, either through medical representatives or as mailing campaigns or distributed on occasion of scientific congresses could be object of this procedure. A borderline between medical information and promotion is not always clear. Generally medical information is reactive (information provided in response to an enquiry) and promotion is proactive (information provided without health professionals having asked first). Even the borderline between educational activities and promotion is not an easy one to draw: proportion of the publication dealing with company product, the overall look of the item, the authorship could help to define the nature.

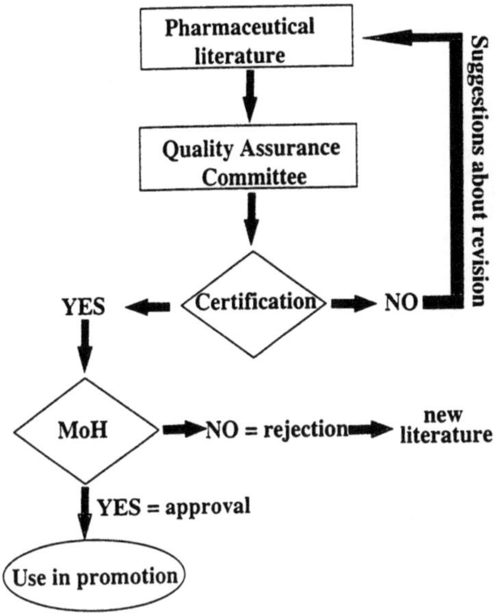

Figure 2. Responsibilities and process within the Quality Assurance Committee

Quality and drug information professionals

Ethical quality of pharmaceutical literature is important particularly in those countries, like Italy, where other forms of medical professional updating are less common. In any country however, drug companies could benefit from operating a process to assure quality and ethical standards for their literature and providing support to all the people involved in the creation of promotion material.

Drug information professionals could contribute to the generation of this literature and positively affect promotion, thanks to their familiarity with published evidence.

References

[1] Snell ES. Education,information and promotion. In: Burley DM, Binns TB (eds). Pharmaceutical Medicine. London: Edward Arnold, 1985. p.189

[2] Herheimer A. I bollettini sui farmaci fanno parte della letteratura scientifica. In: Offerhaus L (ed) ISDB Review. Reggio Emilia: Farmacie Comunali Riunite, 1991. p.9

[3] Del Favero A. L'informazione sui farmaci in Italia. In: Strategie ed Efficacia dell'Informazione sui Farmaci. ISDB Review. Reggio Emilia: Farmacie Comunali Riunite, 1989. p.87

INFORMATION DISSEMINATION 100 YEARS AGO: W.C. ROENTGEN AND THE DISCOVERY OF X-RAYS

Peter Morgan, Cambridge University Medical Library, Cambridge, UK

December 28th 1895 - Roentgen's manuscript

Wilhelm Conrad Roentgen first observed the phenomenon of X-rays on 8 November 1895. After six weeks of experimentation he wrote a preliminary communication, the first of his three papers on the subject, and submitted it to the President of the Wuerzburg Physical-Medical Society, Karl Lehmann, on 28 December 1895. Lehmann recognized the importance of the paper and arranged for it to be printed immediately. Though this paper, "Ueber eine neue Art von Strahlen" ("On a new kind of rays"), was ultimately published in the Society's proceedings for 1895,[1] Roentgen did not deliver his lecture to the Society until 23 January 1896, there being no meeting during the Christmas period.

At the end of the nineteenth century, scientific communication was largely dependent on publication through scientific journals, on personal correspondence and distribution of offprints, and on presentations at scientific meetings. In the developed world the normal method of public long-distance communication was the postal service, via horse-powered vehicles, rail and steamship. Cable telegraphy was well-established for the rapid communication of text, though it could not transmit pictures. The telephone was still in its infancy as a public service, and radio communication was only in the experimental stages.

January 1st 1896 - distribution of offprints

The offprints of his paper were delivered to Roentgen very quickly, and on Wednesday, 1 January 1896, he posted copies to scientific colleagues both in Germany and abroad, in some cases also enclosing copies of selected X-ray plates, including one showing the hand of his wife Bertha, to illustrate the paper. The offprint originally had an extra headline, "Professor Roentgen's Important Discovery!", but Roentgen - a very modest and reticent man - objected to this sensationalism, and the headline was deleted from subsequent printings.

S. Bakker (ed.), Health Information Management: What Strategies?, 317-320.

January 4th 1896 - first reactions

The first recorded reaction took place in Berlin, where Emil Warburg received a copy of Roentgen's communication on 4 January 1896. That same day he added the photographs to an exhibition at Berlin University's Physical Institute, but the photographs were not prominently displayed or explained, and attracted little attention.

The same day Roentgen's paper also reached Franz Exner, Professor of Physics in Vienna. He immediately showed his copies of Roentgen's X-ray prints to a group of friends. One of those present was Ernst Lecher, whose father, Z.K. Lecher, was editor of the Vienna newspaper *Die Presse*. The father, given the story by his son, published it as a front-page story - "A Sensational Discovery" - on Sunday, 5 January 1896. Other newspapers had their own correspondents in Vienna, who duly reported the story to their editors. First to react was the London *Daily Chronicle*, which published its version on 6 January (with the misspelling "Routgen"). On 7 January reports appeared in the London *Standard* (again with the misspelling "Routgen", which was repeated in various other reports for some time thereafter), and in the *Frankfurter Zeitung*, which printed the first X-ray photographs. News agencies which obtained the story by cable telegraphy could receive only text and not pictures, so most early reports, and especially those overseas which relied on slower postal services for photographic material, were not illustrated and therefore prompted more scepticism among their readers.

January 7th 1896 - replication of experiment

The report in the *Standard* was seen by an ingenious electrical engineer, A.A. Campbell Swinton. Acting on the information gleaned from this article, he assembled the necessary equipment and repeated Roentgen's experiment. His results on 7 January were poor, but those on the following day were better and he was able to write to the *Standard* anouncing this, in a letter published on 10 January: his experiments provided the first recorded successful replication of Roentgen's work.

While the popular press had ensured that the news became public very quickly, scientists also began to learn more of Roentgen's discovery, and to see examples of X-ray photographs, at meetings of scientific societies. The first such meeting was that of the Berlin Society for Internal Medicine on 6 January, where M. Jastrowitz reported on the communication he had received from Roentgen. Meetings reports from this period typically follow a common pattern: to begin with, they often include a short item recording that after the main business was concluded, one of the members present gave a brief presentation concerning Roentgen's interesting new discovery. As the weeks passed, these gave way to more substantial contributions, and soon to whole sessions devoted to X-ray research. However, the written reports of these meetings were generally slow to appear in print, and those not present would have needed to rely on other sources for more up-to-date information.

January 8th 1896 - scientific journal publication

The first report in a scientific journal did not appear until 8 January 1896. The journal in question was the New York *Electrical Engineer*, which ran the story under the heading "Electrical Photography through Solid Matter". It was closely followed by the London *Electrician*, the first European scientific journal to cover the story, which on 10 January contained a short front-page item.

The first reports in medical journals appeared on 11 January, when the *Lancet*, the *Medical Times and Hospital Gazette*, and the *New York Medical Record* all noted the discovery. Within a week of the initial article in *Die Presse* the story had been reported worldwide in a wide variety of scientific and popular journals. Translations of Roentgen's paper soon started to appear, beginning with an English translation in *Nature* on 23 January. By 20 February *Nature* was commenting that "so numerous are the communications being made to scientific societies that it is difficult to keep pace with them, and the limits of our space would be exceeded if we attempted to describe the whole of the contributions to the subject, even at this early stage". While physicists and electrical engineers concentrated on investigating the underlying science of X-rays, the medical profession - like the general public - were more interested in potential applications. There was initially a widespread tendency to regard X-rays as a branch of photography, and much of the early literature appeared in photographic journals.

May 1896 - the start of an X-ray journal

Although the *British Medical Journal* did not report Roentgen's work until 18 January, it soon began to cover the topic at some length, and on 8 February it announced that it was commissioning Sydney Rowland, a young English doctor, "to investigate the application of Roentgen's discovery and to study practically its applications". Rowlands' reports monitored research activity (including his own) and became an important source of information. The need to focus on the subject in greater depth soon led to the publication, in May 1896, of *Archives of Clinical Skiagraphy*, with Rowland as editor. This, the first journal devoted to X-ray science, was the forerunner of the present-day *British Journal of Radiology*. ("Skiagraphy", meaning "shadow-pictures", was one of a number of terms employed to describe the new science. Roentgen himself had suggested the term "X-rays", but at his Wuerzburg lecture on 23 January the term "Roentgen's rays" was proposed and adopted, leading eventually to the widespread use of "Roentgenography" to describe the science.)

Public discussion and scientific impact

The popular press continued to devote much attention to Roentgen's work in these early weeks. Their reports ranged from the accurate and objective to the misleading, cynical, and speculative, sometimes in the same paper. The science correspondent of the *Pall Mall Gazette*, for example, provided a series of carefully-considered reports on investigations into the new technology, while on 14 January the same newspaper published a sensational and dismissive description of a demonstration given by Swinton. Elsewhere, humorous poems, songs, and cartoons appeared, reflecting a growing scepticism and boredom. But as public interest began to decline, the scientific, technical and medical press reflected an ever-greater preoccupation with X-rays, underlining the impact created by Roentgen's discovery.

The speed with which Roentgen's preliminary report became known around the world, and the rapid sequence of developments and associated publicity, can be attributed to a number of factors. The paper was published quickly, and offprints were available for distribution, because the president of the Wuerzburg Physical-Medical Society recognized that the paper was too important to be delayed by the normal interruption in the Society's meetings programme caused by the Christmas holiday; the printer was able to produce offprints of the paper within four days of Roentgen submitting his manuscript on 28 December 1895; Roentgen's reputation as a gifted and meticulous researcher ensured that his findings would command respect; his experiments were an extension of research interests already familiar to other physicists, and the equipment he used (induction coil, Hittorf-Crookes vacuum tube, and photographic plate) was already widely available, making it easy for others to experiment further; photography was a popular hobby, with enthusiastic devotees eager to investigate the X-ray phenomenon; Roentgen did not patent his discovery, and his detailed description of his methods allowed others to follow his lead; and some of the reports in the popular daily press were sufficiently accurate and detailed to disseminate information that scientists could utilise without waiting for the slower, more considered channels of publication available through the weekly and monthly professional journals.

Perhaps most significant to the early promotion of Roentgen's work, though, was the immediate strong public interest. The nature of X-rays - with a powerful visual impact and sensational implications in many aspects of life - generated immense interest, both professional and popular. Although Rontgen's preliminary communication reached fellow-physicists rapidly by post, and could then have been expected to be publicised, discussed, and investigated further through the standard channels of scientific communication, the speed with which the news reached a far wider and more public audience was due, ultimately, to the sequence of chances that led to the first newspaper report in *Die Presse*. The sensational aspects of the announcement, and the credibility given to it by Roentgen's name, ensured that other newspapers and agencies which routinely used cable telegraphy would quickly repeat it and seek follow-up stories. This meant in turn that the public, alerted to the medical applications (both real and imagined) of X-ray technology, developed the expectation that their doctors would utilise it for the benefit of their patients, thus making it increasingly necessary for the medical profession to demonstrate its awareness of the new technology and its readiness to employ it.

Bibliography

[1] Roentgen WC. "Ueber eine neue Art von Strahlen". Sitzungsberichte der Physikalisch-medizinischen Gesellschaft zu Wuerzburg 1895;29:132-141

EVOLUTION DU FRONTISPICE DANS LES OUVRAGES DE MEDECINE DU XVIème au XVIIIème SIECLE

Hélène Fauré and Danièle Roberge, Bibliothèque interuniversitaire de Médecine, Paris, France

Frontispieces of medical books from the XVIth century to the XVIIIth century

Although described as part of general illustration, few studies have been published about the frontispieces themselves. From the XVIth to the XVIIIth century, the importance of medical frontispieces within the books changed: not often seen in medical books from the XVIth century, the frontispiece became highly notorious in the XVIIth century and declined in the XVIIIth century. Two connected evolutions took place: the way from an illustrated title-page to an independant illustration and the growing role of iconography in the frontispiece.

Introduction

Le frontispice est une partie de l'ouvrage qui a été peu étudiée en tant qu'élément original. Un certain nombre de frontispices médicaux ont déjà été analysés d'un point de vue purement iconographique, au même titre que d'autres planches mais il nous a semblé qu'ils méritaient une étude particulière pour mettre plus précisément en évidence la fonction du frontispice dans l'ouvrage.

Avant d'aborder les caractéristiques du frontispice, il serait bon de considérer d'abord les différentes définitions que l'on donne du frontispice. La plupart des dictionnaires, actuels ou anciens, proposent deux sens: la page de titre illustrée ou l'illustration, elle-même dégagée de la page de titre et la précédant généralement. Une troisième définition apparaît dans certains dictionnaires, à savoir la vignette surmontant le titre d'un chapitre. Cette dernière acception ne sera pas retenue dans cette étude.

Page de titre illustrée ou illustration séparée, le frontispice tire ses deux significations de l'évolution qu'il a connue dans le temps. La répartition par siècle sera retenue bien qu'artificielle mais nous essaierons de dégager des tournants significatifs.

De la page de titre illustrée à l'illustration indépendante

EVOLUTION CHRONOLOGIQUE

Une constatation s'impose: le frontispice médical du XVIème siècle est avant tout une

S. Bakker (ed.), Health Information Management: What Strategies?, 321-323.

page de titre illustrée; en effet, sur 53 recensés, 51 sont des pages de titre comportant une gravure (sont exclus les marques typographiques et les simples motifs décoratifs), soit 96%. Les deux pages illustrées indépendantes de la page de titre sont d'ailleurs tardives, l'une de 1586 et l'autre de 1597.

Sur l'ensemble du XVIIème siècle, les pages de titre ne représentent plus que 26% des frontispices recensés et au XVIIIème siècle 30%, soit une proportion à peu près similaire au XVIIème siècle si l'on considère que le recensement des frontispices est loin d'être exhaustif; mais on observe un léger déclin des pages illustrées au fil du XVIIIème siècle, trop faible toutefois pour en tirer de véritables conclusions. C'est plus particulièrement entre 1650 et 1675 que la proportion de pages de titre illustrées a le plus baissé par rapport aux pages illustrées indépendantes; on remarque la quasi absence de ces dernières dans le premier quart du XVIIème siècle, sans changement par rapport au XVIème siècle et, inversement, la très faible proportion de pages de titre illustrées dans le dernier quart du XVIIème siècle.

L'illustration s'est ainsi peu à peu détachée des mentions bibliographiques pour acquérir sa propre autonomie.

STRUCTURE DU FRONTISPICE

On peut relever dans les frontispices trois grandes compositions; la première est le portique ou l'arche, fondée sur la symétrie et généralement divisée en trois bandeaux: le socle avec habituellement les indications d'impression, l'étage central composé très souvent de deux statues encadrant les mentions d'auteur et de titre et le fronton supportant des figures allégoriques. Autre type de frontispice, des petites scènes insérées dans des cartouches, chaque cartouche représentant un thème particulier, et enfin le frontispice composé d'une scène unique, occupant soit toute la page soit une partie seulement sous forme de vignette. D'une manière générale, le portique et la scène unique sont les plus représentés dans les frontispices médicaux, le premier plus présent dans les pages de titre et la seconde dans les illustrations indépendantes. Mais la structure du portique devient moins fréquente vers le milieu du XVIIème siècle (comme l'a déjà constaté Th. Moyne[1]).

Rôle de l'iconographie dans le frontispice

LE "SEUIL" DE L'OUVRAGE

Le frontispice a été souvent assimilé aux arcs de triomphe des Entrées solennelles ou aux portails des façades des églises. Quoi qu'il en soit, sa fonction est double, esthétique en donnant une façade illustrée au livre et intellectuelle en présentant un résumé synthétique de l'ouvrage. L'intention, dans les deux cas, est de donner envie de passer ce seuil symbolique et de lire l'ouvrage.

UN FRONTISPICE DE PLUS EN PLUS CONCENTRÉ SUR L'IMAGE

Disparition progressive de toute mention bibliographique. Chronologiquement, le frontispice se confond au départ avec la page de titre illustrée. Comme nous l'avons vu, il s'en sépare ensuite tout en gardant, au milieu de l'image autonome, certaines mentions bibliographiques (rappel de l'auteur ou du titre ou de l'imprimeur ou de plusieurs de ces éléments). Au début du XVIIIème siècle, toute mention bibliographique va peu à peu disparaître complètement du frontispice: alors que les illustrations autonomes représentent moins de 10% au XVIIème siècle, la proportion augmente rapidement pour atteindre près de 95% des frontispices recensés entre 1750 et 1775.

Mais en même temps que les mentions bibliographiques disparaissent du frontispice (et que le frontispice lui-même connaît un déclin), l'illustration retrouve un nouvel essor sur la page de titre avec la multiplication de vignettes, certains ouvrages comportant à la fois une page de titre illustrée et une illustration indépendante.

Un frontispice visuellement rapproché de la page de titre. Lorsque l'illustration s'est détachée de la page de titre, elle a commencé par occuper le recto d'une feuille précédant cette page de titre; puis on la trouve de plus en plus, depuis la fin du XVIIème siècle, au verso, donc en regard de la page de titre. Le premier frontispice que nous ayons recensé, ainsi mis sur le même plan visuel que la page de titre, date de 1630. C'est à partir du deuxième quart du XVIIIème siècle qu'ils représentent plus de 70%.

Une évolution favorisée par l'utilisation de la taille-douce. La gravure sur cuivre permettant plus de richesse et de précision dans le dessin, son adoption accompagna le passage de la page de titre gravée à l'illustration indépendante. Le premier frontispice en taille-douce que nous ayons trouvé dans les ouvrages médicaux date de 1560;[2] à titre d'exemple, pour l'Angleterre, M. Corbett fait remonter le premier frontispice en taille-douce à 1545, mais tous domaines confondus.[3]

De plus, même si son coût de revient est supérieur à celui du bois, l'utilisation du cuivre est plus souple car c'est une technique qui permet aux dessinateurs de faire leur propre gravure, sans l'intervention d'un artiste (réducteur, graveur) spécialisé. Par ailleurs, la taille-douce permet les jeux d'ombre et de lumière.

Ainsi, après avoir connu une évolution ascendante jusqu'à la deuxième moitié du XVIIème siècle, le frontispice médical a décliné au cours du XVIIIème siècle, pour être, au XIXème siècle, plus exceptionnel.

Notes

[1] Moyne T. Les livres illustrés à Lyon dans le premier tiers du XVIIème siècle. Grenoble: Ed. Cent pages, 1987

[2] Valverde de Amusco J. Anatomia del corpo humano. Rome: Ant. Salamanca et Antonio Lafreri, 1560

[3] Corbett M, Lightbown RW. The comely frontispiece: the emblematic title-page in England, 1550-1660. London [etc.]: Routledge and K. Paul, 1979

LA GRAVURE SCIENTIFIQUE DU XVème AU XVIIIème SIECLE DANS LE PROJET DIOSCORIDES DE L'UNIVERSITE COMPLUTENSE DE MADRID

Aurora Miguel-Alonso, Pilar Moreno, Mercedes Cabello and Alberto Morcillo, Biblioteca Universidad Complutense de Madrid, Spain

Abstract. The medical historic engraving is a fundamental source of information for the history of medicine and science. One of the goals of the project Dioscorides developed by the Universidad Complutense de Madrid and the Fundación de Ciencias de la Salud is the reproduction and diffusion of a significant collection from the 15th to 18th centuries. The project Dioscorides includes the digitisation of 15.000 relevant medical books from the period between the 15th and 18th centuries. This electronic library is devoted to art and science historians, bibliographers, iconographers, and researchers interested in the evolution of books and engravings. The program also allows the creation of an independant illustrations data base. The search can be made through three different fields: artists, subjects, and chronological period. Standarization tools as artist authorities lists, subject headings, and special thesauri for iconografic material are required to treat the information.

Introduction

La gravure médico-historique est une source d'information particulièrement intéressante pour l'histoire de la médecine et de la science. La reproduction et la diffusion d'une importante collection qui va du XVème au XVIIIème siècle constituent quelques-uns des buts du Projet Dioscorides réalisé par l'Université Complutense de Madrid, la Fondation de Ciencias de la Salud et les Laboratoires Glaxo-Welcome.

La technique de la gravure permet, à partir d'une matrice, de reproduire avec exactitude des images ou des signes autant de fois que besoin s'en fait. Ainsi, grâce à cette possibilité de reproduction, la gravure va donner lieu à l'un des changements les plus importants de l'évolution de l'Humanité. Désormais le monde ne sera plus seulement perçu de façon différente grâce aux textes diffusés massivement à travers l'imprimerie, mais il pourra également être vu de façon différente à travers les images transmises par la gravure dans tous les coins du monde. De par leur nouveauté, ces nouvelles habitudes visuelles sont comparables à celles que nous avons acquises au cours de notre siècle depuis l'apparition de la photographie, du cinéma, et plus récemment avec celle des multimédias.

Pour le livre scientifique, la gravure n'est pas seulement une question de décor ou un élément qui aide à la compréhension du texte, c'est bel et bien une formule complémentaire, souvent irremplaçable, pour que le message transmis soit correctement compris. Même la meilleure et la plus minutieuse description du corps

S. Bakker (ed.), Health Information Management: What Strategies?, 324-329.

humain, des plantes médicinales ou des animaux, des appareils de distillation, etc..., n'est rien en comparaison de l'image reproduite par les artistes qui suivent scrupuleusement la description de l'auteur.

L'illustration des livres scientifiques à l'aide de gravures offrait une telle possibilité de diffusion qu'elle élargit les termes de la discussion scientifique à une échelle internationale, ce qui permit la naissance définitive de la science moderne au début du XVIIeme siècle. L'association du livre imprimé et de l'estampe scientifique doit être considérée comme l'un des facteurs décisifs pour le progrès de la science moderne.[1]

Dans le livre biomédical, les motifs iconographiques apparaissent tôt et reviennent avec une certaine fréquence: le corps humain et ses différentes variantes d'origine gréco-romaine comme "l'homme zodiacal", ou "l'homme grenouille", qui représente un être humain à demi assis qui montre les différents organes; "l'homme blessé" sur lequel on peut voir les principales blessures de guerre et comment les soigner ou "l'homme saignée" qui indique les meilleurs endroits où pratiquer les saignées, et la série des différents systèmes: le système veineux, le système artériel, le système nerveux, le système osseux, le système musculaire, auxquels s'ajoutent assez fréquement le corps et les organes féminins, et, parfois, la grossesse.

Cette iconographie puise ses origines dans les manuscrits alexandrins, et ne varie pratiquement pas au cours du Moyen Age ni pendant la période des incunables. Elle ne disparaîtra que progressivement à partir du moment où divers artistes de la Renaissance s'efforcent de mieux connaître le corps humain et son fonctionnement. Le premier à le faire, fut Léonard de Vinci, mais n'oublions pas les italiens Pollaiolo, Raphaël, Michel Ange et l'allemand Dürer.

A partir de ces grands dessinateurs, le livre d'anatomie change radicalement, le dessin s'inspire de l'observation du corps humain, sur l'homme vivant bien sûr, mais surtout, sur la table de dissection. En 1538, Vésale publie son premier ouvrage d'anatomie et par la suite, et pendant deux siècles, tous les anatomistes étudieront ses dessins et s'en serviront pour leurs travaux.[2]

Dans le domaine de l'histoire naturelle, le processus fut similaire. Les herbiers, les bestiaires et les lapidaires du Moyen Age reproduisent des plantes, des animaux ou des minéraux que l'artiste n'a en général jamais vus, car le texte ancien, grec ou latin, qu'ils transcrivent, décrit des formes de la nature qui n'existent pas dans son environnement. Plus tard d'autres imprimeurs recopieront ces illustrations sans faire non plus le rapprochement image-texte.

Lorsqu'au début du XVIème siècle, les premières descriptions des plantes du Nouveau Monde commencèrent à arriver, les livres d'histoire naturelle subissent un sérieux revers. Les modèles iconographiques du Moyen Age ne pouvaient être utilisés pour les nouvelles espèces, alors que les naturalistes tenaient à les décrire et dessiner minutieusement. Christophe de Acosta ou Nicolas Monardes, sont quelques-uns de auteurs qui voyagèrent et découvrirent le continent américain pour la science.

Les artistes Weiditz, Bock et Fuchs, collaborateur assidu de Plantin, arrivèrent à donner aux illustrations de leurs ouvrages de botanique une exactitude qui donna le ton aux auteurs suivants, car leurs ouvrages eurent une énorme diffusion dans l'Europe entière. Signalons en dernier lieu, l'italien Andrea Mattioli qui accompagne ses *Commentarii in Dioscoridem* de gravures tout à fait nouvelles qui elles aussi serviront de modèle à d'autres éditions postérieures, parmi lesquelles se trouvent celles du médecin espagnol Andrés Laguna.

Tous ces ouvrages, qui au fil des siècles ont été utilisés par les professeurs et les élèves pour transmettre les nouveaux savoirs, sont actuellement déposés dans les bibliothèques des universités européennes, dont l'histoire remonte au Moyen Age.

L'Université Complutense de Madrid est l'une de ces universités centenaires, elle possède une collection bibliographique qui conserve entre ses pages une information iconographique de la plus haute importance. Etudiée dans son ensemble cette collection constitue un instrument de travail indispensable pour l'histoire de la médecine et de la science en général. C'est précisement, dans le cadre du Projet Dioscorides, ce qui a conduit une équipe de travail de cette Université à récupérer l'ensemble des illustrations pour les mettre à la disposition des chercheurs.

LA COLLECTION BIBLIOGRAPHIQUE INCLUE DANS LE PROJET DIOSCORIDES

La collection biomédicale de l'Université Complutense est extrêmement représentative de la littérature de cette spécialité publiée au cours des siècles qui concernent le projet, et permet de suivre avec attention l'évolution de l'enseignement médical dans les universités européennes. De plus, il s'agit sans aucun doute du principal fonds historico-médical de l'ensemble des pays d'influence hispanique, par conséquent la récupération électronique sera particulièrement utile pour tous les historiens de la science de ces pays.

La provenance de la collection est très diverse et reflète l'histoire des différents établissements qui convergèrent jusqu'au XIXeme siècle pour former l'organigramme actuel de l'Université. Nous y trouvons des livres ayant appartenus aux différents collèges de l'Université d' Alcalá, mère de notre Université, à des centres de la Compagnie de Jésus, aux Collèges Royaux, prédécesseurs de nos Facultés de Médecine et de Pharmacie, ainsi que des livres qui proviennent d'importants legs de professeurs et de particuliers.[3]

En tout la collection biomédicale que l'on pense numériser représente approximativement 15.000 volumes, qui vont du XVème au XVIIIème siècle. Pour le moment on a déjà reproduit la collection du XVème siècle, les incunables, en tout 104 volumes, ainsi que la collection de traités d'anatomie du XVIème siècle, 50 volumes, et l'on s'occupe actuellement des éditions hippocratiques, constituées par 83 volumes. Les séries réalisées jusqu'à présent ont été selectionnées en fonction des intérêts prioritaires des chercheurs, ainsi que pour des besoins de conservation.

Le fonds incunable. La bibliothèque du Collège Mayor d'Alcalá fut créée du temps du Cardinal Cisneros, fondateur de l'Université, et en 1512, elle réunissait déjà mille soixante dix volumes de théologie, de philosophie, de droit et de médecine. Une partie des incunables digitalisés dans le cadre de notre projet furent acquis à cette époque par l'Université d'Alcalá, en tant que livres auxiliaires de l'enseignement qui y était dispensé. Ils nous permettent par conséquent de connaître quel genre de livre était utilisé pour enseigner la médecine au XVème siècle et au début du XVIème.

Si nous étudions les matières les plus communes de la collection des incunables, nous trouvons plusieurs séries, qui correspondent clairement au genre d'enseignement du bas Moyen Age. Ce sont: (a) Des ouvrages d'auteurs classiques: grecs, romains, arabes, hébreux, etc...., et leurs commentateurs; (b) Des ouvrages d'auteurs chrétiens du Moyen Age, en particulier du XIIIème siècle; (c) Des ouvrages d'auteurs comtemporains de l'édition de l'ouvrage; (d) Des compilations médiévales, telles que "Speculum mundi" ou "De propietatibus rerum"; (e) Des ouvrages sur l'histoire naturelle, prise dans son sens le plus large: des herbiers, des bestiaires, des lapidaires, des ouvrages de matière médicale; (f) Des ouvrages populaires ayant un certain rapport, d'un point de vue de la culture médiévale, avec la santé et le bien-être, comme des calendriers ou des livres d'astrologie.

L'illustration des livres de notre collection présente les caractéristiques de cette première période de l'imprimerie: estampe xylographique, traits robustes et schématiques, sans pratiquement de clair-obscur et utilisation d'une même gravure pour différentes situations. Les figures anatomiques sont rares. Il faut dire que le Pape Sixte IV n'autorisa la dissection des cadavres qu'en 1480 et que, d'autre part, dans le domaine artistique, il faudra attendre que la Renaissance soit bien avancée pour que le nu réapparaisse.

Plus que de traiter d'anatomie, la médecine du XVème siècle s'occupait de l'hygiène et de la botanique médicale, par exemple dans notre collection de cent trois incunables, seuls vingt et un ouvrages sont accompagnés d'illustrations, et, seulement huit présentent des illustrations médicales à proprement parler.

Le fonds du XVIe siècle. A cette époque le traité de médecine se situe entre le livre d'art et le livre d'étude. La gravure en taille douce fait son apparition, mais on continue à utiliser la gravure sur bois; on réduit les formats, à *in cuarto* et *in octavo*, sauf pour la plupart des ouvrages d'anatomie qui continuent à être édités en format *in folio* afin de laisser suffisamment de place pour les gravures. D'autre part, le XVIème siècle est marqué par l'étude des organes internes, grâce aux possibilités offertes par la dissection ainsi que par la diffusion des dessins anatomiques d'artistes tels que Léonard de Vinci et Dürer. C'est l'époque de Vésale et de ses grandes séries de gravures, et son influence se fait sentir dans de nombreux traités d'anatomie.

Le fonds ancien de la bibliothèque compte environ treize mille livres du seizième siècle, dont vingt pour cent peuvent être considérés comme étant des livres de biomédecine, dans le sens le plus large du terme. Comme il s'agissait de réaliser la numérisation d'un fonds aussi important, les responsables du Projet Dioscorides ont choisi de numériser en premier la série des gravures anatomiques, d'abord parce que l'oeuvre anatomique dans le livre illustré du XVIème siècle est très importante, ensuite parce que les gravures sont d'une grande beauté, et enfin à cause de l'intérêt qu'elle pouvait susciter auprès des divers groupes de chercheurs, en particulier auprès des historiens de la science et de la gravure. La série "anatomie" compte en tout cinquante livres, dont quarante quatre sont illustrés, et de ceux-ci vingt contiennent en moyenne cinquante illustrations.

Le projet Dioscorides: une bibliothèque numérique

Une bibliothéque numérique est une collection d'informations électroniques qui a été organisée de façon à permettre un accès facile pendant un grand laps de temps. Son implantation est directement liée aux changements que les nouvelles technologies sont en train de faire entrer dans les bibliothèques.

Actuellement les progrès de la technologie des images permettent de coder sur un ordinateur les documents sélectionnés grâce à un scanner afin de les stocker, les transmettre ou les récupérer aussi bien en ligne qu'à distance. La numérisation est sans doute la solution pour que des collections qui sont d'une grande utilité pour la recherche soient accessibles directement, sans que leur conservation soit mise en danger. D'autre part, le grand développement et la diffusion du réseau Internet, et en particulier le grand succés obtenu par l'outil WEB, a entraîné en peu de temps la multiplication de projets qui utilisent précisemment la technologie des images.

Avec l'augmentation de la capacité de stockage et la prolifération des réseaux de communication, les bases de données d'images commencent à être économiquement viables. Les bibliothèques ont commencé à offrir l'accés 'online' à des collections d'images. Les usagers peuvent d'ores et déjà faire apparaître sur leur écran des images d'oiseaux étranges, des collections botaniques, les fonds du Musée du Louvre, les manuscrits de la Bibliothèque Vaticane ou encore le *De humani corporis fabrica* de Vésale, numérisé par notre bibliothèque.

Digitalisation: dans le processus de numérisation on doit aboutir à un compromis entre le degré de qualité, c'est à dire la résolution, et les possibilités de mémoire dont on dispose, plus la résolution est grande, plus la mémoire est grande, et par conséquent plus le programme mettra de temps à lire et à traiter les images.

Pour ce projet, étant donné que la plus grande partie du fonds est constitué par des ouvrages imprimés en noir et blanc, on a commencé avec des paramètres de numérisation de 400 ppp. de résolution. Lorsque cette communication sera présentée nous aurons commencé un processus de scannérisation qui utilisera jusqu'à 256 niveaux de gris et 300 ppp. Les images numérisées sont codées en format TIFF et on utilise les algorythmes de compression du Groupe IV.

La saisie des images est réalisée à l'aide d'un scanner Kodak Imagelink 200 à caméra numérique haute spécialement conçue pour un fonds ancien et qui permet de récupérer l'image sans endommager la structure du livre.

Application: On a conçu une application fondée sur des systèmes ouverts avec une architecture client-serveur. Le système développé permet la connexion entre la base de données bibliographique de la bibliothèque et les archives d'images. Actuellement la liaison entre les deux systèmes est réalisé moyennant l'émulation de terminale installée sur les postes de travail. A l'avenir on prévoit de développer une interrogation unifiée à l'aide des outils WWW et du protocole standard Z39.50.

Méthodologie de travail: La séquence de travail est essentiellement formée de: sélection, catalogage, numérisation, indexation, contrôle de qualité, et enfin interrogation par l'usager.

L'indexation consiste à organiser les images résultantes du livre numérisé en différents modules ou parties, de façon à ce que le chercheur puisse avoir accès aussi bien aux images séquentielles qu'aux parties différentiées qui le constituent. Le système a prévu l'accés direct au dos, à la couverture, aux pages de garde, à la page de titre, aux préliminaires, aux chapitres ou livres, aux gravures, aux index généraux, aux index de gravures et aux pages numérotées.[4]

Dans la section "illustration" nous avons inclu toutes les illustrations contenues dans un ouvrage sauf les lettres capitales et les orles décorées. C'est la raison pour laquelle on a numérisé en tant qu'illustration toutes les pages de titre contenant une gravure ou des marques typographiques, et dans ce cas c'est le nom de l'imprimeur qui permettra d'y accéder. A l'avenir ceci nous permettra de récupérer tous les exemplaires de cet imprimeur par ordre chronologique. De même sous les vedettes "pages de titre" et "pages de titre architecturales" nous pourrons récupérer les ouvrages qui contiennent ce genre d'illustration dans la période chronologique que nous avons choisie.

Les images marquées comme illustrations peuvent être récupérées sous quatre entrées différentes, permetter ainsi de sélectionner les illustrations grâce à une recherche combinée par auteur, par matière et par date.

1) Le *titre* ou le nom de l'illustration: c'est la principale entrée d'identification et la seule que le système oblige à remplir. Pour la période qui a été numérisée, rares sont les illustrations qui sont identifiées par un nom, c'est pourquoi on a eu recours au nom de l'auteur de l'ouvrage, au titre abbrévié et au numéro de l'illustration, soit celui sous lequel elle figure dans l'ouvrage original, soit, si elle n'en a pas, une

numérotation corrélative assignée par l'indexeur. Par exemple: "Aristote. De caelo et mundo, fig. 12".
2) L'*auteur* ou les auteurs des illustrations. Cette entrée requiert une certaine recherche dans les répertoires ou les monographies spécialisées.[5-9] En effet, le plus souvent les illustrations ne sont pas signées ou sont signées d'initiales énigmatiques ou de monogrammes.
3) La *matière* ou les matières assignées à chaque illustration.
4) Les *périodes chronologiques* des illustrations, en tenant compte que la date qui figurera sera la date d'impression des ouvrages qui contiennent les gravures, sauf dans le cas des illustrations qui sont datées.

L'entrée "vedette-matière" est sans aucun doute la plus problèmatique et la plus complexe des quatre au moment de l'indexation, car il faut assigner des matières normalisées capables de décrire toutes les illustrations des livres numérisés, ce qui demande la création d'un language contrôlé qui permettra à l'usager de réaliser la recherche avec les mêmes termes que ceux qui ont été utilisés précédemmment pour la description.[10-12] C'est pourquoi nous sommes en train de créer une liste de vedettes-matière, avec des sous vedettes qui permettent de mieux concrétiser la vedette principale grâce à une organisation hiérarchique des concepts. Pour essayer de décrire les illustrations dans leur totalité, nous utilisons presque toujours deux vedettes et, en général, sur les deux, une vedette plus générale et une autre plus spécifique.

Actuellement l'extension de ce fichier est en train de nous faire considérer la possibilité de le rendre indépendant, dans la mesure où l'application le permet, pour donner aux illustrations un traitement encore plus différencié.

L'Université Complutense a introduit dans son serveur WEB des renseignements supplémentaires sur ce Projet (**http://www.ucm.es/BUCM/diosc/00.htm**)

L'idée de collaboration entre les établissements qui partagent l'information est en train de devenir une réalité, mais le problème à résoudre ne consiste pas seulement à surmonter les barrières techniques, qui commencent à disparaître, mais bel et bien de décider comment le contenu doit être traité pour être distribué à travers les réseaux nationaux et internationaux.

Bibliographie

1 Checa Cremades E. La imagen impresa en el Renacimiento y el Manierismo. En: Carrete Parrondo J, et al. El grabado en España (siglos XV-XVIII). Madrid: Espasa Calpe, 1987
2 Herrlinger F. History of medical illustration from antiquity to A.D. 1600. London: Pitman, 1970
3 Miguel Alonso A. El libro ilustrado en la biblioteca de la Universidad Complutense de Madrid. En: La Universidad Complutense y las Artes: VII Centenario de la Universidad Complutense. Madrid: Universidad Complutense, 1995
4 Moreno Garcia P et al. El Proyecto Dioscórides: una biblioteca electrónica en la Universidad Complutense de Madrid. Documentos de Trabajo UCM, 96/1. Madrid: UCM, 1996
5 Bartsch A. The illustrated Bartsch. New York: Abaris Books, 1978-
6 Benezit E. Dictionnaire critique et documentaire des peintres, sculpteurs, dessinateurs et graveurs de tous les temps et de tous les pays. Paris: Grüd, 1976
7 Hollstein FWH. Hollstein's Dutch and Fleming etchings, engravings and woodcuts 1450-1700. Amsterdam: Memmo Hertzberger, 1949-
8 Paez Rios E. Repertorio de grabados españoles en la Biblioteca Nacional. Madrid: Min. de Cultura, 1981
9 Silvestre MLC. Marques typographiques. Bruxelles: Culture et civilisation, 1966
10 Garnier F. Thesaurus iconographique: système descriptive des représentations. Paris: Léopard d'Or, 1984
11 Waal H van de (dir). Iconclass: an iconographic classification system. Amsterdam: North-Holland, 1974-
12 Library of Congress. Thesaurus for graphics materials. Washington: Library of Congress, 1995

DOCTOR, CHEMIST AND PROFESSIONAL ETHICS IN XI AND XII CENTURY

Brunella Sebastiani and Giuseppe Salvatori, Consiglio Nazionale delle Ricerche, Rome, Italie

Medicine, in the distant past, had magical, religious and empirical aspects all mixed together. In fact the works of Hippocrates - considered to be the basis of scientific medicine and the beginning of medical science based on observation and reasoning, as well as of the ethical principles governing the profession - are written in the Ionic dialect; using sacred language hard to understand for the profane, they were kept in the temple of Apollo.

This mixture of science and magic also occurred in the Middle Ages, when the study and practice of medicine in Europe were characterised by (a) lay medicine based on the ancient Greek and Roman traditions, strictly following the teachings of the classics, which were often little or poorly known; and by (b) ecclesiastical medicine established in the monasteries, where the classical literary heritage was recovered, maintained and passed down in the form of compendia and commentaries, or texts in a broader context which may be considered encyclopaedic and which was used for teaching purposes.

In the XII century, compendia were considered to be highly important and useful; for example, Constantine Africanus (also known as Constantine of Montecassino, the abbey where he spent the latter part of his life) wrote that *"Unde ego, evolutis omnibus bonis medicorum auctoribus ... contraxi in arctum quae nimium fuse isti habent omnia quae possunt perfectum medicum efficere. Quoniam multa prolixius, multa brevius mihi vedebantur ab illis scripta. Et non omnes possunt omnium libros emere"*. For Constantine, books in the form of summaries or commentaries are of decisive importance in the training of physicians, with *"lectio"* and *"memoria"* being the essential elements in the teacher-pupil relationship for learning what is defined as *"prestantissima artium"*.

Medicine summarises the contribution of other sciences and arts, and so physicians, whether in contact with books or with *"opera naturae"* will benefit from *"traditio, ratio, experimentum"*. In fact, *"Non tradimus autem nisi vel a nobis vel ab aliis experimento comprobata, et ratione certe cognita"*. Orderico Vitale, referring to people who lived in the same period, confirms the growth in medical studies and the broadening of the basic culture of physicians. For example, referring to Gilberto Maminot, he states that *"Artis medicinae peritissimus erat"*, and referring to Raoul Malacorona *"... neminem in medicinali arte ... sibi parem inveniret"*.

Nevertheless, before the time of Constantine, the study and cultivation of medicine in Italy existed, e.g. Cassiodorus, minister of Gothic king Theodoricus, made revive on the basis of the principles of Roman law the ethical and deontological values to be

S. Bakker (ed.), Health Information Management: What Strategies?, 330-333.

respected by physicians; later, there were the measures of Charlemagne.

The decline in the standard of living highlighted utilitarian techniques rather than study; furthermore, oriental mysticism and magic had made incursions. The decline of hygienic and health monitoring and overall impoverishment also led to the appearance and spread of epidemics. Thus we have the constant appearance of ill people who are *"infirmi"* or *"aegroti"*, overlapping and identifying with the poor *"pauperes"*, since poverty and disease more or less coincided. The stubbornness of the disease - interpreted as a clear sign of divine displeasure - increased with the impoverishment which had caused it, and in the end spread to the whole family. The term *"infirmi"* therefore refers to a widespread condition including all categories of the less well-off, whatever the cause of this poverty. This mixed category of *"paupertas"* and *"infirmitas"* is clearly related to the religious aspect which was also manifested in the temporary communities formed during journeys to religious sanctuaries. Pilgrimage was one of the most typical aspects of medieval society, where *"peregrini, pauperes et aegroti"* joined in common devotion, as well as benefitting from the charity and assistance provided above all by the monks. This *"vagatio"* brought the ill in search of healing to the monasteries which were therefore crowded not only with the ill and penitents, but also by physicians, who moved by the spirit of charity, *"curiositas"* - a desire to extend their knowledge - or more simply the desire to increase their earnings. They joined the others and travelled between the monasteries and courts, acquiring and selling knowledge. This itinerant medicine also followed the trade routes between cities and villages, acquiring both positive aspects but also negative values, especially before the standards of the profession were restored. In these cases, the physician was considered to be like the other types of wanderers for whom *"vagatio"* was the source of income. Illness can be converted into deception (both by patients simulating an illness and by physicians), a way to gain handouts or fees. There was a degeneration in the basics of medical activity to such an extent that Church Councils issued condemnations and prohibitions against the monks and the clergy.

For medical science, however, the point of departure is the patient who shows the symptoms to be cured, signs which only the physician can interpret. Since at that time the link between body and soul was very much felt, the first condition for achieving a cure was to ensure that feelings of hope and trust arose in the patient. Therefore, as we can see from the *"De instructione Medici secundum Archimataeum"*, the ritual gestures of the physicians when examining the patient were aimed at stressing the distance between those who know and the others, as well as comforting and inducing confidence. The text recommends physicians to follow the entire course of the illness and provide every type of service, including the preparation and serving of meals, becoming involved in *"varietatis operarius"*. Many authors cite sexual prohibitions with regard to patients and their family members, as well as recommendations to happily accept the food, however modest, offered to them, as one can see in the *"De instructione"* and the *"De adventu"*. Much importance is attributed to gestures, dress and external behaviour, so that these rules of behaviour may also have been emulated by the charlatan healers. Charlatans were quite widespread, and Egidius of Corbeil refers disparagingly to the *"pharmocopolae"*, men who wandered about preparing and selling drugs which were sometimes harmful. They usurped the title of physician, throwing it into disrepute. In any case, it is obvious that educated physicians, charlatans, popular physicians and healers flourished side by side, practising with a mixture of magical and technical elements.

The degeneration of the profession involved both laymen and the clergy (in the year 1131 the clergy were prohibited by the Church authorities from engaging in any medical practice) and was in a certain way encouraged by the increase in trade with the east and the importation of drugs and plants which were added to the simpler ones in the preparation of medicine. We can recall that, as early as the year 1000, the Italian Maritime Republics were expanding eastwards, first with Amalfi towards Constantinople, and then with Pisa, Venice and Genoa. In the XI and XII centuries, Venice imported large amounts of products to be used for drugs including cloves, nutmeg, saffron, hyssop, cinnamon, ginger, indago, tamarind, sandalwood and pepper. *"Piper et incenso et ... omnibus speciis indago et verzi"*.

Pharmacology, which started as an obscure subject full of cabalistic and astrological elements (men such as Dante Alighieri, Saint Bernard, Avicenna and Albertus Magnus, for example, still believed in magic) based on the medicinal properties of the plants known since ancient times, thus acquired important elements. With regard to the development of pharmacology, the foundation of the Monastery of Montecassino and the Benedictine Order were highly important, since St. Benedict laid down that the study of medicine and the preparation of remedies were two of the main purposes of the order (article 36 of the Rules) together with instructions for a hospital for the poor to be set up in the monastery, a place where it was obligatory to prepare drugs and test their properties. This led to an increase in studies and texts on the therapeutic qualities of herbs, thus considerably increasing knowledge in this field. (At the same time, however, the monks were prohibited from taking these drugs without authorisation from their superiors). When the old monastic school became public, especially after the Thionville capitularies of the year 805, the study of preparations increased so much that Alcuin commented: *"Accurrunt medici, mox ippocratica tecta hic venas fundit, herbas hic miscet in olla ille coquet pultes ..."*.

However, it was not until the Salerno School and the X-XII centuries that the study of drugs became more complete, with the description of medicinal herbs and the preparation of medicines. The Salerno *"Collectio"* shows that Gariopontus, who lived around the year 1040, had written a work called *"Passionarius"* which referred to *"laxum"* and *"strictum"*, i.e. the relaxing and astringent effect of medicines and drugs. He is also considered to be the author of the *"Liber Dinamidiorum"*, the *"De simplicibus ad Paternianum"* and the *"De Catarticis"*. These texts provide a detailed list of known drugs together with their place of origin, and include arsenic used internally to cure malaria.

A number of doctresses of the Salerno School were also well known for their preparations, including Trotula who lived in the XI century. Works by Trotula, *"De morbis mulierum"* and *"De compositione medicamentorum"*, have recommendations to nurses to abstain from leeks, onions and mustard, on the use of pepper and rue for toothache, on sand-baths for eliminating harmful substances. In the *"Regimen sanitatis"*, one can also find rules of hygiene together with the therapeutic information provided by the School. One distich lists famous antedotes (*"Allea, nux, ruta, pira, raphanus et theriaca heac sunt antidotum contra mortale venenum"*) elsewhere advice on diet (*"Pellibus ablatis est bona pisa satis est inflativa, cum pellibus atque nociva"*) as well as the exceptional qualities of sage (*"Salvia salvatrix naturae consolatrix"* - *"Cur moriatur homo cui salvia crescit in horto"*). In the *"Tabulae Salernitanae"* by master Salerno medicinal products are arranged and classified according to their properties. This book is taken up and commented by a certain Bernard who lived in the middle of the XII century.

At that time the Salerno pharmacists were spreading throughout Europe, bringing their complicated preparations everywhere. Bernard (of Provence) attacked them, proposing a simplification of the *"Materia medica"*. Why use dried exotic drugs which have lost all their qualities except for being expensive? Greedy spice merchants falsify and adulterate them. Tuthia (impure zinc oxide) is adulterated with dogs' bones and asphodels are transformed into myrobalans.

Then, Roger II, king of Sicily, took measures against the charlatans and false physicians who palmed off adulterated drugs; in the year 1134, he obliged everyone wishing to practice medicine to come before government officials and judges, failing which they would undergo imprisonment and the confiscation of their property. The same obligation applied to those who wished to practice the profession of preparing medicines. He condemned those who sold harmful drugs: *"Mala et noxia medicamenta et ad alienandos animos, seu venena qui dederit vendiderit vel habuerit, capitali sententia feriatur. Rex Rogerius"*. Roger's decrees also applied to the clergy, prelates and other ecclesiastics who openly practised the art of healing with very little knowledge of pharmacology thus striking a blow against the widespread practice of the art of healing unaccompanied by real medical knowledge (*"Autem consuetudo et detestabilis inolevit quoniam monachi et regulares canonici, medicinam, gratiam lucri, addiscunt; avaritiae flammis accensi, neglecta animarum cura, pro detestanda pecunia sanitatem pollicentes humanorum curatores se faciunt corporum"*).

Conclusions

All of these considerations have been made on the basis of an analysis of the criteria governing the spreading and utilisation of medical tradition which inevitably reflected the social context in which it flourished. For the period described, if we lose sight of the component linking the illness of the soul with the illness of the body, we tend to underestimate the goals of the medicine of the body. The defence of vocational skills actually started in the XII century, as we can see in Gerson's praise of university-trained physicians as compared to charlatans and false healers. The growing call for vocational standards around the year 1100 was also a clear indication of the increase in unqualified doctors. On the positive side, there was the beginning of the organisation of health care, with a distinction being made between illness and poverty, leading to the increase in the number of Hospitaller Orders in the XIII century. A dialectical analysis is required on the new situation regarding the profession and teaching in the XIII century, together with the legal ratification of the distinction between the profession of physician and pharmacist.

Bibliography

[1] Agrimi J. Malato medico e medicina nel medioevo. Torino: Loescher, 1980

[2] Agrimi J. Medicina del corpo e medicina dell' anima. Note sul sapere del medico fino all'inizio del secolo XIII. Milano: Episteme, 1978

[3] Benedicenti A. Medici, malati, farmacisti. Milano, 1947-1951.

[4] Betri ML. L'arte di guarire. Aspetti della professione medica tra medioevo ed eta' contemporanea. Bologna: CLUEB, 1988

[5] Companion encyclopedia of the history of medicine. London: Routledge, 1993

[6] Costantini Africani. Prologus libri De Communibus medico cognitu necessariis locis. PL.150 1564 B

[7] De Renzi S. Collectio Salernitana. Napoli, 1852-59

[8] Firpo L. Medicina medievale. Torino, 1972

[9] Garrison FH. An introduction to the history of medicine with medical chronology. Philadelphia: Saunders, 1929

[10] Loria E. Salute e magia attraverso i secoli. Padova: Piccin, 1994

[11] Mc Kinney. Medical ethics and etiquette in the early Middle Ages: the persistence of Hippocratic ideals. Bull Hist Med 1952;26:22

[12] Pazzini A. Storia dell'arte sanitaria dalle origini ad oggi. Torino: Minerva medica, 1973

[13] La scuola medica salernitana. Napoli: Electa, 1987

[14] Simili A. Considerazioni storico-critiche sulla medicina monastica. Minerva medica 1974;65

[15] Sournia JL. Storia della medicina. Bari: Dedalo, 1994

[16] Wickersheimer H. L'evolution de la profession médicale au cours du Moyen Age. Le Scalpel 1924;42:44

AUTHOR INDEX

MIX
Papier aus verantwortungsvollen Quellen
Paper from responsible sources
FSC® C105338

If you have any concerns about our products,
you can contact us on
ProductSafety@springernature.com

In case Publisher is established outside the EU,
the EU authorized representative is:
Springer Nature Customer Service Center GmbH
Europaplatz 3, 69115 Heidelberg, Germany

Printed by Libri Plureos GmbH
in Hamburg, Germany